Frontiers in Aerospace Science

(*Volume 3*)

Conceptual Design of Green Transport Airplanes

Authored by

Bento S. de Mattos
José A. T. G. Fregnani
Paulo Eduardo C.S. Magalhães

Aircraft Design Department, Instituto Tecnológico de Aeronáutica (ITA), São José dos Campos, São Paulo, Brazil

Bentham Science Publishers Ltd.
Executive Suite Y - 2
PO Box 7917, Saif Zone
Sharjah, U.A.E.
Email: subscriptions@benthamscience.org

BENTHAM SCIENCE

CONTENTS

PREFACE

Aircraft manufacturers and aviation are very important industries, both in social and economic aspects. According to the International Air Transport Association (IATA), aviation transported around 6.6 billion passengers in 2015 and provides approximately 62.7 million related jobs worldwide. Aircraft boost local and global growth with its civil and defense sector activities.

In particular, aircraft design has also a major impact on the society due to its safety record that inspires other industrial segments and technological spin-off effects. On the environmental side, in times of global warming, efficient aircraft will insert considerably fewer pollutants into the atmosphere and will consume less trip fuel. Most aircraft development programs make use of extensive and intensive research performed by academy as well as with the help of investments of the private sector in innovative technology. Few countries can develop, certify, market and support medium-to-large commercial airliners. This exemplifies the high level of effort, knowledge, and money involved in the aircraft manufacturing industry. Recycling of decommissioned aircraft and proper handling of the industrial processes to avoid environmental damage is part of the aircraft industry nowadays.

It is unfortunate that in the academic world few universities worldwide have a dedicated chair in airplane design, and even fewer in rotorcraft design. Most universities consider only basic disciplines such as aerodynamics, aeronautical structures, flight physics and space technologies as the fundamentals to provide higher education to aeronautical engineering undergraduate students. They disregard aircraft design as a specific discipline worthy of creating a specific chair. However, aircraft design enables the proper integration and practical application of all aeronautical disciplines. The authors of the present book have together over 60 years of experience working for one of the largest aircraft manufacturers in the world, major airlines and institution of superior education.

The present work is not intended to be or become a textbook, but to be complementary to the existing ones while highlighting environmental aspects on aircraft design. There are already several good books that were written with this purpose. Although these books have established some design practices and offer considerable data and information, most of them were mainly issued in the years 1980 to 1990. Also at that time, aircraft design was a sequential process starting with aerodynamics, followed by weight breakdown, load calculation, defining wing and tailplane areas and checking stability and controllability. Some of the methodology of these books is simple due to the lack of computer power in the past. However, aircraft design in the aircraft industry evolved from a sequential process in the past to the current utilization of high-fidelity multi-disciplinary design and optimization frameworks, where all disciplines are considered simultaneously and where everything depends upon everything. Therefore, today´s aircraft manufacturers are aware of the fact that modern engineers need to understand the whole aircraft as one complex system. There is a necessity for understanding the multi-disciplinary aspects of aircraft design also considering environmental aspects. Aircraft design disciplines are the best way to incorporate this philosophy. Books written in the past were unaware of these aspects. In the meantime, aircraft systems have evolved considerably. For instance, fly-by-wire systems have changed the way commercial and military aircraft are designed and flown. Aircraft with fly-by-wire systems are safer, more reliable, easier to fly, more maneuverable and fuel efficient with reduced maintenance costs. A fly-by-wire command and control system is already present in 9-seat business jet airplanes. All these new systems must be taken into consideration during the conceptual design phase, where the aircraft sizing is carried out as well as other important tasks.

The proper understanding of the aviation and manufacturing business is very important for engineers. In this context, the present work provides the process and information for the elaboration of a business plan for a transport airplane project that includes information on how to conduct a market survey, undertake technological assessments as well as financial and risk analysis, and shows establishment of requirements. It is very important that the aeronautical engineer not restrict himself/herself to his/here discipline where he/she carries out his work but that, he/she can also understand the context of the aeronautical industry.

The continuous increase in computer speed and capacity has allowed finite-element methods for all structural layout, cabin configuration, and CFD methods to be incorporated in the conceptual design phase already. It is possible to integrate the different design boundaries, such as high-speed and low-speed aerodynamics, and as a follow-up step, today the multidisciplinary methods permit an aircraft to be designed by integration of aerodynamic, structural and flight mechanics design constraints and by using multidisciplinary optimization methodologies. Multi-disciplinary design and optimization is the modern design methodology for many aircraft design features and aspects and nearly all papers on aircraft design now use some sort of multidisciplinary optimization approach.

Future airplanes need to comply with new and more stringent environmental rules. New challenges with regard to performance and energetic efficiency may reshape the today's airplanes entirely. The exploration of new business opportunities for aviation, which may also affect airplane configuration, is addressed. This book presents emission and noise models that were employed for optimal design airliners of distinct categories. There is a trend to power ground vehicles with electric engines. This will change the share of aviation in emissions and the way public deals with it.

Finally, post design techniques and devices to improve aircraft performance and efficiency by improved and rethought aircraft operations are presented. Mitigation of design flaws are analyzed and discussed.

Bento S. de Mattos
Aircraft Design Department
Instituto Tecnológico de Aeronáutica (ITA)
São José dos Campos, São Paulo
Brazil
E-mail: greenfutureaviation@gmail.com

CONSENT FOR PUBLICATION

Not applicable.

CONFLICT OF INTEREST

The authors declare no conflict of interest, financial or otherwise.

ACKNOWLEDGEMENTS

We thank Financiadora de Estudos e Projetos (FINEP) a support technology agency belonging to Brazilian federal government for the Project CAPTAER II, which provided resources and equipments utilized in the present work.

NOTICE

We thank institutions like NASA and United States Air Force Museum that release to the public domain, a large photo collections. This kind of initiative contributes enormously to widespread aerospace knowledge and help to inspire young hearts.

Part of the computations used in the present work were carried out with hardware and software purchased with support of the Brazilian federal agency Financiadora de Estudos e Projetos (FINEP) through the project CAPTAER II.

CHAPTER 1

Aviation and the Environment

Abstract: The present chapter contains information about the impact of aviation on global warming and describes the industry commitments to reduce greenhouse gas emissions. This chapter also analyses ICAO's efforts in establishing goals and timeframe - carbon neutral by 2020 and 50% reduction on 2005 baseline - to states and industry to reduce aviation pollution. A solid "Four Pillar" initiative was set by the industry with the objective to address such a target, considering investments in operational procedures, infrastructure, technology and market-based measures. According to the recent studies, operational procedures and improvements in infrastructure may not be sufficient to accomplish the ICAO goals with current technological state of art. Innovative technological developments, mainly related to new airframe and engine designs and concepts are indeed considered the most effective and promising measures with potential to lead to fuel efficiency improvements up to 25% when compared with 2005 levels. With this perspective, fuel efficiency is becoming more and more relevant in aircraft design techniques. Electrical vehicles may be a considerably, if not entirely, a part of the ground transportation fleet in coming decades. A study was undertaken in the present work to estimate the percentage of aviation in CO_2 emissions and noise levels considering a steadily increasing fleet of electrical vehicles over time. The evident conclusion is that even when introducing biofuels in aviation operations, their share in pollution compared to present levels will still steadily increase and take up a huge percentage of all transportation pollution. This will be an ongoing process up to the year 2050 despite the overall emission reductions. In other words, there is considerable evidence that aviation will be more and more in focus (and social-political pressure) throughout the years regarding the GHG emissions. This fact obviously reinforces the necessity for improvements in aircraft/engine designs, alternative motorization, and other sources of energy to empower aircraft systems and improve operational efficiencies.

Keywords: Aviation, Aircraft design, Aircraft emissions, Electric car, Environment, Fuel efficiency, Global warming.

AVIATION AND ENVIRONMENT

The Climate Change and Air Transport

Transportation plays a vital role for world economy. Within the transportation sector, commercial aviation has evolved from the 1960s to present days into the fastest, safest means of transport and a global transportation mode. Nowadays,

Bento S. de Mattos, José A. T. G. Fregnani & Paulo Eduardo C. S. Magalhães

over 3 billion people, nearly half the world's population, use the regular air transport, whose industry generates on a worldwide scale 56 million jobs, both direct and indirect [1]. Aircraft carry only 0.5% of the world trade shipments, which represents about 35% of the value of all world trade. This productivity is achieved by consuming just 2.2% of the world energy [1].

Regardless of the world's dependency on air transport, the pollution it causes just as much as other means of transportation, is a matter of great concern, especially in view of increasing global warming [2] and major concerns for the impact on people's health. Aircraft, cars, trucks, and other vehicles operating at airports create emissions because of the combustion of fuel. Aircraft engines produce carbon dioxide (CO_2), which comprises about 70% of their exhaust, and water vapor (H_2O), which comprises about 30% [1]. Less than 1% of the exhaust is composed of pollutants like nitrogen oxides (NOx), oxides of sulfur (SOx), carbon monoxide (CO), partially combusted or unburned hydrocarbons (HC), particulate matter (PM), and other trace compounds. In general, about 10 percent of pollutant emissions by aircraft take place close to the surface of the earth (less than 1000 meters above ground level), the remaining 90 percent of aircraft emissions are released at altitudes above 1 km. The pollutants CO and HCs are exceptions to this rule as they are produced when aircraft engines are operating at their lowest combustion efficiency (aircraft ground switch is on), which makes their split about 30 percent below 1000 meters, and 70 percent above 1000 meters [1].

Significant efforts of the aviation and aeronautical community have been made to lower aviation-related emissions. Alternative fuels, improved airplane designs, new aircraft concepts, and fuel-saving operational procedures are among them. The International Civil Aviation Organization (ICAO) proposed a "Four Pillar" initiative to the aviation and aeronautical industry with the objective to address some targets of emission reduction [3]. This initiative considers investments as well as efforts on operational procedures, infrastructure, technology and market-based measures.

Besides ICAO, there are several governments that have been issuing policies to address pollution caused by aircraft. In 2011, the European Commission established several goals concerning the protection of the environment intended to be accomplished by 2050 [4]. According to these targets, technologies and procedures available by 2050 are supposed to enable a 75% reduction in CO_2 emissions per passenger-kilometer and a 90% reduction in NO_x emissions; the perceived noise emission of flying aircraft is supposed to be reduced by 65%; in addition, aircraft movements are supposed to be emission-free when taxiing. All these targets are relative to the capabilities of typical new aircraft in 2000.

However, according to the recent studies, operational procedures, improvements on infrastructure, and biofuels may not be sufficient to accomplish the ICAO and European Commission goals with the current technological state of art. New, innovative radical designs may be needed to accomplish the envisaged emission reductions that were set by governments of several nations. In addition, aviation share of overall pollution could change significantly if electric road vehicles gain a more widespread use. There are only few studies on the impact of electrical road vehicles in the emission picture on the transport sector, and they disagree significantly with each other regarding their conclusions on the subject.

Electrical car serial production is not new; an article from the 1904 Motor Age Magazine published a conservative estimate of the probable output of the different factories for that year. A total production of 30,000 cars was estimated that was supposed to be divided roughly as follows: Licensed gasoline cars, 16,000; unlicensed gasoline cars, 8,000; electric cars, 3,000; steam cars, 2,000; miscellaneous, 1,000. Columbus Electric from Ohio was one of the electric car manufacturers. Its 1905 electric car weighed 635 kg and had a range of 75 miles before requiring battery recharge [5].

Many researchers claim that the electrical road vehicles will not contribute to lower emission levels in the whole chain, considering that the energy necessary to produce batteries and to power those vehicles will be higher than the current levels. However, a recent report from Electric Power Research Institute (EPRI) and Natural Resources Defense Council (NDRC) affirms that the electrical vehicle emission levels are far lower than the pollution caused by conventional vehicles, and could be even lower if the electric power sector cleans itself up over the next few decades [6]. In addition, cities will become cleaner, avoiding billions of money being spent on health care of people affected by pollution.

For the EPRI-NRDC study, some potential scenarios for the electricity sector in the future and the potential emission impact of widespread electrification displacing petroleum consumption in the transportation sector were well considered. To address the first issue, two potential greenhouse gas scenarios of the future electric power sector were considered: namely the "Base GHG" and "Lower GHG" scenarios. Both revealed that grid emissions will decrease over time, in part because of existing and potential regulations and plausible economic conditions. In the Lower GHG scenario, an increasing price on carbon is supposed to further reduce carbon emissions, as it could result in faster deployment of low-emission generation technologies [6]. In the Base GHG scenario, the study estimates that, by 2050, the electricity sector could reduce annual greenhouse gas emissions by 1030 million metric tons relative to 2015 levels, which represents a 45% reduction. In the Lower GHG scenario, the study estimates that, by 2050, the electricity sector could reduce annual greenhouse gas emissions by 1700 million metric tons relative to 2015 levels, representing a 77% reduction.

The EPRI-NDRC report also analyzed electric sector and transportation sector emissions with and without widespread utilization of electric road vehicles to determine the effect of electrification of light-duty personal vehicles, some medium-duty commercial vehicles like local delivery trucks and certain non-road equipment, like forklifts. It was found that electrification could displace emissions from conventional petroleum-fueled vehicles for each scenario:

- In the Base GHG scenario, carbon pollution is reduced by 430 million metric tons annually in 2050 -equivalent to the emissions from 80 million of today's passenger cars [6].
- In the Lower GHG scenario, carbon pollution is reduced by 550 million metric tons annually in 2050 -equivalent to the emissions from 100 million of today's passenger cars [6].

Independent from these results, there are good perspectives that the electrification of road vehicles will change the emission panorama of the transportation sector. This will turn the cities less polluted and quieter, changing the public standard for acceptable noise and emission levels. The present work therefore performs an analysis of the increasing electrification of road vehicles on the CO_2 emission and how this could change aviation and redirect the efforts to comply with future emission reduction policies.

Aviation in a Global Warming Environment

The Climate Change and Air Transport

Pollution generated since the industrial revolution is changing dramatically the average global temperature (Fig. **1.1**). Global warming and climate change can both refer to the observed century-scale rise in the average temperature of the Earth's climate system and its related effects [2]. Multiple lines of scientific evidence show that the climate system is warming [7]. More than 90% of the additional energy stored in the climate system since 1970 has gone into ocean warming; the remainder has melted ice, and warmed the continents and atmosphere. Many of the observed changes since the 1950s are unprecedented over decades to millennia [7]. Despite emission reductions from automobiles and more fuel-efficient turbofan and turboprop engines, the rapid growth of air travel registered from the 1978 Deregulation Act to the present contributed to an increase in total pollution attributable to aviation. In the European Union, greenhouse gas emissions from aviation increased by 87% between 1990 and 2006 [8].

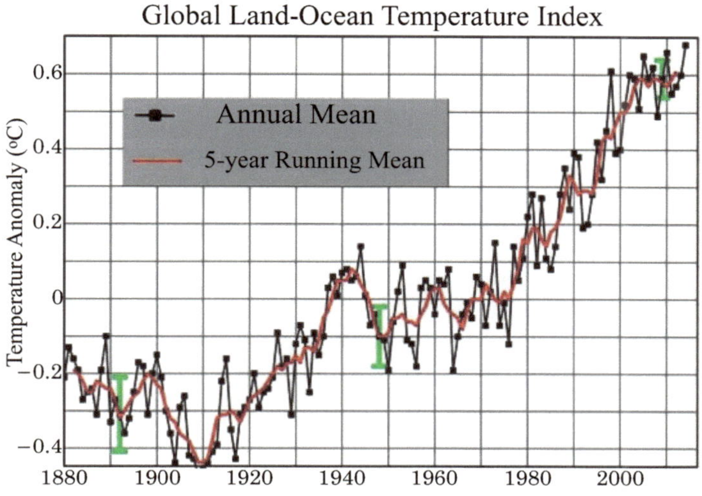

Fig. (1.1). Atmospheric CO_2 concentration and global air surface temperature (Source: NASA Goddard Institute for Space Studies, Graph released to public domain).

Ice cores provide evidence for greenhouse gas concentration variations over the past 800,000 years. Both CO_2 and CH_4 vary between glacial and interglacial phases, and concentrations of these gases correlate strongly with temperature (Fig. **1.2**) [9 - 11]. Direct data does not exist for periods earlier than those represented in the ice core record because the earth internal heat melts the ice. Data indicates CO_2 mole fractions stayed within a range of 180 ppm to 280 ppm throughout the last 800,000 years, until the increase of the last 250 years.

The power stations presented in 2000 the bigger contribution in world energy use and emissions of greenhouse gases (GHGs) with the transport sector coming into third place (Table **1.1**). In 2004, transport energy use amounted to 26% of total world energy use and the transport sector was responsible for about 23% of world energy-related GHG emissions [12]. The 1990–2002 growth rate of energy consumption in the transport sector was highest among all the end-use sectors. Road vehicles account for more than three-quarters of a total of 77 exajoules (EJ) of total transport energy use, with light-duty vehicles and freight trucks having the lion's share. Virtually all (95%) of transport energy comes from oil-based fuels, largely diesel (23.6 EJ, or about 31% of total energy) and gasoline (36.4 EJ, 47%). One consequence of this dependence, coupled with the only moderate differences in carbon content of the various oil-based fuels, is that the CO_2 emissions from the different transport sub-sectors are approximately proportional to their energy use.

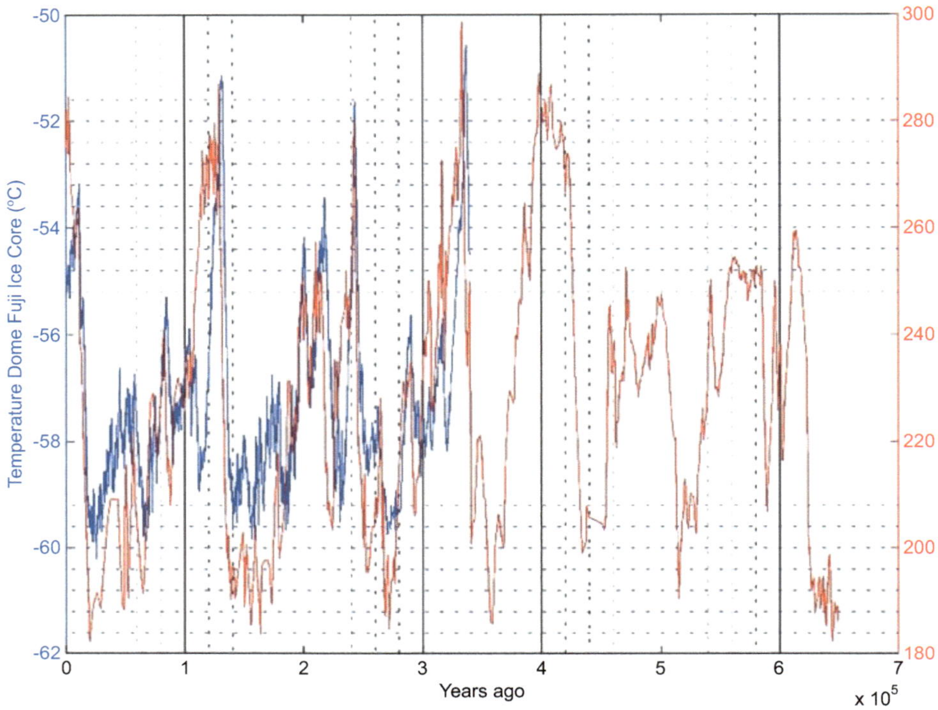

Fig. (1.2). 700 thousand years of ice core data indicates a strong correlation between temperature and CO_2 concentration [9, 11].

Table 1.1. Relative fraction of man-made greenhouse gases (CO_2, CH_4 and N_2O) coming from each of eight categories of sources [13].

Sector	Percent Share Overall	Percent Share CO_2 only
Industrial Processes	16.8	20.6
Power Stations	21.3	29.5
Waste disposal and treatment	3.4	< 1%
Land use and biomass burning	10.0	9.1
Residential commercial, and other sources	10.3	12.9
Fossil fuel retrieval, processing, and distribution	11.3	8.4
Agricultural byproducts	12.5	< 1%
Transportation fuels	14.0	19.2

In fact, aviation contribution to world's pollution is controversial. Contrails represent one of these controversies. Contrails are clouds formed when water vapor condenses and freezes around small particles (aerosols) that exist in aircraft exhaust (Fig. **1.3**). Some of that water vapor comes from the air around the plane; and, some is added by the exhaust of the aircraft. The exhaust of an aircraft contains both gas (vapor) and solid particles. Aircraft contrails can spread into cirrus-like clouds high in the atmosphere. Like natural clouds, they are thought to have an overall warming effect on the planet. But they can also moderate daily temperature extremes by trapping heat that escapes from the ground and reflecting sunlight [14]. This raises the lowest overnight temperatures and, to a lesser degree, reduces the higher recordings during daylight hours.

Noise disturbance is a complicated issue to evaluate, as it is open to subjective reactions. Its impact is not a lasting one on the actual environment, but it can have significant adverse effects on people living close to an airport, including: interference with communication, sleep disturbance, annoyance responses, learning acquisition, performance effects and cardiovascular and psycho-physiological effects.

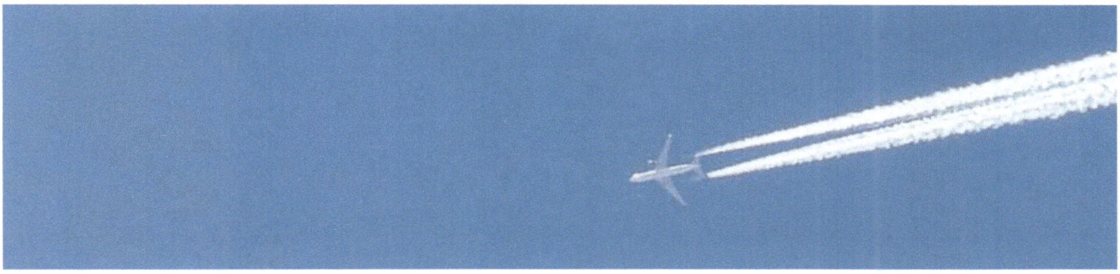

Fig. (1.3). Airplane contrails (Photo: courtesy of Paulo Eduardo Cypriano).

The October 2006 report by Nicholas Stern [15] states that the largest contributor to human-induced CO_2 is power generation (24%), mostly produced in electricity stations burning gas and coal. Land use hits 18%, then agriculture, industry and transport at 14% each (aviation contribution is in the 2-2.5% range). Buildings (8%), other energy related activities (5%) and waste (3%) make up the rest.

Carbon dioxide is not the only greenhouse gas emitted by aircraft, however. The exhaust from aircraft engines is made up of: 7% to 8% CO_2 and water vapor; around 0.03% nitrogen oxides, unburned hydrocarbons, carbon monoxide and Sulphur oxides; traces of hydroxyl family and nitrogen compounds and lesser amounts of soot particles, despite of the industry has managed to eliminate soot emissions over the past few decades. Between 91.5% and 92.5% of aircraft engine exhaust is normal atmospheric oxygen and nitrogen.

The International Civil Aviation Organization has defined a set of conditions for the assessment of local emissions, termed Landing-Takeoff (LTO) cycle, which covers NO_X ($NO+NO_2$), CO, UHC, and smoke emissions. These conditions are detailed in the volume II (Emissions) of the Annex 16 (Environmental Protection) to the Convention on International Civil Aviation [16]. The LTO cycle considers the airplane engine operating at the takeoff, climb, approach and taxi (idle) settings. These settings are defined as a percentage of the rated engine thrust (F_∞): 100% F_∞ (takeoff), 85% F_∞ (climb), 30% F_∞ (approach) and 7% F_∞ (idle). The engine is supposed to operate at each setting for a definite time as follows: 42 s (takeoff), 132 s (climb), 240 s (approach) and 1,560 s (idle/taxi). Fig. (**1.4**) shows the scheme of the LTO cycle.

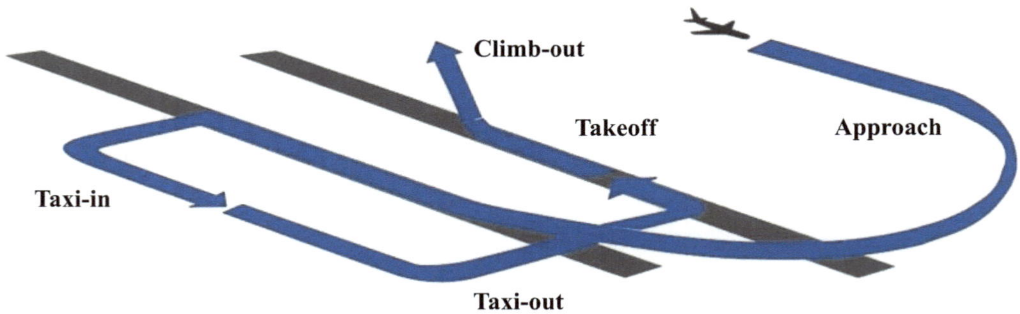

Fig. (1.4). LTO-cycle for evaluation of engine emissions.

Based on the LTO cycle, the ICAO Committee on Aviation Environmental Protection (CAEP) sets forth the limits for engine certification [16]. These limits consider the total pollutant emission parameterized by the total reference engine thrust (F_∞) which enables the comparison of engines of varied sizes. Table (**1.1**) provides values of emissions and fuel used in the LTO phase for aircraft types frequently operated for domestic and international routes [16]. Concorde figures lays well above those of the other airplanes. The values for CO_2 and NO_x emissions per passenger for the aircraft of Table (**1.2**) are displayed in Table (**1.3**).

The impact of NO_x emissions from aircraft, which, although representing only 1–2% of the total emissions of NO_x from human and natural sources in the early 1990s [17] may have a pronounced impact on the chemical composition of the atmosphere. Numerous studies have focused on the different implications of NO_x emissions from aircraft [18 - 22]. Most importantly, NO_x emissions from aircraft are expected to increase ozone in the upper troposphere and lower stratosphere region [22].

Table 1.2. Default fuel and emission factors for some aircraft types in LTO cycle (kg/LTO) [16].

Aircraft	CO_2	CH_4	N_2O	NO_x ($NO+NO_2$)	CO	SO_2*	Fuel
A300	5470	1.0	0.2	27.2	34.4	1.7	1730
A320	2560	0.04	0.1	11.0	5.3	0.8	810
BAe 146	1800	0.16	0.1	4.2	11.2	0.6	570
Boeing 707	5880	9.8	0.2	10.8	92.4	1.9	1860
Boeing 727	4455	0.3	0.1	12.6	9.1	1.4	1410
Boeing 737-300	2905	0.2	0.1	8.0	6.2	0.9	920
Boeing 747-200	10680	3.6	0.3	53.2	91.0	3.4	3380
Boeing 747-400	10710	1.2	0.3	56.5	45.0	3.4	3390
Boeing 757	4110	0.1	0.1	21.6	10.6	1.3	1300
Boeing 767-300	5405	0.4	0.2	26.7	20.3	1.7	1710
Boeing 777-200ER	7346	-	-	55.8	12.6	2.3	2332
Fokker 100	2340	0.2	0.1	5.7	13.0	0.7	740
SAAB 340	945	1.4	0.03	0.3	22.1	0.3	300
Concorde	20290	10.7	0.6	35.2	385	6.4	6420
* The Sulphur content of the fuel was assumed to be 0.05%.							

Table 1.3. CO_2, NO_x, and fuel per passenger for the LTO cycle (kg of LTO/PAX) [16].

Airplane	Pax capacity (single class)	CO_2/PAX	Fuel/PAX	NO_x/PAX
A300	345	15.85	5.01	0.08
A320	180	**14.22**	**4.50**	0.06
BAe 146	112	16.07	5.08	0.04
Boeing 707	189	31.11	9.84	0.06
Boeing 727	189	23.57	7.46	0.07
Boeing 737-300	140	20.75	6.57	0.06
Boeing 747-200	480	22.25	7.04	0.11
Boeing 747-400	565	18.96	6.00	0.10
Boeing 757	239	17.19	5.44	0.09
Boeing 767-300	290	18.63	5.90	0.09
Boeing 777-200ER	440	16.69	5.30	0.127
Fokker 100	107	21.87	6.92	0.053
SAAB 340	34	27.79	8.82	**0.01**
Concorde	120	**169.08**	**53.5**	**0.29**

Emission Control Policy

The mitigation of environmental impact is one of the key challenges for aviation and a main driver for research and technology in the sector. While the focus in the past was on noise and pollutant emissions, aviation greenhouse gas emissions have become the predominant environmental topic for the aviation community in the last years. Modern airliners are powered by turbofan or turboprop engines burning kerosene, which is a mixture of hydrocarbons and contains a large variety of carbon chain molecules, generally with chain lengths of nine to sixteen atoms. This is the case with JET A-1, fuel produced according to international standard specifications for use in civil aviation. Engine emissions can be divided into two basic groups: those proportional to engine fuel burn and those proportional to engine thrust setting. The fuel-burn proportional emissions as seen before are essentially carbon dioxide (CO_2), water vapor (H_2O), and sulfur oxides (SO_X), whereas those proportional to thrust setting comprise carbon monoxide (CO), unburnt hydrocarbons (UHC), nitrogen oxides (NO_X), soot, and smoke. From all these combustion products, carbon dioxide (CO_2) is the main greenhouse gas that occurs naturally in the environment and the single most important waste product of industrialized economies. It is produced in the engine at a rate of approximately 3.15 grams per kilogram of fuel burnt in the engine. It is relatively abundant and has a very long life in the atmosphere, having, therefore, a leading importance in the global climate system. Per Intergovernmental Panel on Climate Change (IPCC) in 2007 [23], the CO_2 emissions from global aviation were increased by a factor of about 1.5, from 330 $MtCO_2$/year in 1990 to 480 $MtCO_2$/year in 2000, and accounted for about 2% of total anthropogenic CO2 emissions. Considering also other relevant exhaust emissions from aircraft engines including contrails and cirrus, the contribution of air transport to the total anthropogenic greenhouse effect has been estimated at around 3%. IPCC [23] also concluded that, in the absence of additional measures, projected annual improvements in aircraft fuel efficiency of the order of 1–2% are likely to be overlapped by traffic growth of around 5% each year, despite of political and economic turmoil, leading to a projected increase in emissions of 3–4% per year. IPCC also forecasts that by 2050 aviation contribution to global anthropogenic carbon emissions could grow to 3%, representing 5% of the total greenhouse effect [23]. While aviation is a relatively small contributor of greenhouses gases, the scientific findings of the IPCC [24] indicate a clear urgency for action from all sectors to achieve their medium and long-term objectives. Therefore, emissions reduction measures were perceived by the industry as a real need for compensation of the effect of the traffic growth forecasted.

The Aviation Industry Initiatives

Considering the above scenario, at the United Nations Climate Conference in Copenhagen in 2009 (two years after the IPCC report), the aeronautical and aviation industry (airlines, manufacturers, airports and air navigation service providers) finally announced its commitment to a global approach to mitigating aviation greenhouse gas emissions, setting the following objectives [25]:

1. Improvement in fuel efficiency of 1.5% per year from 2009 to 2020 (measures under industry control, linked to operational procedures and basic infrastructure improvements).
2. Carbon-neutral growth at 2020 (fuel CO_2 emissions are neutralized).
3. Reduction in CO_2 emissions to 50% of 2005 levels by 2050.

It was noticeable that this is a very ambitious roadmap where the aviation industry would invest hard and continuously on innovative technologies. Focus on fuel efficiency turned therefore the main goal for the industry, not only driven by fuel prices, but now in the environmental impact. Opportunities continue to exist for addressing aviation emissions through further air traffic management and operational measures, but clearly not sufficient to push the ambitious 50% reduction by 2050. From Fig. (**1.5**) it is widely perceived by the aviation industry has and must continue to pursue a range of opportunities in new areas [26].

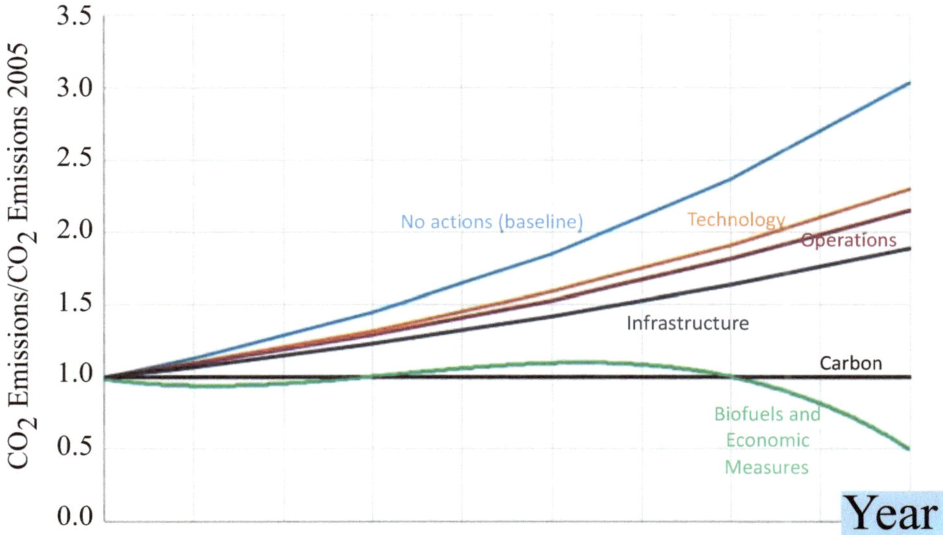

Fig. (1.5). Emissions reduction roadmap.

Advances on new aircraft design technologies as well as the development of "drop-in" bio fuels to replace fossil-based fuels could offer further gains in the future to reach the targets. In addition, a range of market-based measures (MBM), including purchase of offsets from other sectors could further mitigate the climate impact of CO_2 emissions from international civil aviation. Based on this industry commitment, to achieve the above high-level goals, the aviation industry, led by the International Air Transport Association (IATA), announced the so-called "Four-pillar Strategy" [26] with the objective to commit the industry stakeholders on such emissions reduction goals, which are resumed in Table (**1.4**)

Table 1.4. Global strategies for reducing aviation fuel uses and emissions [26].

Technology	Operations	Infrastructure	Biofuels and Economic Measures
New airframe and engine technologies	Improved operational procedures	More efficient air traffic management	Global offset mechanisms
Retrofits	More efficient flight procedures	More efficient airports	Positive economic incentives
Sustainable aviation fuels	Weight reduction		Public-private initiatives

In fact, at the Third Aviation and Environment Summit in Geneva (April 2008) a global declaration was signed across the air transport industry (ACI, CANSO, IATA, ICCAIA, Airbus, Boeing, Bombardier, CFM International, EMBRAER, General Electric (GE), Pratt and Whitney (PW), Rolls Royce (RR), ATAG) which committed the industry to a four-pillar strategy based on technological progress, infrastructure enhancements, operational improvements and suitable economic instruments to work towards the vision of zero net carbon emissions.

Following such initiative, at the 36th Session of the International Civil Aviation Organization (ICAO) Assembly in 2009, Contracting States adopted the statement of continuing ICAO policies and practices related to environmental protection. Under this scope, the Group on International Aviation and Climate Change (GIACC) formalized ICAO Council these initiatives from the industry commitment and recommendations, mostly based on the Four Pillars proposal. GIACC was therefore tasked with developing and recommending to the Council an aggressive program of Action on International Aviation and Climate Change and a common strategy to limit or reduce greenhouse gas emissions attributable to international civil aviation. The group has recommended the following potential areas of development and investments to Contracting States defined as follows [27]:

1. **Investment in innovative technologies:** Measures in this category may include purchase of new aircraft, retrofitting and upgrade improvements on existing aircraft, innovative designs in aircraft/engines, fuel efficiency standards and alternative fuels. Some of these measures have the potential for very high gains in fuel efficiency/emissions reduction but the costs are likely to be high with a long timeframe for implementation.
2. **Development of efficient operations:** These measures include minimizing weight, improving load factors, reducing speed, optimizing maintenance schedules, and tailoring aircraft selection to use on routes or services. This area is essentially a matter for aircraft operators who will make their decisions based on commercial factors in their operational scenarios.
3. **Investment on effective infrastructure:** These measures mean more efficient air traffic management planning, ground operations, terminal operations (departure and arrivals), en-route operations, airspace design and usage, and air navigation capabilities are measures with potential for relatively short to medium-term gains although the scale of potential relative gains is low to medium. In addition, more efficient planning and use of airport capacities, construction of additional runways and enhanced terminal facilities, and clean fuel operated ground support equipment to be implemented in the short to medium-term, but potential emission reduction gains are likely to be low. Increased airport capacity may also encourage increased emissions from aircraft unless appropriate actions are taken to address the emissions.
4. **Positive economic measures:** These measures include voluntary carbon offsetting, emissions trading schemes (MBM, Market Based Measures), emissions charges and positive economic incentives. Measures in this category have potential for achieving gains in term of reductions in net emissions.
5. **Regulatory and others:** Measures that include regulatory enforcements on carbon emissions reduction (*i.e.* aircraft movement caps/slot management) and other initiatives such as enhanced weather forecasting, transparent carbon reporting and education/training programs.

Finally, the governmental meeting at ICAO in its Climate Change Resolution 17/2 at the 37th General Assembly in October 2010 set out a fuel efficiency goal to 2% per year (from former 1.5%) and reinforced the carbon-neutral growth to the 2020 goal, which represents a real challenge for the aviation industry. This new goal now considers comprehensive government controlled measures at State Level, such the development of Air Traffic Management programs, mainly focused on Performance Based Navigation (PBN) implementation. In this session, the Assembly also decided to develop an ICAO aircraft certification standard for CO_2 emissions, like the existing standards for noise and engine emissions (nitrogen oxides, carbon monoxide, unburned hydrocarbons and smoke). With this ICAO would foster development and use of fuel-efficient technologies and designs by aircraft and engine manufacturers. With ICAO's engagement, all levels of the industry and States were finally committed with the new emissions reductions targets the focus turned significantly to fuel efficiency programs.

Historically, the development of aviation has always been driven by fuel efficiency (fuel burn per seat), and over the last 50 years the fuel burn (and the carbon emissions) per passenger kilometer has been reduced by over 70%. Fuel is the most important single cost element for airline operators; and the high and strongly volatile oil prices of the last years have even more increased their need for more fuel-efficient aircraft. In addition, an aircraft certification standard limiting carbon emissions is currently being developed under ICAO, which is intended to drive forward the development and encourage the use of more low-emissions aircraft.

The fuel efficiency of civil aviation can be improved by a variety of means including the incorporation into airplanes of innovative technologies, operations techniques and air traffic management. Per IPCC [24], technology developments might offer a 20% improvement in fuel efficiency over 1997 levels. By using data from Ref [28], a graph containing fuel efficient of transport airplanes was elaborated (Fig. **1.6**). This graph contains some airplanes due to enter service in the next coming years like the Boeing 737MAX. It is noticeable that over the past 40 years, since the first generation of jet transport aircraft, fuel efficiency has improved considerably, considering the 4th generation of jet engines and airplanes made of CFRP (Carbon-fiber Reinforced Polymer).

The development of new operational procedures and techniques are relevant, but limited to the current technological limitations. Fuel conservation programs are widely se by airlines and improvements are set observed on the magnitude of 5% to 10% at most. This represents a significant improvement with relatively lesser amounts of investments and airlines are constantly encouraged to optimize their operations on Fuel Conservation initiatives.

However, the first of the four pillars (innovative technologies) is considered nowadays as the main potential contributor for achieving the desired ICAO objectives in emission reduction. Its achievement strongly depends on the development and implementation of innovative technologies by aircraft, engine and equipment manufacturers, using higher fidelity aircraft design tools. The principal areas have direct impact on fuel efficiency are envisioned to be airframe (aerodynamics, structures, equipment systems and new configurations) and engines technologies. Nowadays, many individual technologies are under consideration for implementation in future aircraft and engines. For example, a study conducted in 2013 by IATA [26], the German Aerospace Center (DLR) and the Aircraft System and Design Laboratory (ASDL) of the Georgia Institute of Technology launched the Technology Roadmap for Environmentally Sustainable Aviation (TERESA) [27]. The objective was to quantify the expected benefits of the implementation of individual technologies in an operational framework, considering a typical world fleet. Current NASA's readiness levels [29] are considered to estimate the availability of each proposed technology. Tables (**1.5**) and **1.6**) contain the list of proposed technological improvements (airframe and engines related) and their associated fuel efficiency reduction. It is noticeable that up to 30% reduction on 2005 levels on fuel efficiency may be achievable after 2020, most of them related to engines technologies.

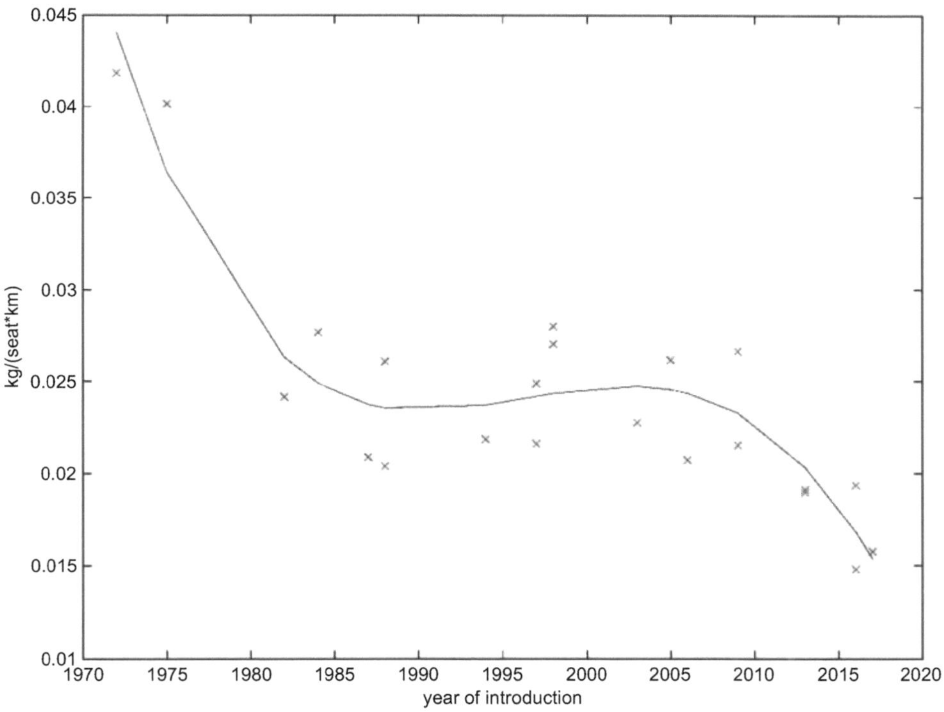

Fig. (1.6). Fuel efficiency gain since the early jet age [28].

Finally, it is valuable to mention that environmental benefits of innovative technologies (through a better fuel efficiency and thus lower carbon emissions) will become effective through airline fleet modernization and, to a minor degree, retrofits to in-service aircraft. There is an underlying challenge to select the appropriate technologies as this selection are driven by uncertain factors such as their current development status, benefits, risk and their research and development costs.

Table 1.5. Airframe technologies development impact and expected availability for introduction. TRL means Technology Readiness Level [29].

Group	Concept	Technology	Applicability	Fuel Reduction Benefit	TRL in 2014	Expected Availability
Aircraft Configuration	Truss braced wing		After 2020	10 to 15%	2	2028
	Hybrid wing-body		After 2020	10 to 15%	4	2026
	Cruise efficient stall		After 2020	< 1%	3	2027
	Flying without landing gear		After 2030	10% to 20%	1	2032
Aerodynamics	Advanced Wingtip	Wingtip fence	Retrofit	1% to 3%	9	2012
		Blended winglet /Sharklets	Retrofit	3% to 6%	9	2012
		Racked wingtip	Retrofit	3% to 6%	9	2012
		Split winglets (scimitar tips)	Retrofit	2% to 6%	7	2022
		Spiroid wingtip	After 2020	2% to 6%	7	2022
	High Lift Devices	High lift / Low Noise	After 2020	1% to 3%	4	2026
		Variable Camber Trailing Edge	Before 2020	1% to 2%	9	2012
		Dropped spoiler	Before 2020	1% to 2%	9	2012
		Hingeless flap	After 2030	1% to 2%	3	2027
	Drag reduction	Drag coating	Retrofit	< 1%	9	2012
		Turbulent flow coating (riblets)	Retrofit	1%	8	2015
		Graphic Films	Retrofit	1%	9	2012
	Natural Laminar Flow		After 2020	5% to 10%	7	2022
	Hybrid Laminar Flow		After 2020	10% to 15%	7	2022
	Variable Camber		Before 2020	1% to 3%	8	2015
	Variable Camber with new control surfaces		After 2020	1% to 5%	5	2024
Structures	Active Load Alleviation		Before 2020	1%to 5%	9	2012
	Composite Primary Structures		Before 2020	1% to 3%	9	2012
	Smart wing/actuators		After 2020	< 1%	6	2023
	Morphing wings		After 2030	2% to 8%	5	2024

Table 1.6. Engine technologies development impact and expected availability for introduction. TRL means Technology Readiness Level [29].

<table>
<tr><th>Group</th><th>Concept</th><th>Technology</th><th>Applicability</th><th>Fuel Reduction Benefit</th><th>TRL in 2014</th><th>Expected Availability</th></tr>
<tr><td rowspan="6">New Engine Architecture</td><td colspan="2">Geared Turbofans</td><td>Before 2020</td><td>10%-15%</td><td>7</td><td>2016</td></tr>
<tr><td colspan="2">Advanced Turbofans</td><td>Before 2020</td><td>10%-15%</td><td>7</td><td>2016</td></tr>
<tr><td colspan="2">Counter rotating fan</td><td>After 2020</td><td>15%-20%</td><td>3</td><td>2019</td></tr>
<tr><td colspan="2">Open Rotor</td><td>After 2020</td><td>15%-20%</td><td>5</td><td>2019</td></tr>
<tr><td colspan="2">New engine core concepts</td><td>After 2030</td><td>25%-30%</td><td>2</td><td>2026</td></tr>
<tr><td colspan="2">Embedded Distributed Fan</td><td>After 2030</td><td>Less than 1%</td><td>2</td><td>2026</td></tr>
<tr><td rowspan="10">Advanced Concepts</td><td rowspan="4">Fan</td><td>Component Improvements</td><td>Before 2020</td><td>2%-6%</td><td>8</td><td>2013</td></tr>
<tr><td>Zero Hub</td><td>Before 2020</td><td>2%-4%</td><td>7</td><td>2016</td></tr>
<tr><td>High BPR</td><td>Before 2020</td><td>2%-6%</td><td>7</td><td>2016</td></tr>
<tr><td>Variable Nozzle</td><td>After 2020</td><td>1%-2%</td><td>7</td><td>2016</td></tr>
<tr><td rowspan="3">Combustor</td><td>Variable Flow Splits</td><td>After 2020</td><td>1%-2%</td><td>5</td><td>2020</td></tr>
<tr><td>Ultra compact low emission</td><td>Before 2020</td><td>1%- 2%</td><td>5</td><td>2020</td></tr>
<tr><td>Advanced</td><td>Before 2020</td><td>5%-10%</td><td>8</td><td>2013</td></tr>
<tr><td rowspan="2">Compressor</td><td>Bling concept</td><td>After 2030</td><td>1%-3%</td><td>3</td><td>2023</td></tr>
<tr><td>Bisk Concept</td><td>After 2020</td><td>1%-3%</td><td>7</td><td>2016</td></tr>
<tr><td colspan="2">Variable Geometry Chevron</td><td>After 2020</td><td>Less than 1%</td><td>5</td><td>2020</td></tr>
<tr><td rowspan="2">Nacelles and Installation</td><td colspan="2">Buried engines</td><td>After 2020</td><td>1%-3%</td><td>5</td><td>2020</td></tr>
<tr><td colspan="2">Reduced nacelle weight</td><td>Before 2020</td><td>1%-3%</td><td>7</td><td>2016</td></tr>
<tr><td rowspan="2">Engines Cycles</td><td colspan="2">Adaptive Cycles</td><td>After 2030</td><td>5%-15%</td><td>2</td><td>2030</td></tr>
<tr><td colspan="2">Pulse Detonation</td><td>After 2030</td><td>5%-15%</td><td>2</td><td>2030</td></tr>
<tr><td rowspan="3">Others</td><td colspan="2">Boundary Layer Ingestion Inlet</td><td>After 2020</td><td>1%-3%</td><td>3</td><td>2023</td></tr>
<tr><td colspan="2">Ubiquitous Composites</td><td>After 2020</td><td>10%-15%</td><td>3</td><td>2023</td></tr>
<tr><td colspan="2">Adaptive flow control</td><td>After 2020</td><td>10%-20%</td><td>2</td><td>2026</td></tr>
</table>

In summary, aircraft design techniques under the environmental perspective became significantly relevant throughout the last decade, driven by the industry commitment on emissions reductions set by ICAO goals. The inclusion of fuel efficiency focus on the design framework is a key parameter on the next aircraft generations.

AERONAUTICAL INDUSTRY FACING THE ENVIRONMENTAL CHALLENGES

The Clean Sky Project

Within Europe, public and governmental positions increasingly point towards a desire to regulate the climate impacts caused by aircraft. The report by the UK Royal Commission on Environmental Protection (RCEP) noted that without regulatory control, the rapid growth of air transport would proceed in fundamental contradiction to the British government's stated goal of sustainable development [30]. Europeans have a great concern with sustainable growth. The UK position on climate regulation is shared with many others European countries. In 2001, the report of the Group of Personalities "European Aeronautics: A vision for 2020" pioneered an integrated vision of the European Air Transport System for the next 20 years. It established, as its top-level objectives, the need to respond to society needs and to secure European leadership in the aeronautics, encompassing significant reductions in pollution and noise emission levels. The report also recommended the creation of the Advisory Council for Aeronautics Research in Europe (ACARE).

ACARE is the first European technology platform, which produced a set of strategic research objectives (SRA1) in 2002 and a second updated edition (SRA-2) in 2004. SRA-1 is built around five challenges for technology development. It has been used as a reference guide for several national and institutional bodies for establishing their research programs. SRA-2 describes six high-level target concepts (HLTCs) and their associated technologies with respect to different socio-economic scenario. Each HLTC stresses an aspect of the Air Transport System. The Clean Sky project was created to address of ACARE HLTCs. In fact, Clean Sky is one of the most ambitious aeronautical research program ever launched in Europe. Its mission is to develop breakthrough technologies to reduce environmental impacts of aircraft and aerial vehicles developing aircraft that are quieter and more fuel-efficient. CS1 was created as a public-private partnership. Clean Sky 1 (CS1) started in 2008. Clean Sky 2 (CS2) will enable a natural continuation to the progress achieved in the first Clean Sky Program launched under the EU's 7th Framework Program for Research and Technological Development (FP7), which will end in 2017. CS2 extends the public-private partnership to 2024, and expands it to encompass large-scale high-bypass propulsion, hybrid laminar flow control, integrated cabin systems and structures, and next-generation cockpits. The program will fly both compound and tiltrotor high-speed rotorcraft, and show technologies for a 90-seat turboprop and a 19-seat transport.

The Clean Sky project intends to investigate key aircraft technologies:

Large Passenger Aircraft: This Clean Sky component includes new propulsion systems and their integration in future aircraft; advanced fuselage and aircraft systems concepts for possible next generation cabin architectures; and innovative cockpits. Large-scale demonstrators, test rigs and flight test demonstration are planned activities.

The Green Regional Aircraft (GRA): The future green regional aircraft features considerably less empty weight, more energy efficiency, lower drag, and higher level of operative performance. All this must be in pace with reduced pollutant emissions and lower noise signature.

The Fast Rotorcraft initiative: consists of two separate demonstrators, the NextGenCTR tilt-rotor and the LifeRCraft compound helicopter. These two fast rotorcraft concepts aim to deliver superior vehicle productivity and performance.

Airframe: Investigation of advanced and innovative airframe structures like a more efficient wing with natural laminar flow, optimized control surfaces, control systems and embedded systems highly integrated in metallic and advanced composites structures. It will also test novel engine integration strategies and investigate innovative fuselage structures.

Engines: Clean Sky will build on the work done in the Sustainable and Green Engines activity to validate more radical engine architectures.

Systems and equipment are crucial for aircraft operation, flight optimization and air transport safety. Thus, the Clean Sky project will investigate innovative aircraft architectures, such as more electrical aircraft and bleed-less engines rely on new system technologies to improve global aircraft performance.

The Small Air transport represents the research and technology for small aircraft in the 19-passenger category or for freight transport. This component of Clean sky project aims to develop, validate and integrate key technologies on demonstrators that can revitalize an important segment of the aeronautics sector that can bring key new mobility solutions.

Eco-Design will coordinate research geared towards high eco-compliance in air vehicles over their product life. It will heighten the stewardship in intelligent Re-use, Recycling and advanced services. This activity is critical to obtain excellence in materials, processes and resources; supporting the manufacturing base and supply chain competitiveness and sustainability.

The ERA initiative

The United States has also established a policy for improvement of airplanes considering environmental aspects. Created in 2009, as part of NASA's Aeronautics Research Mission Directorate's Integrated Systems Research Program, the Environmentally Responsible Aviation (ERA) Project explores and documents the feasibility, benefits and technical risk of vehicle concepts and enabling technologies to reduce aviation's impact on the environment. ERAs goals include slashing aircraft level fuel burn by 50%, drag by 8%, weight by 10%, emissions by at least 70% and noise by up to 42 EPNdB. The main grounds for starting ERA are [31]:

Fuel Efficiency

- In 2008, North American major carriers burned 19.6 billion gallons of jet fuel. Department of Defense alone burned 4.6 billion gallons. Considering an average price of US $3.00/gallon, fuel cost amounted US$ 73 billion. Even small reductions in fuel burn would result in significant lesser money spending.

Emissions

- Majority of U.S. airports are in non-attainment areas that do not meet Environment Protection Agency (EPA) local air quality standards for particulate matter and ozone.
- The fuel consumed by U.S. commercial carriers and Department of Defense releases more y than 250 million tons of CO_2 into the atmosphere each year.

Noise

- Aircraft noise continues to be regarded as the most significant hindrance to airspace capacity growth.
- FAA made several attempts to reconfigure New York airspace, which resulted in 14 lawsuits by 2010.
- Since 1980, FAA has invested over US$ 5 billion in airport noise reduction programs.

Market outlook from airplane manufacturers and forecasts from U.S. governmental agencies predict that the air transportation system will expand significantly within the next decades. Considering that such an expansion will bring negative environmental impacts, it makes imperative neutralize or reduce them. This is the goal of the ERA Project and its focused research. The project is organized to [31]:

- Mature promising technology and advanced aircraft configurations that meet mid-term goals for community noise, fuel burn and nitrogen oxides (NOx) emissions as described in the National Aeronautics Research and Development Plan and;
- determine the potential impact of these advanced aircraft designs and technologies if successfully implemented into the air transportation system.

To mature technologies and study vehicle concepts ERA Project is working on technologies in these research areas, called integrated technology demonstrations (ITC):

- Innovate Flow Control Concepts for Drag Reduction.
- Advance Composites for Weight Reduction.
- Advance UHB Engine Designs for Specific Fuel Consumption and Noise Reduction.
- Advance Combustor Designs for Oxides of Nitrogen Reduction.
- Advance Airframe and Engine Integration Concepts for Community Noise and Fuel Burn Reduction.

The ERA Project is comprised of three subprojects: Airframe Technology, Propulsion Technology and Vehicle Systems Integration. Work within the project is coordinated with research performed by other programs within NASA's Aeronautics Research Mission Directorate as well as other federal government agencies. NASA has also put mechanisms in place to engage academia and industry, including working groups and technical interchange meetings; Space Act Agreements for cooperative partnerships; and the NASA Research Announcement process that provides for full and open competition for the best and most promising research ideas. The ERA Project disseminates all its research results to the widest practical extent. Teams from The Boeing Company in Huntington Beach, Calif., Lockheed Martin in Palmdale, Calif., and Northrop Grumman in El Segundo, Calif., have spent time and effort studying how to meet NASA goals to develop technology to meet ERA'a targets (Fig. **1.7**).

A modified 757 is being employed as technology demonstrator by Boeing to investigate AFC. The airplane is called ecoDemonstrator. The airplane was fitted with devices that will blow jets of air on the vertical tail (VT) and the other involves non-stick coatings to help repel bugs from the leading edge of wings.

The first technology that was tested is called the Active Flow Control Enhanced Vertical Tail Flight Experiment. NASA worked with Boeing to install 31 tiny jets called sweeping jet actuators that can manipulate, on demand, the air that flows over the ecoDemonstrator 757's vertical tail and rudder surfaces [32]. An aircraft's vertical tail is primarily used to add stability and directional control during takeoff and landing, especially in the event of an engine failure. But when the aircraft is cruising at altitude the same large, heavy tail is less utilized. If the size of the VT the size of the vertical tail by using the sweeping jets to generate the same side force during takeoff and landing that a larger tail does. That would reduce the weight and drag of the airplane and decrease its fuel consumption.

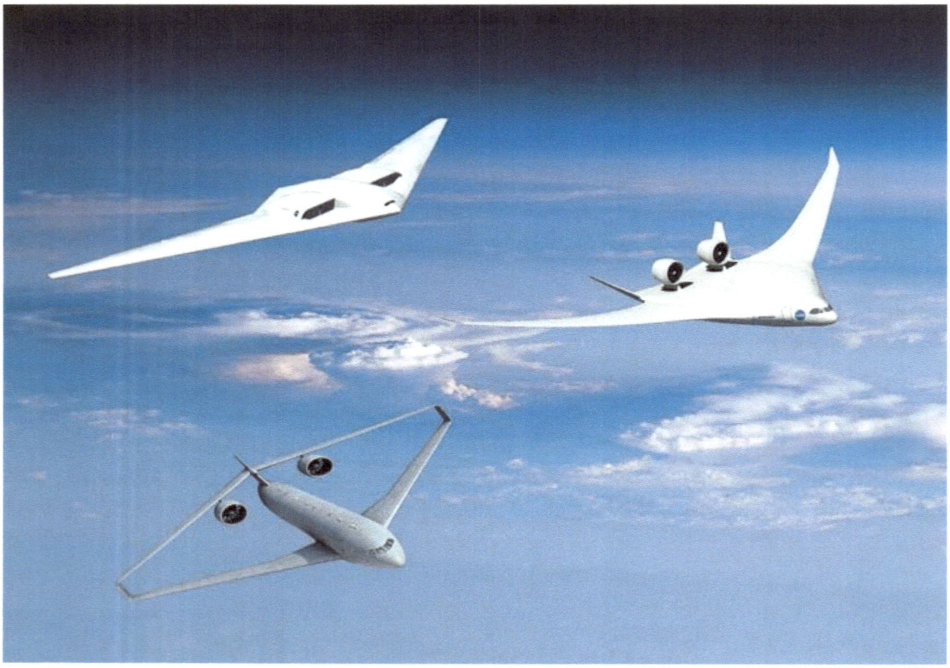

Fig. (1.7). Unusual configurations proposed by Boeing (Blended wing body at right), Lockheed-Martin (joined wings twinjet), and Northrop-Grumman for the ERA Project (Illustration: Courtesy NASA).

ELECTRIC VEHICLES AND AVIATION

Electrical Automobiles

The trend of replacing hydraulic, pneumatic, mechanical systems and sub-systems with electric equivalents, coupled with a call for high passenger comfort and in-flight entertainment systems has resulted in an ever-increasing demand on an aircraft's power requirements. This move requires advances in the areas of power electronics, necessary to provide the technology to improve efficiency and safety of aircraft systems operation. At the same time, an increased use of electromechanical and electro hydrostatical actuation requires the evolution of the electrical power distribution system.

Below, some advantages of electrical road vehicles are listed:

- Higher torque
- Increased propulsion efficiency
- Quieter than vehicles powered by internal combustion engines
- Greater simplicity
- Greater reliability
- Uses regenerative brake
- In use, do not pollute the environment
- Less maintenance
- When stopped and in use, do not consume fuel
- Can be used for energy storage
- Flexibility in relation to power supply sources
- More power per weight unit or volume unit

The automotive industry has made considerable progress towards electrical cars. Tesla and General Motors stand out among automakers. Hence, a deep analysis the Tesla Model S (Fig. **1.8**) and Chevrolet Volt is carried out in this section.

The Chevrolet Volt is a plug-in hybrid electric vehicle manufactured by General Motors. The Volt operates as a pure battery electric vehicle until its plug-in battery capacity drops to a predetermined threshold from full charge [33]. From there its internal combustion engine powers an electric generator to extend the vehicle's range as needed. When the engine is running it may be periodically mechanically linked (by a clutch) to a planetary gear set, and hence the output drive axle, to improve energy efficiency. The Volt's regenerative braking also contributes to the on-board electricity generation. Under the United States Environmental Protection Agency (EPA) cycle, the 2013/14 model year Volt all-electric range is 38 mi (61 km), with a combined electric mode/gasoline-only rating of 62 mpg-US (3.8 L/100 km; 74 mpg-imp) equivalent (MPG-equivalent). The Tesla Model S is a full-sized electric five-door, luxury liftback, produced by Tesla Motors [34]. The all-wheel drive system of Model S employs two motors for the front and rear wheels with a digital-independent control torque, resulting in an unparalleled traction control in all conditions. In July 2017, Tesla started delivery of its more affordable electric car the Model 3. The company intends to reach the goal of making 500,000 in 2018. Fourteen-year-old Tesla has never made more than 100,000 cars in a year. Thus, the envisaged production level is a very challenge task.

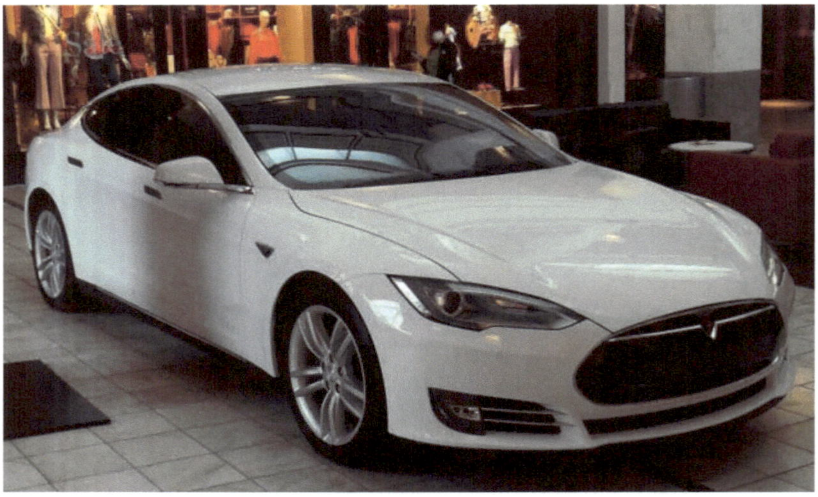

Fig. (1.8). Tesla Model S (Photo: ©2016 Bento Mattos).

What the aeronautical industry is doing towards more electric airplanes? A point to remember: if cars go electric, the aviation share of greenhouse gases generation will rise sharply. The Electric Vehicles Initiative (EVI) is a multi-government policy forum dedicated to accelerating the introduction and adoption of electric vehicles (EVs) worldwide [35]. EVI is one of several initiatives launched in 2010 under the Clean Energy Ministerial, a high-level dialogue among energy ministers from the world's major economies. EVI currently includes 15 governmental members from Africa, Asia, Europe, and North America, as well as participation from the International Energy Agency (IEA) [36]. The initiative seeks to facilitate the global deployment of 20 million EVs, including plug-in hybrid electric vehicles and fuel cell vehicles, by 2020.

EVI will enable progress toward this goal by:

- Encouraging the development of national deployment goals, as well as best practices and policies to achieve those goals;
- Leading a network of cities to share experiences and lessons learned from early EV deployment in urban areas and regions;
- Sharing information on public investment in research, development, and demonstration (RD&D) programs to ensure that the most crucial global gaps in vehicle technology development are being addressed; and
- Engaging private-sector stakeholders to better align expectations, discuss the respective roles of industry and government, and focus on the benefits of continued investment in EV technology innovation and EV procurement for fleets.

Figs. (**1.9** and **1.10**) show cumulative sales and stock targets for the 9 out of the 15 EVI members that have official targets.

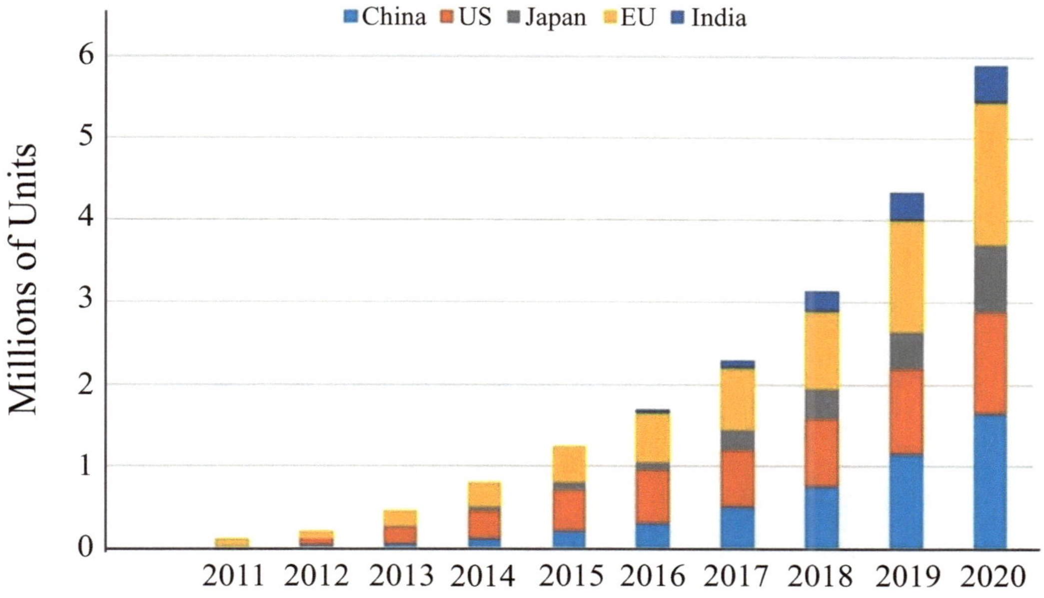

Fig. (1.9). Electric vehicles sales target established by Electric Vehicles Initiative (Source EVI).

Together these targets add up to 5.9 million in sales and 20 million of stock by 2020. There are other countries outside of the EVI member group that have official targets, but the bulk of EV sales until 2020 will likely take place in EVI member countries, which can therefore be considered a useful benchmark for EV deployment in the near term.

National sales and stock targets are not meant to be forecasts, but they can be used for creating national roadmaps that outline steps to be taken to achieve the goals while also tracking progress.

At the end of 2012, total worldwide electric vehicle stock numbered over 180,000, with over 90% of this stock in the EVI membership group. The largest non-EVI stock can be found in Norway, which numbers about 10,000.

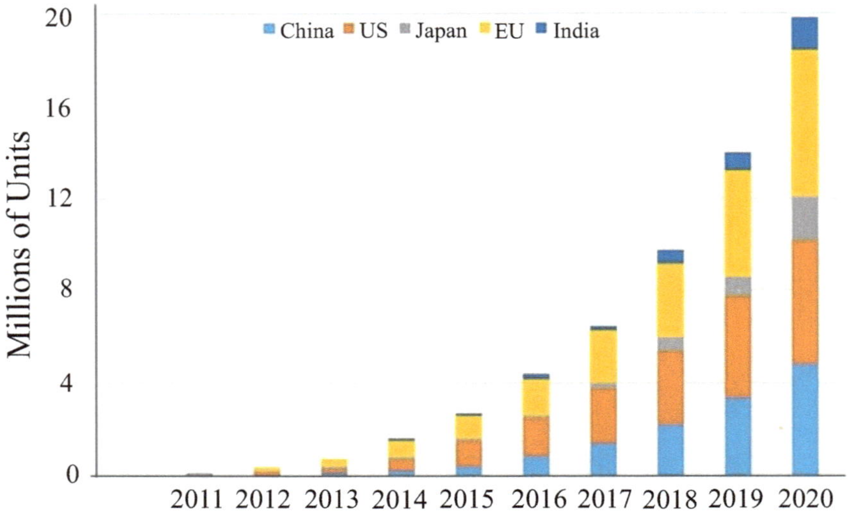

Fig. (1.10). Electric vehicles stocks target established by Electric Vehicles Initiative (Source EVI).

The Future of the Airliners will be More Electric?

Fig. (**1.11**) contains a graph that plots airplane energetic efficiency - the mass of fuel required to move a passenger a mile, for various transport jets. Data from airport planning manuals that aircraft manufacturers made available for the public were used for the calculations of the energetic efficiency. From the graph, it is noted that maximum efficiency occurs with aircraft which have about 3000 nm range, with typical passenger load, such as the Boeing 767-200. From there, the efficiency falls again with increased range up to about 5200 nautical miles. Again, we see an improvement in efficiency until we reach the Boeing 777-200LR. Regional jets typically have reach with typical payload of less than 2000 nautical miles. It is easy to note that regional jets present low energy efficiency compared to aircraft of greater capacity. The Fokker 70 has the same wing of the Fokker 100. For this reason, the wing area of Fokker 70 is oversized to carry 79 passengers in a single class and, therefore, reveals an energy efficiency index relatively poor compared to the airplanes listed in the chart of Fig. (**1.11**).

According to the graph from Fig. (**1.11**), the Boeing 787-9 airliner is more efficient energetically than the larger 777, Airbus A380 and Boeing 747-400. The key to the exceptional performance of the 787 Dreamliner (Fig. **1.12**) is its suite of innovative technologies and its structural design, which includes high flexible wings. Composite materials make up 50 percent of the primary structure of the 787, including the fuselage and wing. Boeing 787 an innovative systems architecture that is simpler, more functional and more efficient than that of other airplanes. For example, onboard health-monitoring systems monitor and report systems maintenance requirements to ground-based computer systems. Advances in engine technology are the biggest contributor to overall fuel efficiency improvements on the Dreamliner. The 787 is fitted with new engines that feature increased by-pass ratio, higher overall pressure ratio, advanced materials, and electric start. The design and build process of the 787 has added further efficiency gains. For example, manufacturing the Boeing 787 fuselage as one-piece sections eliminated 1,500 aluminum sheets and 40,000-50,000 fasteners per section.

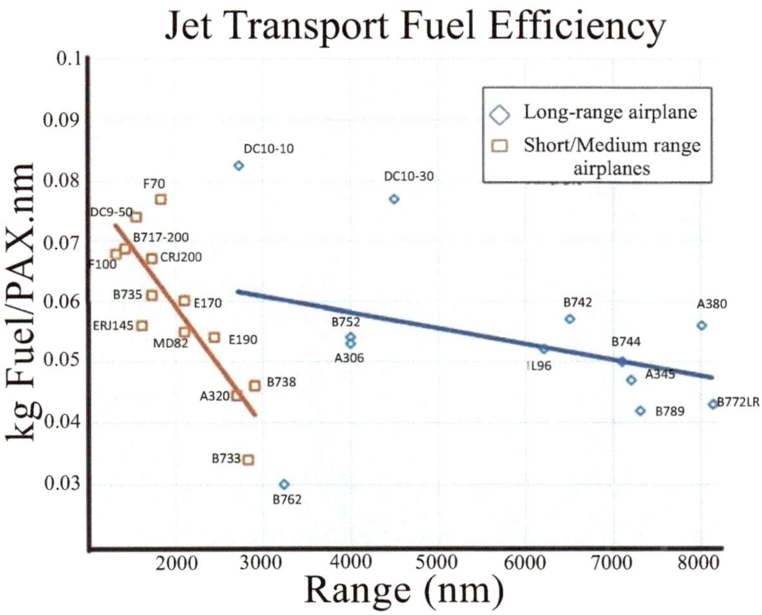

Fig. (1.11). Energetic efficiency for some transport airplanes.

In fact, Boeing 787 reflects a completely novel approach to onboard systems. Virtually everything that has traditionally been powered by bleed air from the engines has been transitioned to an electric architecture. The affected systems include [37]:

- Engine start.
- Auxiliary power unit (APU start).
- Wing ice protection.
- Cabin pressurization.
- Hydraulic pumps.

The only remaining bleed system on the 787 is the anti-ice system for the engine inlets. The auxiliary power unit (APU) provides an excellent illustration of the benefits of the more electric architecture. One of the primary functions of a conventional APU is driving a large pneumatic load compressor. The replacement of the pneumatic load compressor with starter generators results in significantly improved start reliability and power availability. The use of starter generators reduces maintenance requirements and increases reliability due to the simpler design and lower parts count. In terms of inflight start reliability, the 787 APU is expected to be approximately four times more reliable than conventional APUs with a pneumatic load compressor. Another fundamental architectural change on the 787 is the use of variable frequency electrical power and the integration of the engine generator and starter functions into a single unit. This change enables elimination of the constant speed drive (also known as the integrated drive generator, IDG), greatly reducing the complexity of the generator. In addition, by using the engine generator as the starter motor (an approach used with remarkable success on the Next-Generation 737 APU), the 787 has been able to eliminate the pneumatic starter from the engine. When compared to the more complex 767 IDG, the Boeing 787 starter generator is predicted to have a mean time between faults (MTBF) of 30,000 flight hours - a 300 percent reliability improvement compared to its in-service counterpart [37].

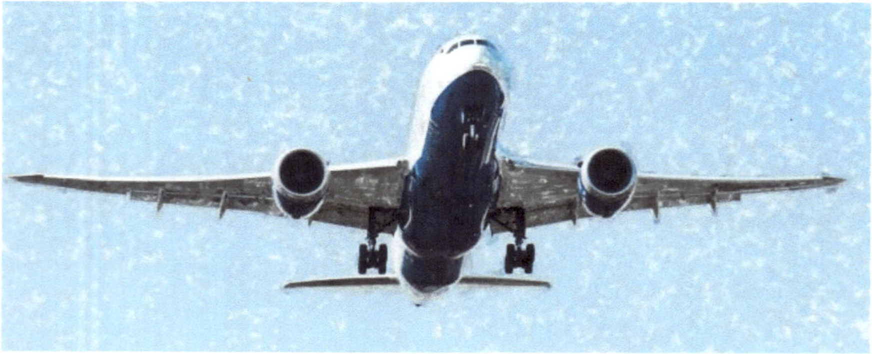

Fig. (1.12). Artistic view of Boeing 787-8.

EMISSION FORECAST CONSIDERING THE INCORPORATION OF ELECTRIC VEHICLES INTO THE GROUND TRANSPORTATION SYSTEM

Road Transportation and Pollution

Electrical vehicles have gained steady acceptance among the public and are being supported by some governmental policies worldwide, namely due to its appeal to lower emissions and almost absence of noise. In California State, Tesla Motors has been developing promising electric automobiles as seen in before in this Chapter. Apple is reportedly looking to go beyond smartphones, laptops and wearables and is current intends to come up with the company's first Apple-branded electric car. According to InsideEVs.com, total sales of EVs in the United States rose 23% annually in 2014.

Boeing forecasts that the demand for airliners ranging from regional jets to wide-body airplanes will grow an average of 3.6% a year in the 2015-2034 timeframe [38]. Airliner fleet will grow from 21,600 in 2014 to 43,560 in 2034 [38]. If in coming decades the sales or electric vehicles soars, considerably replacing internal combustion vehicles, noise and emission percentage caused by road vehicles will drop significantly. In this possible scenario, the contribution of aviation to pollution and noise levels will be then raised to new heights. How the public, government, industry and academy will accept this? To provide insights in this question, the present section presents some estimation of the aviation's contributions to CO_2 emissions in the context of an increasing EV fleet.

To answer the question of the preceding paragraph, it is necessary to utilize existing estimations of the pollution caused by different means of transportation The International Energy Agency (IEA) has worked with the world Business Council for Sustainable Development (WBCSD) in its Sustainable Mobility Project (SMP) to develop a global transport spreadsheet model that can serve both organizations in conducting projections and policy analysis [39]. The SMP transport spreadsheet model is designed to handle all transport modes and most vehicle types. It produces projections of vehicle stocks, travel, energy use and other indicators through 2050 for a reference case and for various policy cases and scenarios. It is designed to have some technology-oriented detail and to allow detailed bottom-up modelling. The SMP emission forecast for air transportation utilizes a simplified approach: passenger kilometers (revenue passenger kilometers, RPK) are multiplied by energy use per RPK (energy intensity) to derive energy use. CO_2 emissions are estimated based on fuel use. Domestic and international air travel in each region is treated together. The road vehicles were supposed to burn fossils fuels or some types of biofuels.

Table **1.7** displays the projection of CO_2 emissions [39] obtained from the SMP project spreadsheet, whose data and projections are summarized in Fig. (**1.13**). Aviation total CO_2 emissions will jump from 13.2% in 2000 to 19.5% in year 2050.

Table 1.7. Projected CO_2 emissions (Gt and percentage) by modes until 2050 (Source: IEA and WBCSD).

Year	Road	Aviation	Maritime	Road Total	Aviation Total	Maritime Total
2000	4.10	0,70	0.50	77.4%	13.2%	9.4%
2005	4.30	0,80	0.60	75.4%	14.0%	10.5%
2010	4.80	0.90	0.60	76.2%	14.3%	9.5%
2015	5.20	1.00	0.80	74.3%	14.3%	11.4%
2020	5.70	1.10	0.80	75.0%	14.5%	10.5%
2025	6.10	1.30	0.80	74.4%	15.9%	9.8%
2030	6.50	1.50	0,80	73.9%	17.0%	9.1%
2035	7.00	1.60	0.80	74.5%	17.0%	8.5%
2040	7.45	1.85	0.90	73.0%	18.1%	8.8%
2045	8.00	2.00	1.00	72.7%	18.2%	9.1%
2050	8.60	2.30	0.90	72.9%	19.5%	7.6%

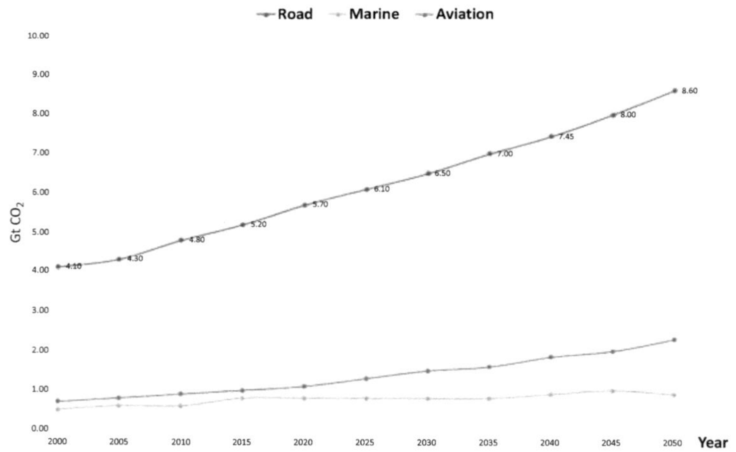

Fig. (1.13). Historical and projected CO_2 emission from transport by modes in the 2000-2050 period (Source: IEA and WBCSD).

Tables **1.8a** and **1.8b** contain the estimation of aviation participation in global CO_2 emissions if electric road vehicles increasingly replace internal combustion engines (ICE), with and without de introduction of aviation biofuels. These kinds of alternative fuels produce, considering the whole logistics value chain, in average 70% less emissions when compared with fossil fuels [40]. In addition, both tables consider that electrical road vehicles will produce 80% less emissions than the ones using conventional fossil fuel engines. For instance, not considering the use of aviation Biofuels, in 2030, 25% of all road vehicles will be electric and the aviation share in emissions will be 20%, 3% above if no EV would compose the fleet of road vehicles. However, if the use aviation biofuels are considered, per IE data, this energetic source is estimated to be used in 5% of the flights in 2030), the aviation emissions share drops to 19.4%.

Table 1.8a. Aviation Contribution on CO_2 Emissions related to Transportation Systems (with and without EV introduction). EV efficiency of 80% and airplanes will not use biofuels.

Year	EV	No EV	With EV	delta
2000	0%	13,2%	13,2%	0,0%
2005	0%	14,0%	14,0%	0,0%
2010	0%	14,3%	14,3%	0,0%
2015	10%	14,3%	15,2%	0,9%
2020	15%	14,5%	**15,9%**	1,4%
2025	20%	15,9%	**18,0%**	2,1%
2030	25%	17,0%	**20,0%**	3,0%
2035	30%	17,0%	**20,7%**	3,7%
2040	50%	18,1%	**25,6%**	7,5%
2045	80%	18,2%	**34,0%**	15,8%
2050	100%	19,5%	**46,7%**	27,3%

Table 1.8b. Aviation Contribution on CO_2 Emissions related to Transportation Systems (with and without EV introduction). EV efficiency of 80% and airplanes will utilize biofuels.

Year	Biofuel use	No EV	With EV	delta
2000	0%	13,2%	13,2%	0,0%
2005	0%	14,0%	14,0%	0,0%
2010	0%	14,3%	14,3%	0,0%
2015	0%	14,3%	**15,2%**	0,9%
2020	1%	14,4%	**15,8%**	1,4%
2025	3%	15,6%	**17,7%**	2,1%
2030	5%	16,5%	**19,4%**	2,9%
2035	11%	15,9%	**19,4%**	3,5%
2040	18%	16,3%	**23,2%**	6,9%
2045	28%	15,1%	**29,3%**	14,1%
2050	43%	14,5%	**38,1%**	23,6%

Tables **1.9a** and **1.9b** consider less efficient electrical road vehicles (20% less emissions than the ones using conventional fossil fuel engines) with and without aviation biofuels utilization. Fig. (**1.14**) plots the data contained in Tables **1.8a**, **1.8b**, Tables **1.9a** and **1.9b**.

Table 1.9a. Aviation Contribution on CO_2 Emissions related to Transportation Systems (with and without EV introduction). EV efficiency of 20% and no aviation biofuels introduction.

Year	EV	No EV	With EV	delta
2000	0%	13,2%	13,2%	9,4%
2005	0%	14,0%	14,0%	10,5%
2010	0%	14,3%	14,3%	9,5%
2015	10%	14,3%	**14,5%**	11,6%
2020	15%	14,4%	**14,8%**	10,8%
2025	20%	15,6%	**16,3%**	10,1%
2030	25%	16,5%	**17,7%**	9,4%
2035	30%	15,9%	**17,8%**	8,9%
2040	50%	16,3%	**19,6%**	9,5%
2045	80%	15,1%	**20,6%**	10,3%
2050	100%	14,5%	**22,8%**	8,9%

Table 1.9b. Aviation Contribution on CO_2 Emissions related to Transportation Systems (with and without EV introduction). Remark: EV efficiency 20% and aviation biofuels utilization.

Year	Biofuels	No EV	With EV	delta
2000	0%	13,2%	13,2%	0,0%
2005	0%	14,0%	14,0%	0,0%
2010	0%	14,3%	14,3%	0,0%
2015	0%	14,3%	**14,5%**	0,2%
2020	1%	14,4%	**14,7%**	0,3%
2025	3%	15,6%	**16,0%**	0,5%
2030	5%	16,5%	**17,2%**	0,6%
2035	11%	15,9%	**16,7%**	0,8%
2040	18%	16,3%	**17,6%**	1,3%
2045	28%	15,1%	**17,2%**	2,1%
2050	43%	14,5%	**17,1%**	2,7%

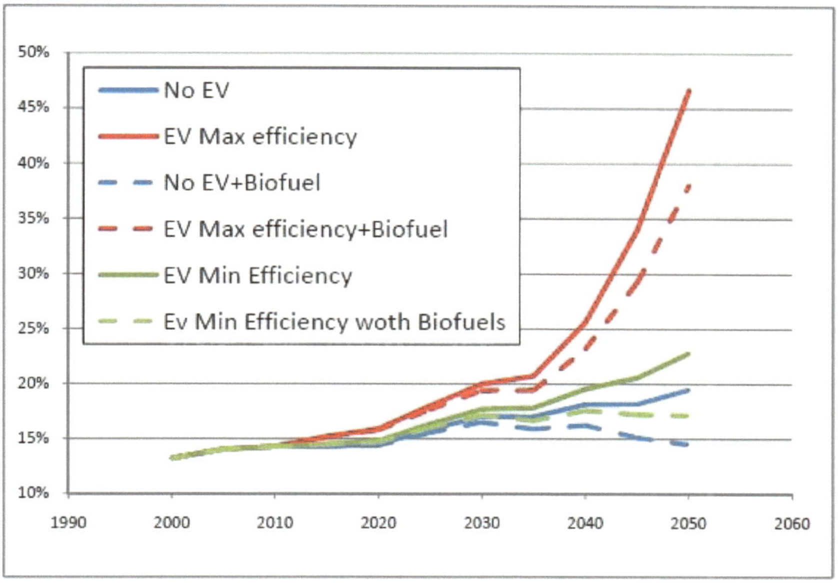

Fig. (1.14). Aviation contribution with global CO_2 emissions considering an increasing EV fleet over time. Maximum electric car efficiency was 80%, minimum efficiency 20%.

Considering the presented data, the following remarks are relevant:

- The aviation biofuels reduction of CO_2 emissions was effective from 2020, according to IEA [31]. For example, by 2050, considering 100% of road vehicles being electrical ones, aviation contribution would be increased by 27.3% if no biofuels are used. If biofuels are utilized, this figure drops to 23.6%, a difference by -3.7%. Improvements up to -5.7% are observed.
- In 2050 under the most "pessimistic scenario" for aviation, when 100% of the road vehicles would be electrical (with maximum efficiency 80%) and no biofuels are used, the participation of aviation on transport CO_2 emissions would be 46.7%, 3.3 times greater than 2005 levels (considering that no EVs and no biofuels are present).
- In 2050, under the most "optimistic" scenario for aviation, if 100% of the road vehicles present only 20% efficiency (technology has not evolved so far...) and aviation biofuel is used on 43% of the flights [40], the participation of aviation on transport CO_2 would be 17.1%, approximately 1.2 times greater than 2005 levels (considering no EVs and no biofuels are present).

The evident conclusion is that even introducing biofuels on aviation operations, the increasing demand for electrical road vehicles would lead aviation to a scaling, increasing its share on transportation emissions throughout the year 2050, despite the overall emissions reduction. In other words, there is substantial evidence that aviation will be more and more in focus (and social-political pressure) throughout the years regarding the GHG emissions. This fact obviously reinforces the necessity of improvements in aircraft/engine design, alternative motorization, and other sources of energy to power aircraft systems and improvements in operational efficiencies.

The Noise Impacts

Noise belongs to the everyday life in urban environments. Transport, industry and neighbors are common sources of noise. Exposure to transport noise disturbs sleep in the laboratory, but not generally in field studies where adaptation occurs. Noise interferes in complex task performance, modifies social behavior and causes annoyance [41]. Studies of occupational and environmental noise exposure suggest an association with hypertension, whereas community studies show only weak relationships between noise and cardiovascular disease. Aircraft and road traffic noise exposure are associated with psychological symptoms but not with clinically defined psychiatric disorder [41]. In both industrial studies and community studies, noise exposure revealed a raise in catecholamine secretion [41]. In children, chronic aircraft noise exposure impairs reading comprehension and long-term memory and may be associated with raised blood pressure [41]. Further research is needed examining coping strategies and the possible health consequences of adaptation to noise.

An experiment in Germany helps to explain how noise interferes with learning. After the old Munich-Riem airport ceased operations in 1992, the new airport in Freising, a distant site from the city, began to operate regular flights from and to Munich. Tests undertaken on third- and fourth-graders -- before that switch, soon after it and again later -- showed that students near the old airport initially scored lower than others in the tests of memory and reading but improved after the airport closed, while their counterparts living near the new airport experienced a decline in scores after the switch occurred [42].

When dealing with a new or proposed noise, LAeq is often used [also written dBA Leq]; this term is the Equivalent Continuous Level. The formal definition is when a noise varies over time; the Leq is the equivalent continuous sound which would contain the same sound energy as the time varying sound. However, it can be though as a type of average, where noisy events have a considerable influence. LAeq is the main unit used for assessing the occupational noise. As with all forms of average, it is important to consider the period over which the average is taken.

A UK Government research indicates that people start being concerned by aircraft noise at 57dB, averaged over 16 hours (57dB LAeq) [43]. They use this as the starting point in airport and aircraft noise policies. The noise contours in the vicinities of Gatwick Airport [43] present an irregular shape because at the ends of the runway (where airplanes take off and land), more noise is generated than at the sides. The map under consideration shows the contours for 2013, combining noise for all flights, regardless of the wind direction and therefore of the direction, the planes were flying.

In the last 20 years, the 57dB noise contour around the Gatwick airport diminished considerably. This can be credited to the new generation quieter aircraft. Thus, the number of people who live within 57-dB noise contour has reduced. In 1993, there were 14,600 people in this noise contour around Gatwick [43]; by 2011, this was reduced to 3,050 [43]. This is despite a rapid growth in air travel at the same time, from around 191,000 flights a year in 1993 to 244,741 in 2011. The data survey about the number of noise complaints by aircraft type against the Gatwick Airport indicates that Airbus A319 records both the higher numbers of complaints and movements [43].

To compare the noise caused by airplanes with that from road traffic, a study carried out in the city of São Paulo provides valuable data: a-weighted sound pressure level (Leq) for the roads with heavy traffic ranged from 70.88 to 80.18 dB(A) and the maximum peak ranged from 102.47 to 108.37 dB(C) [44]. Thus, in large cities, the main source of noise is the vehicular traffic which is frequently characterized by traffic jams. Here, some sources:

- The substantial number of motor vehicles, with many of them in poor conservation conditions.
- Disrespect for traffic laws.
- Loud noises from horns, alarms, and friction of tires on imperfect road surfaces produce an uncomfortable environment and make life quality significantly worse.

Verheijen and Jabben [45] preformed an important study where 90% of passenger road vehicles and 80% of the heavy trucks were substituted with electric vehicles in a city of the Netherlands. A noise reduction map was made of the entire city and an overall noise reduction in order of 3 dB was effectively measured by the first time in several places. This study showed that electric cars could mean a significant reduction in the noise level on urban roads with speed below 30 km/h. At speed above 50 km/h, electric and hybrid cars are not quieter than conventional cars because the tire-road noise increases with speed and becomes the dominant noise source [45]. In addition, Lelong and Michelets [46] showed that replacement of all cars with electric cars would give very little effects at peak hours and noon. This lack of reduction is explained by the fact that at these hours, more buses and trucks populate the streets and these types of vehicles are not expected to be replaced by electric vehicles in short turn. Out of peak hours, during night curfews for example, differences up to 5dBs were observed, revealing that electrical cars have a very good potential to lower noise levels.

With the increasing use of electrical road vehicles, reaching an adherence between 90% and 100% up to 2050, cities will be most likely quieter and the communities will therefore perceive aviation noise on vicinities of airports with more sensitivity. In aviation, noise reductions up to 5 dB magnitudes are hard to obtain with operational mitigations only and therefore, this level of reduction would probably reach on aircraft and engine design improvements.

Although a noise reduction of 3 dB seems to be small at first glance, but this is not. The noise contours (LA_{eq}) around London City Airport [47] reveal that in the area between the 57 dB, the highest acceptable noise level, and 60 dB, it is easily to perceive that a 3-dB noise reduction has a profound impact on regions close to airports [47].

CONCLUSIONS

In 2017, there have been many announcements making the future of electric road vehicles very promising:

- Porsche is moving away from diesel. the German automaker is preparing for its first foray into the electric space. Porsche is spending US$ 1.16 billion to overhaul its Stuttgart plant to introduce the Mission E in 2019.
- Tesla started delivering its US$ 35,000 model 3.
- Volvo, now a Chinese-owned firm, best known for its emphasis on driver safety, has become the first traditional automaker to signal the end of the internal combustion engine. Volvo plans to launch five fully electric models between 2019 and 2021 and a range of hybrid models.
- After France announced in July 2017 that it plans on banning new petrol and diesel cars by 2040, the British government followed suit announcing similar measures.

Electric road vehicles will certainly become a considerable part of road vehicles in upcoming decades, causing a profound impact on pollutant emission levels and the urban noise.

Urban noise reduction provided by electric road vehicles is small. Electric cars could mean a significant reduction in the noise level on urban roads with speed below 30 km/h. At speed above 50 km/h, electric and hybrid cars are not quieter than conventional cars because the tire-road noise increases with speed and becomes the dominant noise source.

The most significant contribution of electric vehicles will therefore be in pollutant emission reductions. Biofuels can be introduced in thermoelectric power stations to minimize the power demand of electric vehicles.

In 2050, under the most "pessimistic scenario" for aviation, when 100% of the road vehicles supposedly would be electrical (with maximum efficiency 80%) and no biofuels would be used, the participation of aviation on transport CO_2 emissions would be 46.7%, 3.3 times greater than the 2005 levels (considering that no EVs and no biofuels are present).

Introduction of biofuels into commercial aviation is a far cry from compensating the increase in the percentage of aviation in CO_2 emissions due to the introduction of electrical road vehicles. Radical aircraft design targeting emission reductions must thus become reality as the ones envisaged by ERA and CleanSky programs.

REFERENCES

[1] Federal Aviation Administration, *Aviation Emissions, Impacts & Mitigation: A Primer.* FAA Office of Environment and Energy, 2015.

[2] Earth Science Communications Team at Jet Propulsion Laboratory, *Global Climate Change,* NASA, September 2017. [Online]. Available: https://climate.nasa.gov/.

[3] Group on International Aviation and Climate Change (GIACC), "Global Aviation CO2 Emissions Projections to 2050", *GIACC 4th Meeting,* 2009 Montreal.

[4] European Comission, *Flightpath to 2050: Europe's Vision for Aviation.* European Union, High Level Group, 2011.

[5] C.D. Test, *Early Electric Cars*.20. [Online]. Available: http://chuckstoyland.com/ national/ electric/index.html.

[6] Electric Power Research Institute, *Environmental Assessment of a Full Electric Transportation.* Eelectric Power Research Institute: California, 2015.

[7] D.L. Hartman, A.K. Tank, M. Rusticucci, V.L. Alexander, S. Brönnimann, Y. Charabi, F.J. Dentener, E.J. Dlugokencky, D.R. Easterling, A. Kaplan, B.J. Soden, P.W. Thorne, M. Wild, and P.M. Zhai, "Observations: Atmosphere and Surface", In: *Intergovermmental Panel on Climate Change.* New York 2013.

[8] European Commission, *Climate Change: Commission Proposes Bringing Air Transport into EU Tradiging Schemes, Brussels: European Commission Press release,* .

[9] K. Kawamura, F. Parrenin, L. Lisiecki, R. Uemura, F. Vimeux, J.P. Severinghaus, M.A. Hutterli, T. Nakazawa, S. Aoki, J. Jouzel, M.E. Raymo, K. Matsumoto, H. Nakata, H. Motoyama, S. Fujita, K. Goto-Azuma, Y. Fujii, and O. Watanabe, "Northern Hemisphere forcing of climatic cycles in Antarctica over the past 360,000 years", *Nature,* vol. 448, no. 7156, pp. 912-916, 2007. [http://dx.doi.org/10.1038/nature06015] [PMID: 17713531]

[10] E.a. Wolff, I. Basille, P. Jean-Robert, and J. Schwander, "EPICA Dome C Core EDC96 Dielectric Profiling Data", *Ann. Glaciol.,* vol. 29, no. 1, pp. 89-93, 2003.

[11] U. Siegenthaler, T.F. Stocker, E. Monnin, D. Lüthi, J. Schwander, B. Stauffer, D. Raynaud, J.M. Barnola, H. Fischer, V. Masson-Delmotte, and J. Jouzel, "Stable carbon cycle-climate relationship during the Late Pleistocene", *Science,* vol. 310, no. 5752, pp. 1313-1317, 2005. [http://dx.doi.org/10.1126/science.1120130] [PMID: 16311332]

[12] International Energy Agency, *World Energy Outlook 2006.* IEA: Paris, 2006.

[13] Wikipedia, *Greenhouse Gas.*Wikipedia, the Free Encyclopedia, 18 May 2016. [Online]. Available: https://en.wikipedia.org/wiki/Greenhouse_gas.

[14] A. Barnet, *Can Aircraft Trails affect Climate?.* December 2008. [Online]. Available: http://www.nature.com/news/2008/081231/full/news.2008.1335.html. [http://dx.doi.org/10.1038/news.2008.1335]

[15] N. Stern, *The Economics of climate Change: The Stern review.* Cambridge University Press: New York, 2007. [http://dx.doi.org/10.1017/CBO9780511817434]

[16] ICAO, "Annex 16: Environmental Protection", In: *in Convention on International Civil Aviation, Montreal*, 2008.

[17] IPCC, *"WG III Formulation of Response Option Strategies," in International Panel on Climate Change.* IPCC: Geneve, 1990.

[18] D.S. Lee, I. Köhler, E. Grobler, R. Sausen, L. Gallardo-Klenner, J.J. Olivier, and F.D. Dentener, "Estimations of Global NOx Emissions and their Uncertainties", *Atmos. Environ.,* vol. 31, pp. 1735-1749, 1997. [http://dx.doi.org/10.1016/S1352-2310(96)00327-5]

[19] H. Hidalgo, and P.J. Crutzen, "The Tropospheric and Stratospheric Composition Perturbed by NOx Emissions of High-altitude Aircraft", *J. Geophys. Res.,* vol. 82, pp. 5833-5866, 1977. [http://dx.doi.org/10.1029/JC082i037p05833]

[20] C.E. Johnson, J. Henshaw, and G. McInnes, "Impact of Aircraft and Surface Emissions of Nitrogen Oxides on Tropospheric Ozone and Global Warming", *Nature,* vol. 355, pp. 69-71, 1992. [http://dx.doi.org/10.1038/355069a0]

[21] U. Schumann, "The Impact of Nitrogen Oxides Emissions from Aircraft upon the atmosphere at Flight Altitudes - results from the AERONOX Project", *Atmos. Environ.,* vol. 31, pp. 1723-1733, 1997. [http://dx.doi.org/10.1016/S1352-2310(96)00326-3]

[22] M. Gauss, and D.S. Isaksen, "Impact of aircraft NOx Emissions on the Atmosphere - Tradeoffs to reduce the Impact", *Atmos. Chem. Phys.,* vol. 6, pp. 1529-1548, 2006. [http://dx.doi.org/10.5194/acp-6-1529-2006]

[23] B. Metz, O.R. Davidson, P.R. Bosch, R. Dave, and L.A. Meyer, *Contribution of Working Group III to the fourth Assessment Report.* Cambridge University Press: New York, 2007.

[24] Intergovernmental Panel on Climate Change, *Mitigation of Climate Change - Contributionof Working group III to the Fourth Assessment of the IPCC.* Cambridge University Press: New York, 2007.

[25] International Civil Aviation Organization, *Group on International Aviation and climate Change.* ICAO: Montreal, 2009.

[26] International Air Transport Association, *Technology Rodamap.* IATA: Montreal, 2013.

[27] P.a. Nolte, "Quantitative Assessment of Technology Impact on Aviation Fuel Efficiency", *Air Transport Operation Symposium,* 2012 Delft

[28] Wikipedia, *Fuel Economy in Aircraft.*Wikipedia, the Free Encyclopedia, 11 May 2016. [Online]. Available: https://en.wikipedia.org/wiki/Fuel_economy_in_aircraft

[29] J.C. Mankins, "technology Readiness Levels, A White paper", *Office of Space Access and Technology, NASA, 1995.*

[30] Royal Commission on Environmental Pollution, *The Environmental Effects of Civil Aircraft in Flight.* Royal Commission on Environmental Pollution: London, 2002.

[31] F. Collier, "Overview of NASA's Environmental Responsible aviation (ERA): A NASA Aeronautics

Project Focused on Midtrem Environmental Goals", In: *48th AIAA aerospace Sciences Meeting, Orlando, 2010.*, 2010.

[32] K. Barnstorff, *NASA Tests Green Aviation Technology on Boeing ecoDemonstrator.*NASA, April 2015. [Online]. Available: https://www.nasa.gov/aero/nasa-tests-green-aviation-technolo-y-on-boeing-ecodemonstrator.html

[33] Wikipedia, Wikipedia, September 2017. [Online]. Available: https://en.wikipedia.org/ wiki/ Chevrolet_Volt

[34] Wikipedia, "The Free Encyclopedia, "Tesla Model S," Wikipedia", September 2017. [Online]. Available: https://en.wikipedia.org/wiki/Tesla_Model_S

[35] The Clean Energy Ministerial, *Electric Vehicles Initiative (EVI), Energetics Incorporated,*.[Online]. Available: http://www.cleanenergyministerial.org/Our-Work/Initiatives/Electric-Vehicles

[36] Electric Vehicle Initiative, *International Energy agency - Understanding the Electric Vehicle landscape to 2020,* 2013.https://www.iea.org/publications/globalevoutlook_2013.pdf

[37] The Boeing Company, *Boeing 787 from the Ground Up.* Boeing Aero Magazine, 2006.

[38] The Boeing Company, *Current Market Outlook 2015-2034.*2014. http://www.boeing.com/ resources/ boeingdotcom/ commercial/ about-our-market/ assets/ downloads/ Boeing_ Current_ Market_ Outlook_2015.pdf

[39] L. Fulton, and G. Eads, *IEA/SMP Model Documentation and reference case Projection,* 2004.http://oldwww.wbcsd.org/web/publications/mobility/smp-model-document.pdf

[40] International Energy Agency, *Global Energy Outlook.* IEA: Paris, 2009.

[41] S.A. Stansfeld, and M.P. Matheson, "Noise Pollution: Non-auditory Efefcts on health," British medical", *Bulletin,* vol. 68, no. 1, pp. 243-257, 2003.
[PMID: 14757721]

[42] R. Weiss, Noise Pollution Takes Tool on health and Happiness, Washington: Washington Post, 2007.

[43] Gatwick Airport Flight Performance Team, *2014 Annual Report.*. Gatwick Airport, London, 2015.

[44] C. Moura-De-Sousa, and M. Regina Alves Cardoso, "Urban Noise in the City of São Paulo, Brazil: An Important Problem of Public Health", *Noise Health,* vol. 4, no. 16, pp. 57-63, 2002.
[PMID: 12537842]

[45] J. Lelong, and R. Michelet, "Passenger Cars - Power Unit and Tyre-road Noise, Driving behavuour", In: *Inter-Noise 2001, The Hague*, 2001.

[46] E. Verheijen, and J. Jabben, Effect of Electric cars on Traffic Noise and Safety*National Institute for Public health and The Environment, Bilthoven*, 2010.

[47] London City Airport, *London City Action Plan 2010-2015.* London City Airport: London, 2009.

CHAPTER 2

Aeronautical Technology Over Time

Abstract: The present chapter performs an analysis of the aviation from the dawn of aviation to early 2017, highlighting the European pioneering work in many aspects like supersonic flight and innovative aircraft configurations. The work of aviation pioneers is also analyzed. An overview of technological evolution since World War I to the present days is carried out, also addressing some notable events that shaped the commercial aviation. Special attention is given to the development of supersonic civil aircraft and its impact on the environment. Aircraft concepts that used or are currently employing alternative fuels and power are shown and discussed. Alternative means of transportation are also analyzed. The chapter also presents an appendix containing the major advances of aeronautical technology. Throughout this chapter, the reader will notice that some usual historical considerations are reviewed, and news analyses are provided.

Keywords: Aerodynamics, Air transportation, Aircraft design, Aircraft industry, Aircraft technology, Airline, Airliner, Alternative fuels, Commercial aviation, Entropy statistics, Global warming, Supersonic flight, World War II aircraft.

THE FLIGHT PIONEERS

Flying with Style

The beginning of the heavier-than-air flight was possible thanks to the efforts of several pioneers: The Lilienthal brothers, the Brazilian Santos-Dumont, the Wright brothers, Henri Farman, Louis Blériot, Gabriel and Charles Hoisin and many others. Thanks to the spread of the French Revolution ambience among the aviation pioneers in the early XX century, aviation took off in France [1].

The work of Santos-Dumont, a very rich person who settled down in France at the end of the XIX century, provides a good picture of the events that shaped aviation. For this reason, the present chapter carries out a deeper investigation of his masterpiece.

Dumont started his aviation career by designing balloons and airships, the latter making him a worldwide celebrity. After his success with airships, Dumont turned his attention to the airplane design and construction. He soon realized that the

Bento S. de Mattos, José A. T. G. Fregnani & Paulo Eduardo C. S. Magalhães

internal combustion engine would be ideal for powered flight. Several earlier flight attempts had been carried out with electric and steam engines.

Santos-Dumont won the Deutsch de la Merthe Award in 1901. The organizing committee of this award established the challenge of a flight tour starting from the Saint Cloud field encompassing a turn around the Eiffel Tower (Fig. **2.1**). Santos-Dumont accomplished this task with his airship No. 6. He had tried this previously with his airship No. 5, but due to hydrogen leak, he ended up crashing into the Hotel Trocadero (which no longer exists in Paris today). Santos-Dumont continued to develop airships. The smallest of them, was the No. 9, semi-rigid, dubbed La Baladeuse (Fig. **2.2**). It was designed and built to be his personal aerial transport [1] and fulfilled Dumont's expectations in regard to performance and maneuverability. Dumont used to employ this airship to go to public places such as restaurants, shops and snack bars, visiting friends and he was often seen at clubs [1]. He frequently flew over the houses of Paris, almost scraping their roofs. On July 14, 1903, he allowed his friend, Aida de Acosta, a Cuban married woman, to pilot the aircraft on a small trip (Fig. **2.2**).

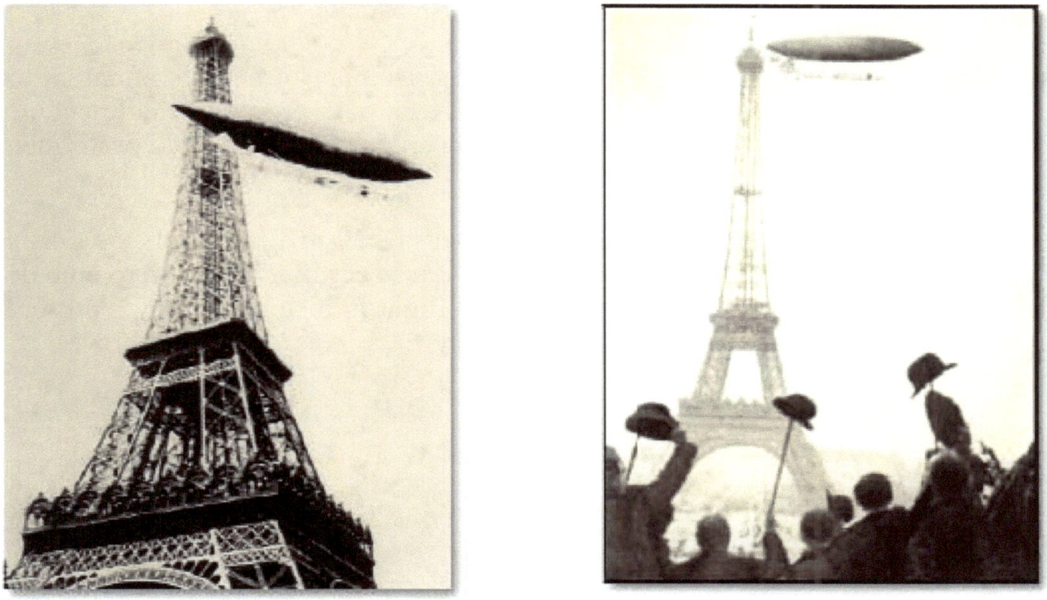

Fig. (2.1). A milestone for aeronautical engineering: Santos-Dumont airships around Eiffel Tower in 1901. *Left* – Number 5 suffered hydrogen leak after flying round the Eiffel tower [1]. Many historians often misinterpret this picture, as they refer to the aircraft in the photo as the number 6. *Right:* Number 6 on the way to win the Deutsch de la Meurthe prize.

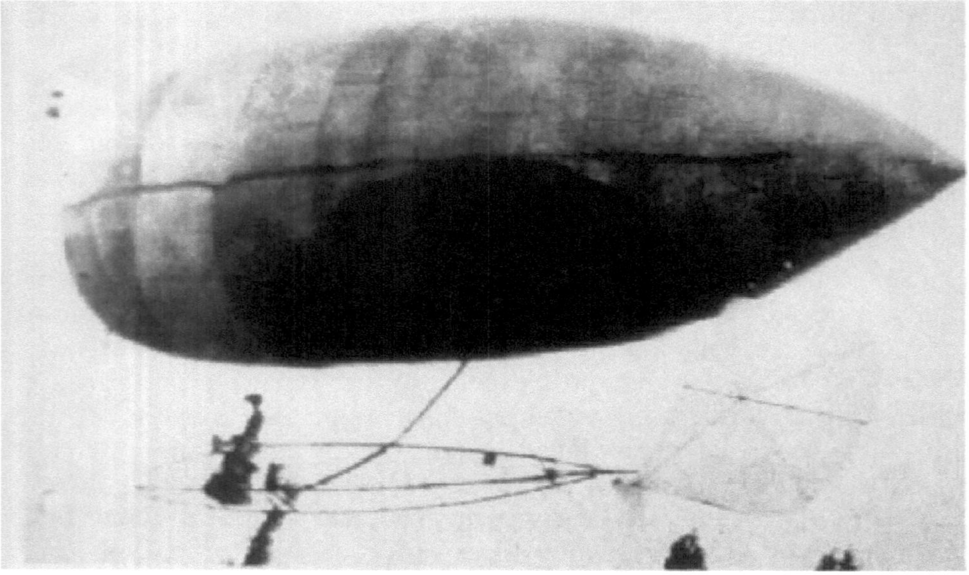

Fig. (2.2). Aida D'Acosta, Dumont's friend, at controls of his No. 9 airship.

After his success designing and flying airships, Dumont turned his attention to heavier-than-air machines. Initially, he conceived a twin-propeller single-engine monoplane but later he built a biplane based on an existing glider and performed some flights with it.

In October of 1906, Santos-Dumont performed a 220-m flight with his 14Bis biplane in France (Fig. **2.3**) [2]. Dumont's flight was certified by an Aero club de France committee as the first heavier-than-air flight in history. A crowd present on the Le Bagatelle field also watched the air ride.

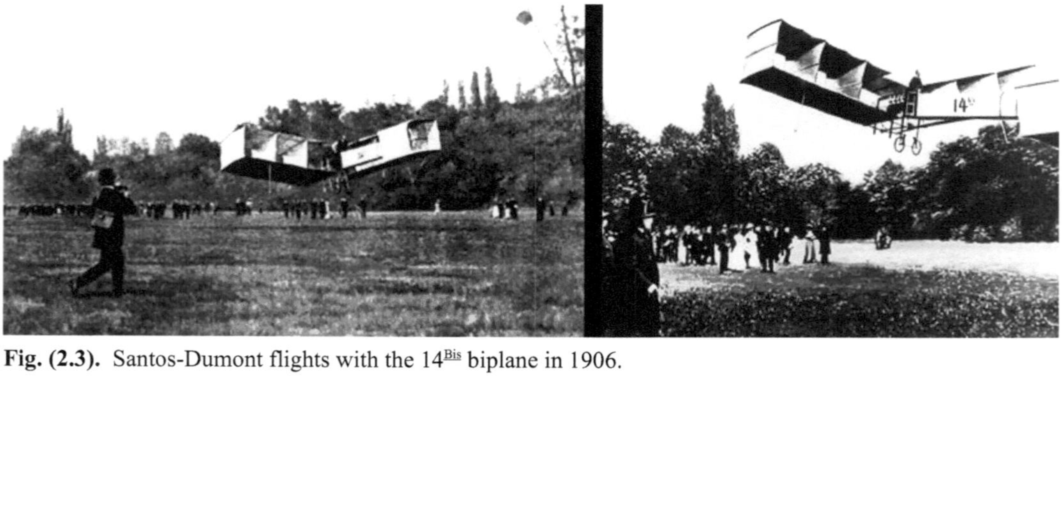

Fig. (2.3). Santos-Dumont flights with the 14$^{\underline{Bis}}$ biplane in 1906.

The First Operational Airplane

In 1907, Santos-Dumont started work on a groundbreaking airplane, going back to the monoplane configuration that he had considered before the flights with his 14Bis biplane [1]. Thus, the Demoiselle high-wing monoplane arose, which was the first practical airplane [1]. Demoiselle shaped things that would come, like the Blériot XI monoplane that crossed the English Channel [2]. The single-engine Demoiselle airplane (Fig. **2.4**) was Dumont's last concept, closing his aeronautical activities in 1909. The Brazilian aviation pioneer performed many experiments with Demoiselle, which received successive designations – Number 19 to 22. The Demoiselle was an extraordinary experience in terms of construction and configuration because Dumont pioneered a geodesic bamboo structure that employed steel piano wiring for its rigidity.

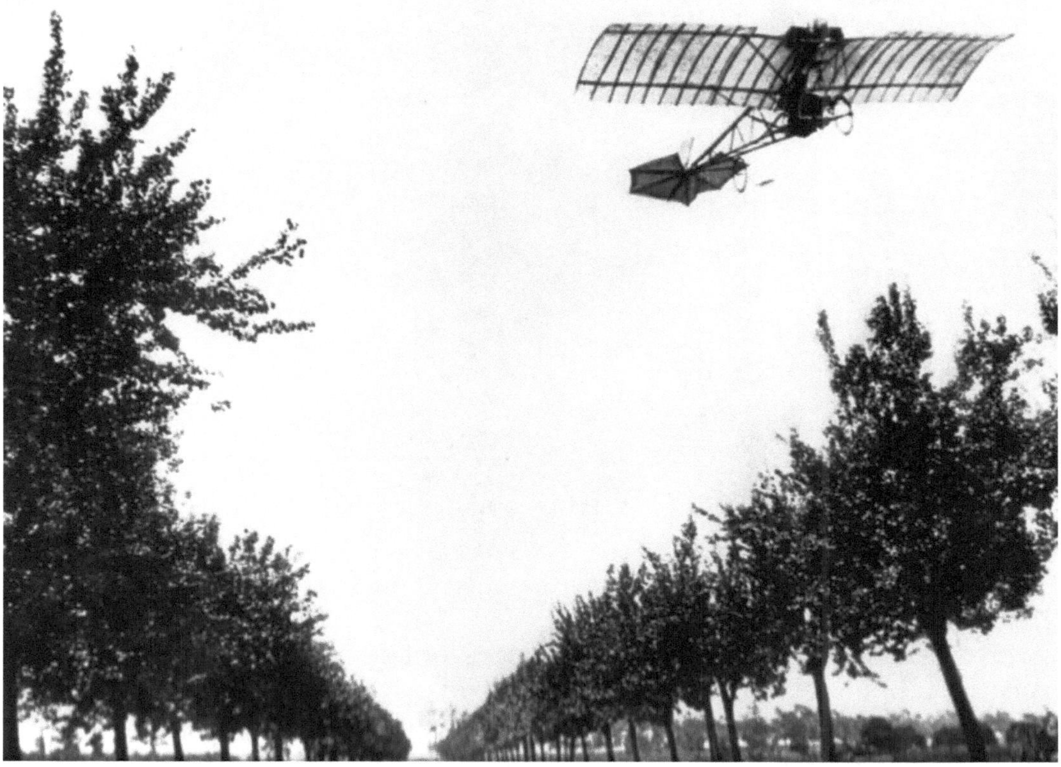

Fig. (2.4). Demoiselle was the first practical airplane [1] [3].

Demoiselle was produced in many countries, including Germany, France (Clément Bayard Company), Holland, and the United States [3]. Dumont employed Demoiselle as his personal means of transportation [2]. The small airplane could be transported in the back of his electric automobile (Fig. **2.5**), which was adapted for this purpose [4]. He let others make use of his design, in agreement with the philosophy of the French Revolution ambience that prevailed at that time in France [1]. The fuselage consisted of a specially reinforced bamboo boom, and the pilot found accommodation beneath the main wheels of a bicycle landing gear. Pitch and directional control was provided by a cruciform tail and roll control by wing warping (Number 20).

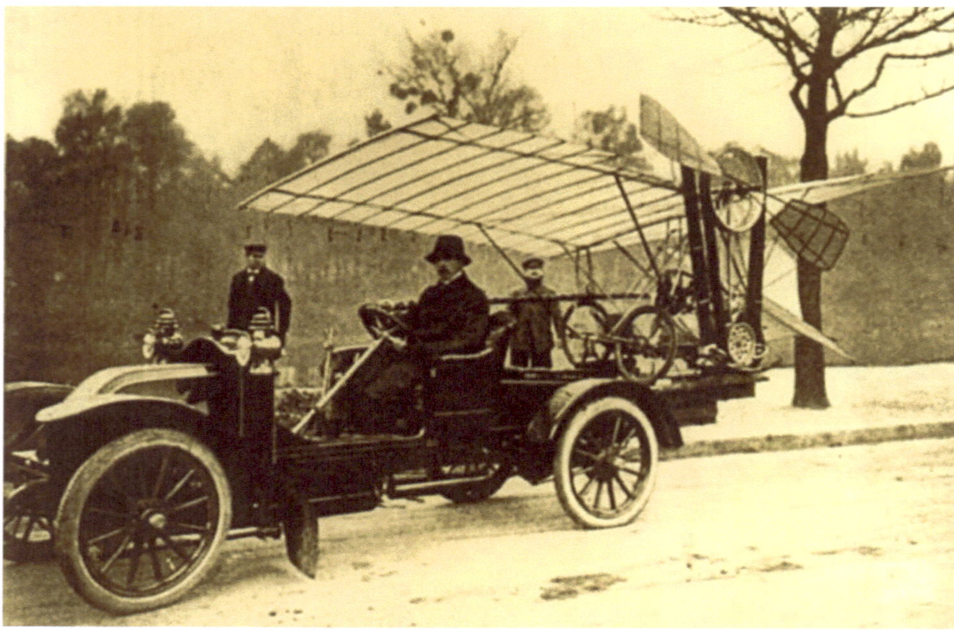

Fig. (2.5). Demoiselle monoplane being transported by electric automobile in 1909 [3].

Demoiselle was produced in many countries, including Germany, France (Clément Bayard Company), Holland, and the United States [4]. Dumont employed Demoiselle as his personal means of transportation [2]. The small airplane could be transported in the back of his electric automobile (Fig. **2.5**), which was adapted for this purpose [3]. He let others make use of his design, in agreement with the philosophy of the French Revolution ambience that prevailed at that time in France [1]. The fuselage consisted of a specially reinforced bamboo boom, and the pilot found accommodation beneath the main wheels of a bicycle landing gear. Pitch and directional control was provided by a cruciform tail and roll control by wing warping (Number 20).

Dumont steadily increased the wingspan of his airplane. Earlier Demoiselle versions presented a wingspan of 5.10 m and an overall length of 8 m. Gross weight of Demoiselle was 110 kg with Santos-Dumont at controls. Take-off run was typically 40 m [3]. The pilot was seated below the fuselage-wing junction, just behind the wheels, and commanded the tail surfaces using a steering wheel [1]. Concerning aerodynamics, Demoiselle featured airfoil with much camber at the wing leading-edge region. Initially, Santos-Dumont employed a liquid-cooled Dutheil & Chalmers engine delivering 20 hp. Later, he repositioned the engine to a lower location, placing it in front of the pilot. He also replaced the former engine by a 24-hp Antoniette and introduced some wing reinforcements [1]. Due to structural problems and continuous lack of power, Santos-Dumont introduced additional modifications into the Demoiselle's configuration: a triangular and shortened fuselage made of bamboo; the engine was moved backwards, but kept its positioning in front of the wing and increased wingspan. This resulted in the configuration designated No. 21 [1]. The design of No. 22 was like No. 21. Santos-Dumont tested opposed-cylinder (he patented a solution for cooling this kind of engine) and cooled-water engines, with power settings ranging from 20 to 40 hp, in both variants [1]. An interesting feature of the water-cooled variant was the liquid-coolant pipeline that followed the wing lower side geometry in order not to cause too much aerodynamic degradation (Fig. **2.6**).

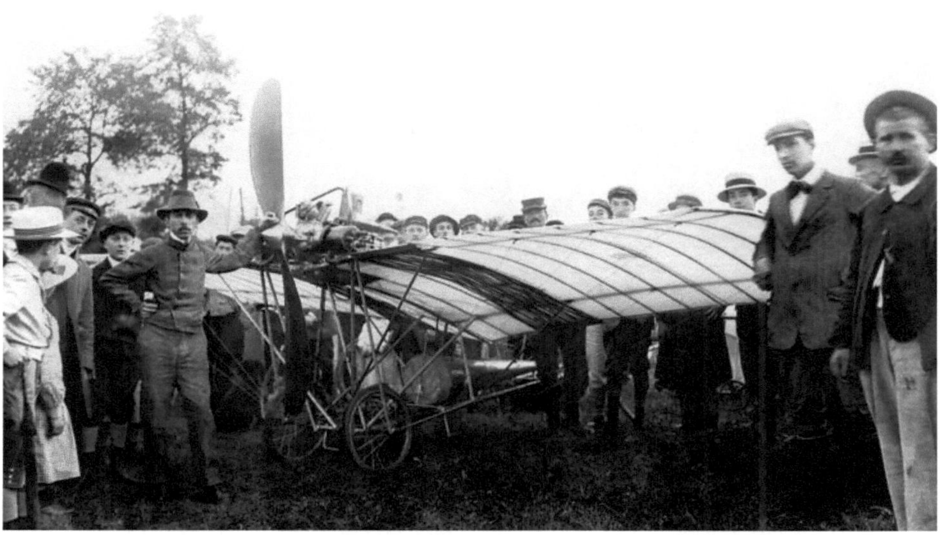

Fig. (2.6). Demoiselle with conformal radiators on wing lower side.

Delivering outstanding performance, demanding a very short takeoff length and being able to fly at speeds higher than 100 km/h, Demoiselle was the last aircraft built by Santos-Dumont. He used to perform flights with the airplane in Paris and to nearby places [3]. Flights were continued at various times through 1909, including the first cross-country flight recorded in history. The Demoiselle that was fitted with a two-cylinder engine became rather popular. Influenced by the spirit of French revolution of 1789, Santos-Dumont released the drawings of Demoiselle free of charge, believing that aviation would be the mainstream of a new era of economic growth [1]. Clément Bayard, an automotive and bicycle maker, constructed several units of Demoiselle, which were sold for 50,000 Francs each. Time required to build an exemplar of Demoiselle was just 15 days. Over 300 Demoiselle exemplars were built, making it a very successful airplane [4].

The design of Demoiselle influenced the configuration of the Blériot XI airplane (Fig. **2.7**), which was used by Dumont's friend Louis Blériot for the British Channel crossing in 1909. Blériot XI was a tractor-configuration monoplane with a partially covered box-truss fuselage built with wire bracing to guarantee rigidity. Wing warping was employed for lateral control. The tail surfaces consisted of a small balanced all-moving rudder mounted on the rearmost part of the fuselage and a horizontal stabilizer mounted under the lower longerons.

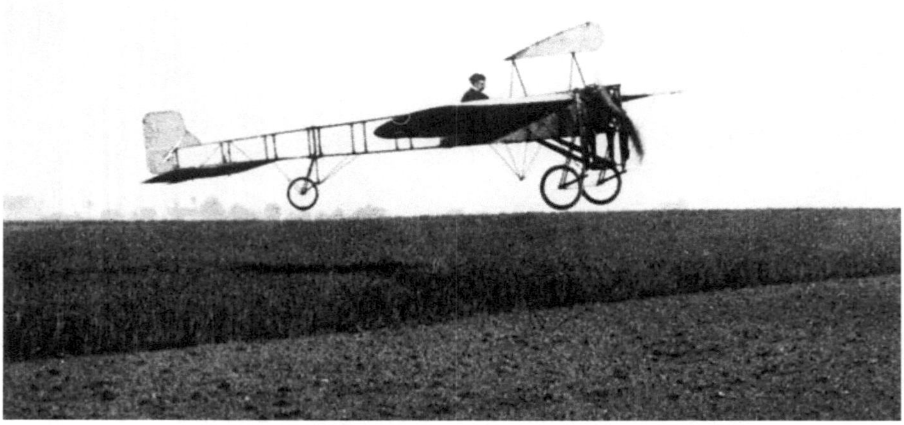

Fig. (2.7). Blériot XI as first built (Photo: Library of Congress, public domain).

THE FIRST AIRLINERS

From War to Peace

Table **2.1** displays the impressive progress of the solution of the problem of heavier-than-air flight [2]. All achievements were recorded by Aéro-Club de France. Although Wilbur Wright had settled down in France in 1907, he was only able to deliver a remarkable performance in late 1908, probably after he incorporated European technology into Flyer`s configuration. The Wrights did not take part in the competition organized by Scientific American in the U.S for the first kilometer flight journey. The Brothers would have been required to install wheels and discard the catapult launch to compete for the 1908 prize. Curtiss won the competition with his "June Bug" biplane in July 1908.

Table 2.1. Progressive flight records [2].

Aviator	Place	Date	Distance/Time
Santos-Dumont	Bagatelle	22 Aug. 1906	Few seconds
Santos-Dumont	Bagatelle	14 Sept. 1906	7-8 m
Santos-Dumont	Bagatelle	23 Oct. 1906	50 m
Santos-Dumont	Bagatelle	12 Nov. 1906	220 m
Henry Farman	Issy	26 Oct. 1907	771 m
Henry Farman	Issy	13 Jan. 1908	1 500 m
Henry Farman	Issy	21 March 1908	2 004 m
Delagrange	Issy	10 April 1908	2 500 m
Delagrange	Issy	11 April 1908	3 925 m
Delagrange	Rome	27 May 1908	5 km
Delagrange	Rome	27 May 1908	9 km
Delagrange	Rome	30 May 1908	12.5 km
Delagrange	Milan	22 June 1908	17 km
Henry Farman	Gand	6 July 1908	19.7 km
Delagrange	Issy	6 Sept. 1908	24.727 km
Orville Wright	Fort Meyer	9 Sept. 1908	1 h 2 min 30 s
Orville Wright	Fort Meyer	10 Sept. 1908	1 h 5 min 57 s
Orville Wright	Fort Meyer	11 Sept. 1908	1h 10 min 50 s
Orville Wright	Fort Meyer	12 Sept. 1908	1h 15 min 20 s
Wilbur Wright	Auvours	21 Sept. 1908	1 h 31 min 25 s
Wilbur Wright	Le Mans	18 Dec. 1908	1 h 54 min 22 s

After many successful flights with Demoiselle, Dumont ceased aeronautical activities in 1909 because he was suffering from multiple sclerosis. However, aviation was in fiber one year before. Henri Farman was one of Dumont's closest friends. In 1908, he performed the first kilometer flight in history [2]. On March 29 of the same year, Henri Farman carried aviation Maecenas Ernest Archdeacon aloft for 134 m on the first airplane passenger flight in the World (Fig. **2.8**) [2]. On May 14, 1908, Wilbur Wright flew mechanic Charles Furnas 600 m in 29 seconds, making him the first airplane passenger in the United States. On June 2, 1908, Farman performed a flight with a single passenger covering 1,241 km [2]. On October 10, 1908, Wilbur Wright held the passenger-carrying record with a flight of 1 h 9 min 45 sec that covered 80 km [2].

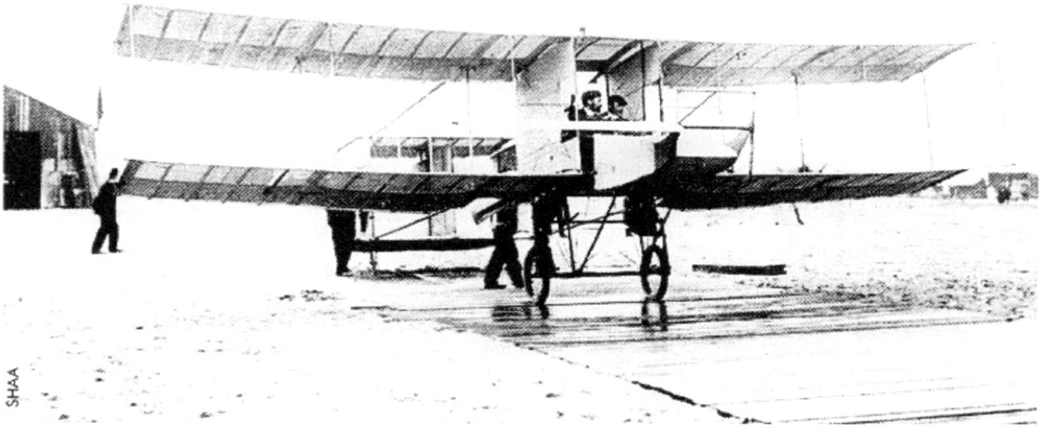

Farman et son passager Archdeacon, Issy-les-Moulineaux 1908.

Fig. (2.8). Henri Farman and his passenger Archdeacon (1908) [2].

Aviation was gaining even greater momentum from 1909 on. The Frenchman Louis Blériot came out of a partnership with the Voisin brothers, with whom he had built gliders. Afterwards, he founded his own aircraft manufacturing company. One of his concepts was the Blériot Aerobus 1911 [4], which performed flights with passengers exposed to the wind (Fig. **2.9**). Sometime later, the Aerobus cabin was closed (Fig. **2.9**), yet providing little comfort to passengers. There are reports of flights up to six passengers. The Avro Type F and the Etrich Luftlimousine, both from 1912, were conceived to carry passengers in an enclosed cabin (Fig. **2.9**) [4].

The Ilya Muromets (Fig. **2.10**) aircraft as it appeared in 1913 [5] was a revolutionary design, intended for commercial service with its spacious fuselage incorporating a passenger saloon and washroom on board [6, 7]. During World War I, it became the first four-engine bomber to equip a dedicated strategic bombing unit [6, 7]. The Ilya Muromets was initially conceived and built as a luxurious aircraft. For the first time in aviation history, an airplane had an insulated passenger saloon, comfortable wicker chairs, a bedroom, a lounge and even the first airborne toilet [8]. The aircraft also had heating and electrical lighting in passenger cabin [5].

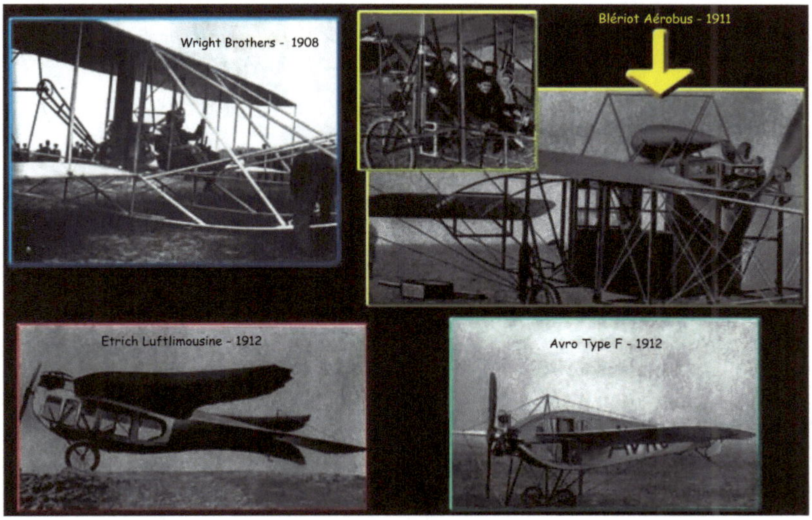

Fig. (2.9). First passenger airplanes [1, 4].

Immediately after World War II, many transport aircraft were derived from combat aircraft used in that conflict, especially bombers. There have been major technological leaps arising from the war like the use of thick airfoils, water-cooled engines, propeller-synchronous machine gun, and aluminum construction; the latter pioneered by the German company Junkers Flugzeug- und Motorenwerke AG. The German electricity company AEG (Allgemeine Elektricitäts-Gemeinschaft (AEG) also manufactured aircraft for the army during the First World War. The AEG JI was used by the Germans in World War I as ground attack aircraft. After the conflict, it represented one of the first conversions of military aircraft for civilian use with the J.II variant (Fig. **2.11**).

Soon after World War I, commercial aviation development experienced an exponential growth. French aviation pioneer Henri Farman set up an airplane manufacturing plant. He designed and built a bomber capable of carrying a bomb load of 1000 kg for a 1500-km distant target [9]. The bomber was undergoing some tests when World War I came to an end. Farman reconfigured the bomber turning it into an airliner, which received F. 60 Goliath designation (Fig. **2.12**). Farman soon put the Goliath into service and made several public flights. On February 8, 1919, the Goliath flew with 12 passengers from Toussus-le-Noble to RAF Kenley, near Croydon [9]. New European airlines were rapidly acquiring the F.60 airliner.

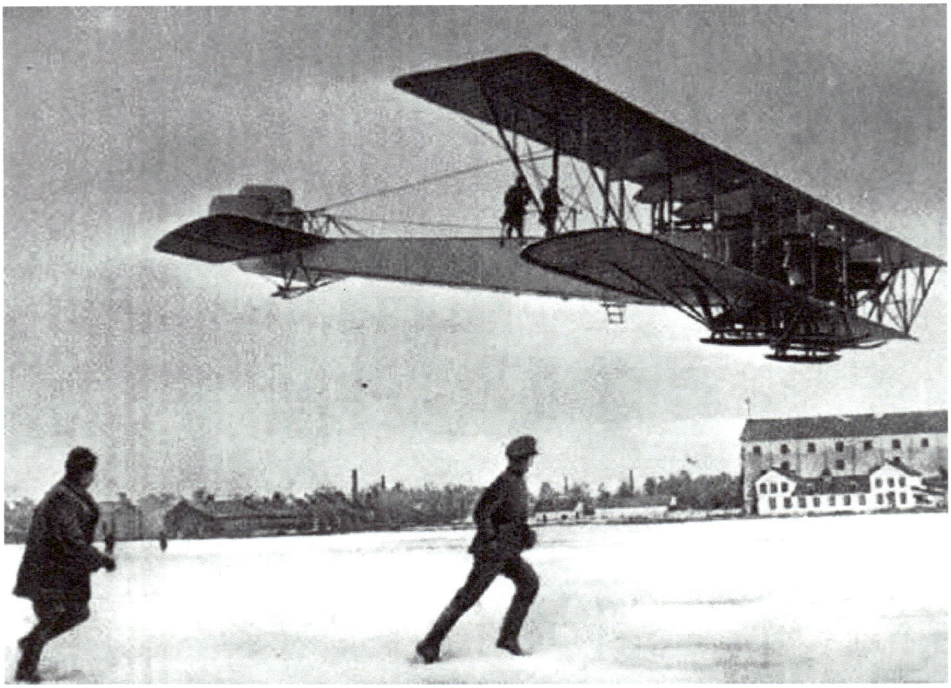

Fig. (2.10). Sikorsky Ilya Muromets in 1913 (Public domain photo).

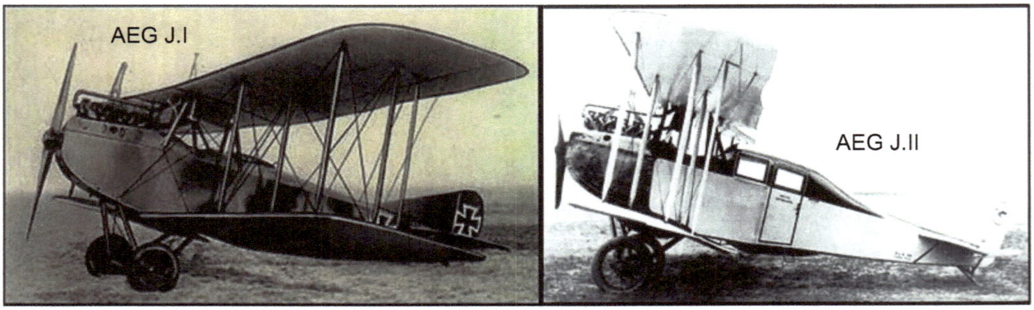

Fig. (2.11). The AEG J.II transport airplane was derived from the military plane J.I.

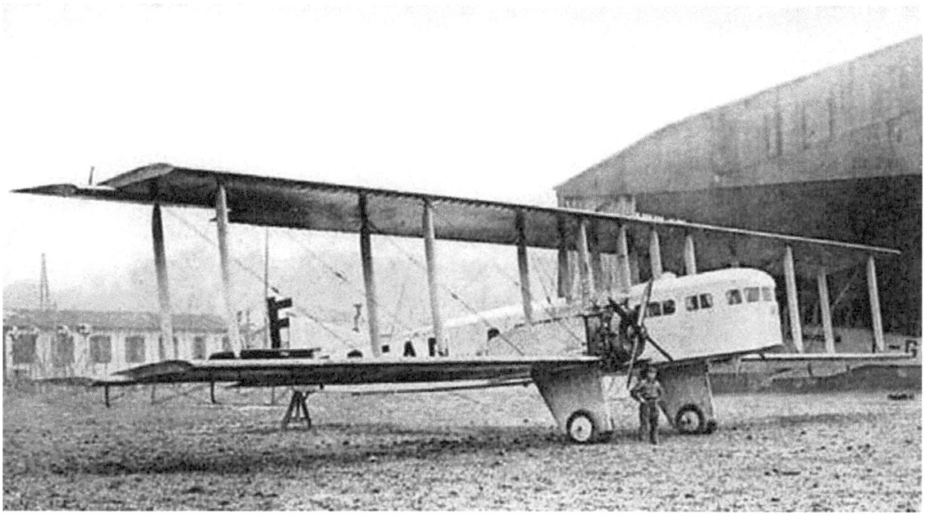

Fig. (2.12). Farman F.60 Goliath.

International Services

On February 8th, 1919, the first regular international commercial route was opened between Paris and London [8] flown by a Farman F.60 Goliath from Farman Airlines. Regular flight service with daily departures began between London and Paris also in 1919. The conditions aboard the airplanes were in certain degree unpleasant, with passengers experiencing freezing cold, vibrations, unbearable noise, and strong turbulence [10]. The 1919 Convention of Paris ended the hopes of early aviation pioneers that the skies would be borderless and without much control [10]. Instead, it was decreed that each country had complete and exclusive sovereignty over the airspace above its territory [10].

In 1920, the Compagnie des Grands Express Aériens (CGEA) began scheduling regular flights between Le Bourget and Croydon. The Compagnie des Messageries Aériennes (CMA) soon followed suit. The Société Générale de Transports Aérien (SGTA) opened a Paris-Brussels route in July 1920, flown by the Goliath. In May 1921, this route was extended to Amsterdam. Belgian airline Société Nationale pour l'Etude des Transports Aériens (SNETA) also opened a Brussels-London route in April 1921.

The Goliath suffered several fatal accidents along its career as airliner. A remarkable accident involving that plane type took place in 1922. The Daimler Airway mail flight from Croydon to Le Bourget operating a De Havilland DH.18A took off early in the morning on April 7 [11]. There was just one pilot on board as well as a young flight attendant. Just after noon, a Farman F.60 Goliath took off from Le Bourget heading to Croydon, flown by its pilot, M. Mire, with a mechanic on board as well [11]. Few passengers had purchased tickets for the trip performed with the Goliath airliner. Clouds at low altitudes, fog and a light drizzling rain marked the weather in that region. Excepting the magnetic compass, navigation instruments did not exist in those days. Because this the pilots of both airliners were flying at the base of the clouds, looking down on the ground for references [11]. Thereby, both aircraft were flying at the same altitude. At the time, as informal practice, pilots should offset from navigational landmarks, based on the road rules. Thus, a French pilot would fly up a roadway, offset to the right side and looking down on the road to the left. Opposing traffic therefore would pass also on the left. The same informal practice was implemented in England, though few considered the potential international conflict based on English roadway rules, cars had right hand drive and drove on the left side of the roads. Thus, the British pilot of the Daimler Airway flight naturally offset to his left, not to the right. This put both airplanes on a collision course with the cloud base dictating their identical altitude [11].

In the wake of Goliath's accident, aviation authorities started to discuss safety measures. Some new rules were then recommended and approved. First, the midair collision resulted in a universal definition of "right of way" in the air, where planes should offset to the right when flying over roads or landmarks that on seeing another aircraft approach head-on that they should each turn to the right to thereby avoid a collision [11]. The accident also spurred the creation of the world's first airway systems, the same ones that we currently use today, combining lower altitude airways with the "J-routes" or airway for jet aircraft at higher altitudes. Check points (usually at navigational aids) are connected by straight line airways between them, enabling aircraft separation by altitudes on the airways and conversely giving rise to the system of westerly headings on even altitudes (8,000 ft, 10,000 ft, *etc.*) and easterly headings on odd altitudes (9,000 ft, 11,000 ft, *etc.*).

In 1926, the German government formed a national airline, Lufthansa. The governments of France (Air France, 1933) and Britain (BOAC, 1939) followed suit. The earliest national airline had been founded by the Netherlands in 1919, KLM. By 1929, KLM was regularly flying the longest scheduled route in the world, which was an eight-day trip from the Netherlands to Jakarta, Indonesia (then the Dutch East Indies). The Queensland and Northern Territory Aerial Services Limited (Qantas) was founded in 1920 as a private company by a couple of pilots. AVIANCA, former national carrier of Colombia, is one of earliest airlines, the first one in South America. It was founded on December 5, 1919, when it was initially registered under the name SCADT.

Advances in Aeronautical Technology

Germany emerged as the world leader of passenger air transport in the 1920s, with the most advanced technology. In 1904, the great researcher Ludwig Prandtl of the Göttingen University delivered a pioneer paper, *Fluid Flow with Very Small Viscosity* [12], in which he described the boundary layer and its importance for fluid dynamics, particularly drag created by streamlined bodies. The paper also described flow separation of the boundary layer, which led to the concept of stall of lifting surfaces. In addition, Prandtl developed the first theories about supersonic shock waves in 1908, placing Germany in the vanguard for the understanding of the supersonic flow before World War II. The Prandtl-Meyer expansion fans allowed for the construction of supersonic wind tunnels. Prandtl had little time to work further on the problem until the 1920s, when he worked with Adolf Busemann and created a method for designing a supersonic nozzle in 1929 [13]. Today, all supersonic wind tunnels and rocket nozzles are designed using the same method [13].

A solid development for the understanding of supersonic flow would have to wait for the work of Theodore von Kármán, a graduate student of Prandtl at Göttingen University. This university also introduced the thick airfoil concept, which was employed for the best fighter airplane of World War I, the Fokker D.VII biplane (Fig. **2.13**). Typically, thick airfoils present better stall characteristics and lift-t--drag ratio than those thinner ones employed in previous airplanes. Since thicker airfoils enable lighter and stronger wing structure, the Fokker D.VII designers could eliminate the external structural bracing, which, in turn, reduced the airplane drag. All this combined reflects on the airplane performance, increasing it considerably.

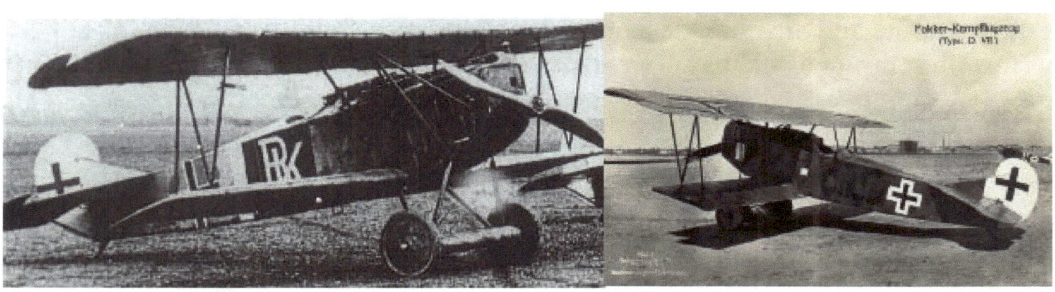

Fig. (2.13). Fokker D.VII (Public domain photos via Wikimedia Commons).

Prandtl also developed the mixing length theory for model the momentum transfer by Reynolds stresses within a turbulent boundary layer [14]. Since a long time, it is of widespread wisdom that the concept of a mixing length does not adequately model the correct physical phenomenon of the detailed structure of turbulence.

Despite this, mixing length theories are nevertheless most useful to engineers as a method for the correlation with experimental data [15].

Junkers revolutionary airplane metal construction during the World War I is the technology that can be considered one of the biggest aviation advances from World War I [16]. Its Junkers D.I monoplane was initially funded by the Junkers company alone [16].

After the four-engine Ilya Muromets, Junkers F.13 was the second airplane that was designed to carry passengers from the beginning. Thus, it was not a civil variant of a military concept like most of its contemporary airplanes according to previous text in this Chapter. This aircraft performed its first flight in June 1919. It was an advanced cantilever-wing monoplane, with enclosed accommodation for four passengers in a heated cabin [17]. Like all Junkers duralumin-structured designs, F.13 used an aluminum alloy for its structure. The airplane was covered with Junkers' patented corrugated and stressed duralumin skin. Internally, the wing was built up on nine tubular cross-section duralumin spars kept in place by transversal duralumin bracing [18]. All control surfaces contained horns that provided lower control forces. Junkers F.13 was produced along thirteen years and saw commercial service for almost twenty years in several countries and over 300 were sold [17]. Rimowa, a traditional German company that produces luggage made of aluminum and polycarbonate presented at Oshkosh air show 2015 a replica of the venerable F.13 [18]. The company is marketing the airplane will sell it from 2017. The “new” F.13 is fitted with a 450-hp Pratt & Whitney R-985 driving a Hamilton Standard adjustable propeller [18].

After World War I, major advancement during the 1920s in the design and technology of aircraft gave aviation new roles. Improvements in wind-tunnel testing, engine and airframe design, and maintenance equipment made for better-performing airplanes. Thus, private planes became less expensive and, in turn, grew in number and popularity. Safer airplanes attract more passengers, increasing the profitability of the airlines.

The development of the autopilot started in 1908, when Elmer Sperry introduced a type of gyrocompass that was later used in ship piloting systems (magnetic compasses were unreliable in steel-hulled ships) [19]. In 1914, Elmer’s son, Lawrence Sperry, demonstrated an automatic gyrostabilizer in New York State. A gyroscope linked to sensors kept the vehicle in level flight, traveling in a straight line without human intervention. Two years later, Sperry and Elmer added a steering gyroscope to the stabilizer gyroscope and developed this way the first automatic pilot. In 1929, Sperry's company tested a similar device for aircraft, as well as another device, the artificial horizon [19]. These instruments, which enabled the pilot to fly without seeing the ground below, were rapidly installed aboard mail and commercial airplanes.

The first in-flight movie that has been recorded was the one that was shown in 1921 aboard an Aeromarine Airways airplane showing a film called Howdy Chicago to its passengers [20]. *The Lost World* motion picture was shown to passengers of an Imperial Airways flight on April 1925 between London (Croydon Airport) and Paris [20]. In the same year, Lufthansa also offered in-flight movies to passengers. The fact is that a silent movie was ideal one at that time because the noise of the engines anyway did not allow the dialogues and music from the movie to be heard.

The Curtiss Condor (Fig. **2.14**) was one of the first aircraft to offer a soundproof cabin [21]. It was considerable quiet inside and people could carry on a conversation or listen to the radio. This was amazing to passengers at that time. In addition, the wide fuselage allowed for 12 sleeping berths. They were operated by Eastern Air Transport, American Airways and Swissair. Condor was made of old-fashioned frame-and-fabric components with a tubular wing spar and was powered by two 750-hp Wright Cyclone SGR-1820-3 engines.

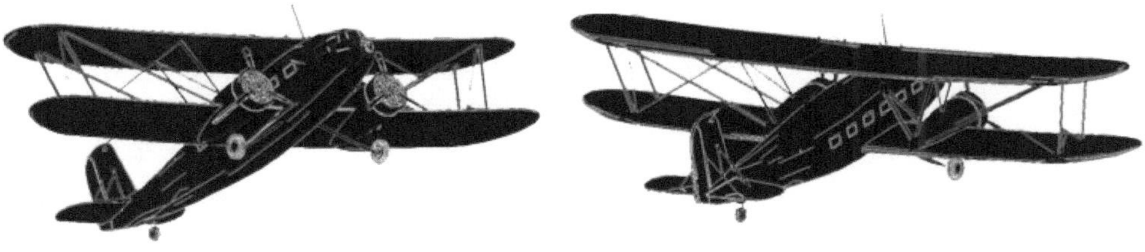

Fig. (2.14). Curtiss Condor.

The primary structural material of World War I aircraft was wood, which was well suited to the small workshops and skilled labor of the period. However, the properties of wood are anisotropic, and strength characteristics can vary depending on supply source. A potential alternative was metal, but it would not be a simple matter of substituting metal for wood. Early attempts to use aluminum and steel did not immediately satisfy the goal of weight reduction. The low stress levels in the airframes of this period required only a fraction of the inherent load bearing capacity of metal.

The late 1920s and early 1930s registered a structural evolution in aeronautics with the widespread manufacturing of streamlined metal aircraft with such features as cowled multiple engines, variable-pitch propellers, retracting landing gear, and stressed-skin aluminum construction [22]. The transition from the wood-and-fabric airplane to the all-metal airplane was essentially completed before World War II with all-metal fighters like the Me 109 and multiple-engine bombers and airliners, whose examples are the Boeing B-17 and the Boeing 307 Stratoliner, respectively.

Metal did indeed allow engineers to extend performance parameters afforded by innovative structural design. Metal construction has enabled aircraft to endure the greater stresses incurring at high speeds and when carrying large payloads and were not affect by moisture and artisanal fabrication. Indeed, it would not be possible to achieve the same performance of a Boeing 777 airliner or an F-18 fighter aircraft if they were constructed of wood instead [22].

The Junkers 52 was an all-metal aircraft designed to transport 17 passengers. It is also one of the most successful transport aircraft in history, with 4,845 units manufactured. Designed by Ernst Zindel of the Junkers factory in the city of Dessau, Germany, the initial model was fitted with a single engine, and was designated Ju 52/1m. The prototype made its first flight in 1931 and was certified in the same year. Due to lack of interest from buyers, mainly from Deutsche Lufthansa, Junkers redesigned the airplane, adding to the aircraft two engines to improve its performance. The modified airplane received the designation Ju 52/3m (Fig. **2.15**). The aircraft was fitted with BMW engines and some export models also used Pratt & Whitney Wasp or Bristol Pegasus engines. The first aircraft with the new configuration, equipped with Pratt & Whitney engines, were delivered to Lloyd Aero Boliviano (LAB). The extinct Brazilian airline VASP (Viação Aérea São Paulo) acquired two Ju-52/3m, dubbed the *Cidade de São Paulo* and *Cidade do Rio de Janeiro*. Assembly parts of the two aircraft were shipped from Germany to Brazil, with the final assembly taking place in Brazil. The two aircraft inaugurate the Sao Paulo-Rio route on August 5, 1936.

The Ju 52 was also a key player in Operation Merkur (The German invasion of Crete) in 1941 as a paratroop transport aircraft. This operation was considered a success because the planned goals have been achieved. However, the loss of airplanes was large and more than half of the 493 aircraft that participated in the action were damaged or destroyed. Due to the high human and material losses of this operation, further offensive using airborne troops was not carried out by Germany anymore in World War II. Even the Allies had initially considered an autogyro as main force to retake continental Europe from Germany. For this role, the Hafner Rotabuggy was conceived, which was a British experimental aircraft, essentially a Jeep Willys MB combined with a rotor kite, developed with the intention of producing a way of air-dropping off-road vehicles [23]. Although initial tests showed that the Rotabuggy was prone to severe vibration at speeds greater than 70 km/h, thanks to improvements the Rotabuggy achieved a flight speed of 113 km/h in February 1944. However, the introduction of gliders such as Airspeed Horsa that were capable of transporting road vehicles made the Rotabuggy superfluous and further development was cancelled.

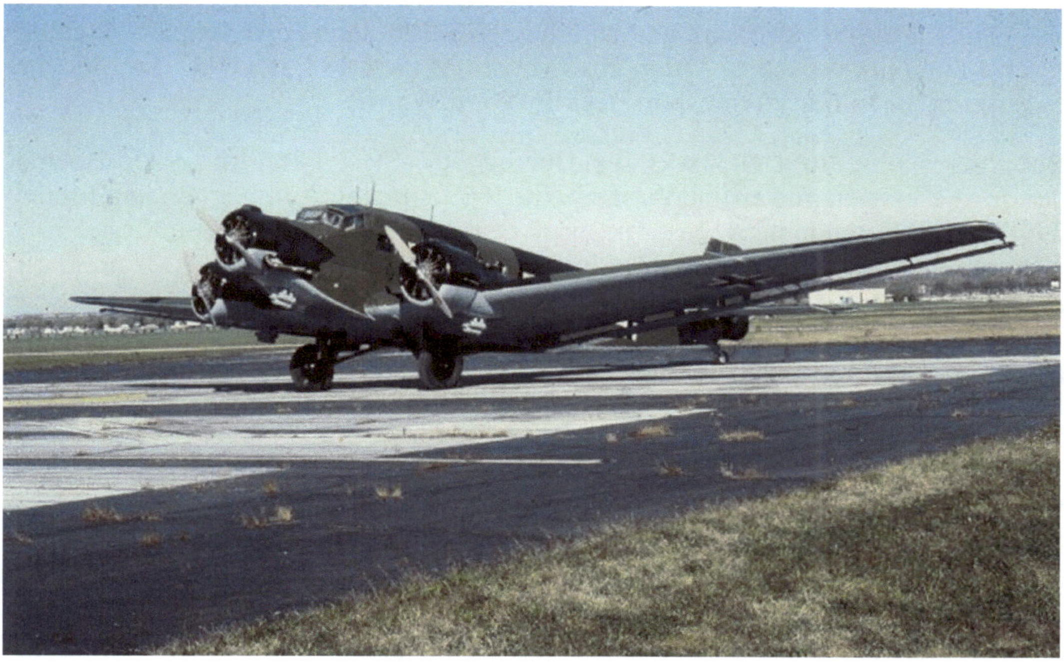

Fig. (2.15). Junkers Ju 52/3m at the National Museum of the US Air Force (Photo: U.S. Air Force, public domain).

The number of Ju52/m delivered to Luftwaffe is unclear [24]. The airplane was versatile, seeing use as bomber, paratrooper transporter, towing gliders, cargo and passenger transport, and advanced trainer. The airplane also saw service as minelayer.

Hugo Junkers, who had pioneered a series of innovation in aviation, once again brought a new concept when decided to employ aileron as flap on takeoff for the Ju 52/3m. The ailerons could also be adjusted to locally change the lift on the wing to generate lower induced drag, the drag related to the lift and that is dependent on the load distribution along the wingspan (chord x lift coefficient).

The Boeing Model 247 monoplane was an important airliner of the interwar period. It entered service in 1933 and brought many advanced technologies at that time like wing deicing boots, cantilever construction, and autopilot [25]. United Airlines and Boeing belonged to the same holding at that time. For this reason, United Airlines was given priority for Boeing 247 deliveries. Thus, TWA approached Douglas to develop an airliner to compete with Boeing 247 and the DC line was then created: DC-1, DC-2, and DC-3. The DC-3, which went into service in 1936, was easy to maintain and it was considered a reliable airplane. It had several innovative design features, a semi-retractable landing gear, flexible wings of simple construction, and with its two 1,200-horsepower engines it could reach a maximum speed of 370 mph. A variant of the DC-3, the C-47, became the flagship of the military's transport fleet in World War II.

Boeing response to DC-3 was the Boeing 307 Stratoliner. In 1935, Boeing designed a four-engine airliner based on its B-17 strategic bomber (Boeing Model 299), then in development [26]. The airplane received the designation Model 307. It combined the wings, tail, rudder, landing gear, and engines from their production B-17C with a new, circular cross-section fuselage, which was designed to allow cabin pressurization [26]. The first order, for two 307s, was placed in 1937 by Pan American Airways; Pan Am soon increased this to six exemplars and a second order for five from Transcontinental & Western Air (TWA), prompting Boeing to begin production on an initial batch of the airliner. World War II interrupted the commercial operation of the Boeing 307 but they were employed as military transport during the war.

The Focke-Wulf 200 Condor (Fig. **2.16**) was a long-range passenger transport designed by Prof. Kurt Tank of the German company Focke-Wulf Flugzeugbau AG. Professor Heinrich Focke, Georg Wulf and Dr. Werber Naumann founded the Fock-Wulf company in 1923. In 1936, Prof. Focke was removed from the company due to pressure from shareholders. in 1937 Prof. Focke redirected the focus of his work to helicopters and founded the company Focke Achgelis in partnership with Gerd Achgelis. Professor Kurt Tank, the Technical Board and those who had worked on the development of the Fw 44 Stieglitz, were also responsible for the design of several other planes Focke-Wulf, among them, the Fw 200 airliner.

The Zeppelin Company had established regular passenger flights with airships between Germany and the South and North America. Most of those flights were performed by the venerable Graf Zeppelin, which was capable to transport 20 passengers. The Hindenburg airship performed ten trips in 1936. The eastern bound legs to North America took 53 to 78 hours and those back to Germany lasted from 43 to 61 hours. Besides being slower than land-based airplanes, passenger capacity of airships is very low regarding their size and they are very expensive to operate.

The first prototype, the Fw 200 V1, was fitted with additional fuel tanks. It performed several record flights and was the first airliner to fly nonstop between

Berlin and New York City [27]. The airplane took off from Berlin-Staaken to Floyd Bennett Field in August 1938 and the flight duration was 24 hours and 56 minutes [28]. The return flight to Berlin was performed in 19 hours. These flights have meant an end of airship era, independently of the Hindenburg disaster in May 1937. The non-stop long-haul flights era began.

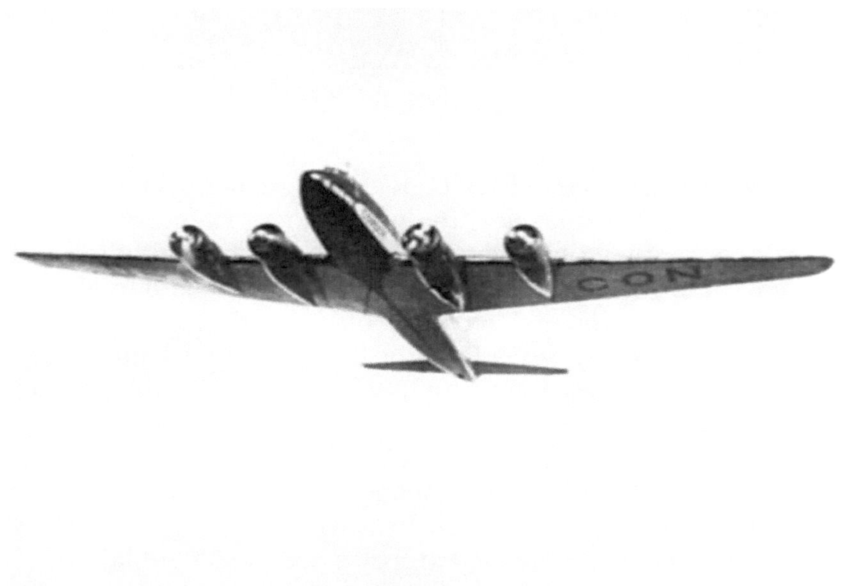

Fig. (2.16). The first Focke-Wulf Fw 200 "Brandenburg" (D-ACON) in flight. This airplane first flew on 27 July 1937 (Photo: Australian War Memorial, public domain).

The Fw 200 was operated by Deutsche Lufthansa, DDL Danish Airlines, and Lufthansa's Brazilian subsidiary Syndicato Condor, the latter was nationalized by Getulio Vargas after Brazil entered the World War II against the Germans [27]. Dai Nippon KK of Japan also ordered Fw 200 airliners. However, these could not be delivered to Japan due to the war outbreak and Lufthansa took delivery of them instead. On April 14th, 1945, an Fw 200 flew Lufthansa's last scheduled service before the end of World War II, from Barcelona to Berlin [27]. Other airlines continued to operate the Fw 200 after the end of World War II.

Military versions of the Focke-Wulf 200 were also developed. The Luftwaffe initially used the aircraft to support the German Navy by conducting maritime patrols and reconnaissance missions, searching for Allied convoys and destroyers that could be targeting German submarines [28]. The Fw 200 could also carry a 900-kg bomb load, rockets and it could lay naval mines. The Fw 200 was also used as a cargo aircraft, notably it provided equipment and supplies to the German forces that were attacking the city of Stalingrad in 1942. However, extra weight introduced by military equipment and higher loads associated to the airplane's new flight envelope led to structural failures of the fuselage at landing, a problem that was never entirely solved by Focke-Wulf. Later models were equipped with Lorenz FuG 200 Hohentwiel low UHF-band Airborne Surface Vessel (ASV) radar in the nose. In 1943, Fw 200 was adapted to carry the Henschel Hs 293 guided missile, which was steered by a gauntlet like current joysticks.

TECHNOLOGICAL LEGACY FROM WORLD WAR II

Fighters

In World War II, the aeronautical technology experienced an incredible boost. Besides the development of rocketry, the war introduced technological leaps in aircraft design and improved considerably their performance. Aerodynamically refined, all-metal high-performance fighters were developed during the conflict, replacing wood and fabric biplanes and monoplanes with fixed landing gear from the period between wars (Fig. **2.17**). Radar also experienced a huge development and its miniaturization enabled that night fighters were equipped with radar equipment to give effective combat to bomber airplanes. By War outbreak, the Bf 109 fighter equipped most squadrons (*Geschwäder)* of the Luftwaffe. The Japanese had developed the extremely maneuverable Zero, in part due to the non-placement of protective shields; the Spitfire was the frontline workhorse of the English Fighter Command and the United States operated the outdated Curtiss P-40 and Grumman Wildcat.

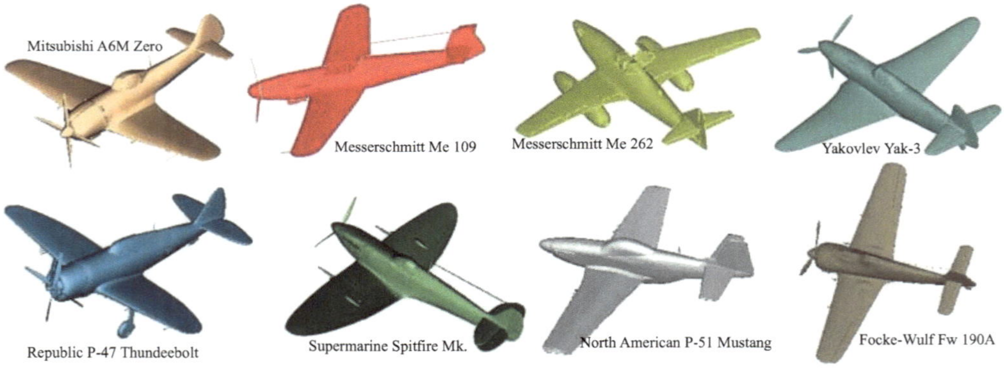

Fig. (2.17). Some allied and Axis fighters of World War II (Not in same scale).

The Messerschmitt Bf 109 (Bf stands for Bayerische Flugzeugwerke), commonly referred as Me 109, was designed by Willhem Messerschmitt and Robert Lusser during the early to mid-1930s [29]. The aircraft constituted the bulk fighter force of the Luftwaffe in World War II, with approximately 35,000 being built [29].

The type saw combat in the Spanish Civil war and continued to be produced along World War II. The fighter was initially fitted with a Rolls-Royce Kestrel engine, later replaced by a Jumo 210 before the beginning of World War II. Airplanes produced during the war received both DB 601 and the liquid-cooled inverted V12 DB 605 engine. The Reichsluftfarhtministerium (RLM) open a competition for a Messerschmitt 109 successor and the Focke-Wulf 190 was the winner.

The background thinking behind the Focke-Wulf 190 was to *Dienstpferd* (workhorse) not a cavalry horse like the Bf 109. For this reason, Focke-Wulf decided for an air-cooled, 14-cylinder BMW 139 radial engine instead of an inline water-cooled one. A water-cooled engine would be more difficult to maintain in the battlefront and more prone to be damaged by enemy fire.

The Bf 109 fighter was fitted with a simple mechanical slat system. Slats are high-lift devices placed at wing leading edges. The slat system of Bf 109 was conceived to count on ram air pressure to keep the slats in their closed position at higher speeds. The ram air pressure exerts a force against the bias of springs, which ensures the slats can be actuated outwards when the airplane is flying at lower speeds or when it performs a flight maneuver. In this latter case, the inner wing faces a lower wind speed that triggers the slat deflection and therefore increases the lift of that wing, with consequent maneuverability improvement of the fighter.

In fact, slats were first developed by the German Gustav Lachmann in 1918. An airplane accident in 1917 caused by stall led Lachman to idealize the slat mechanism. In 1918, Lachmann presented a patent for leading-edge slats in Germany. However, the German patent office initially rejected it because the officials did not believe in the possibility of increasing lift by splitting the wing into two or more pieces.

Independently of Lachmann, Handley Page Ltd in Great Britain also developed the slotted wing to increase the maximum lift coefficient of wings. The process consists in providing high-energy flow from below the wing to the decelerated airflow on the wing upper side after it contoured the leading edge. The English airplane company applied for a patent in 1919 and to avoid a legal dispute, they reached an agreement with Lachmann, which became a De Havilland's employee. In 1919, De Havilland D.H.9, a British bomber from World War I, was fitted with slats and successfully flown. Later, a D.H.4 was modified as a monoplane with a large wing fitted with full span leading edge and ailerons along the entire wingspan, which could be deployed in conjunction with the leading-edge slats to boost field performance [30]. Several years later, having subsequently taken employment at the Handley-Page aircraft company, Lachmann was responsible for several aircraft designs, including the Handley Page Hampden [30]. Licensing the concept became one of the company's major sources of income in the 1920s [30]. The original designs were in the form of a fixed slot in the frontal part of wings, an engineering solution that was employed by Boeing for its four-engine 307 Stratoliner.

Slats are used for both fighter and transport aircraft. Fieseler Fi 156 Storch (Fig. **2.18**) was a small German liaison aircraft built by Fieseler before and during World War II. A fixed slat ran along the entire length of the leading edge of the long wings, while a hinged and slotted set of control surfaces ran along the entire length of trailing edge [31]. The Storch is renowned for its remarkable short takeoff landing field lengths and extremely low stalling speed of 50 km/h. The Fi 156 can take off in less than 45 m and land in 18 m.

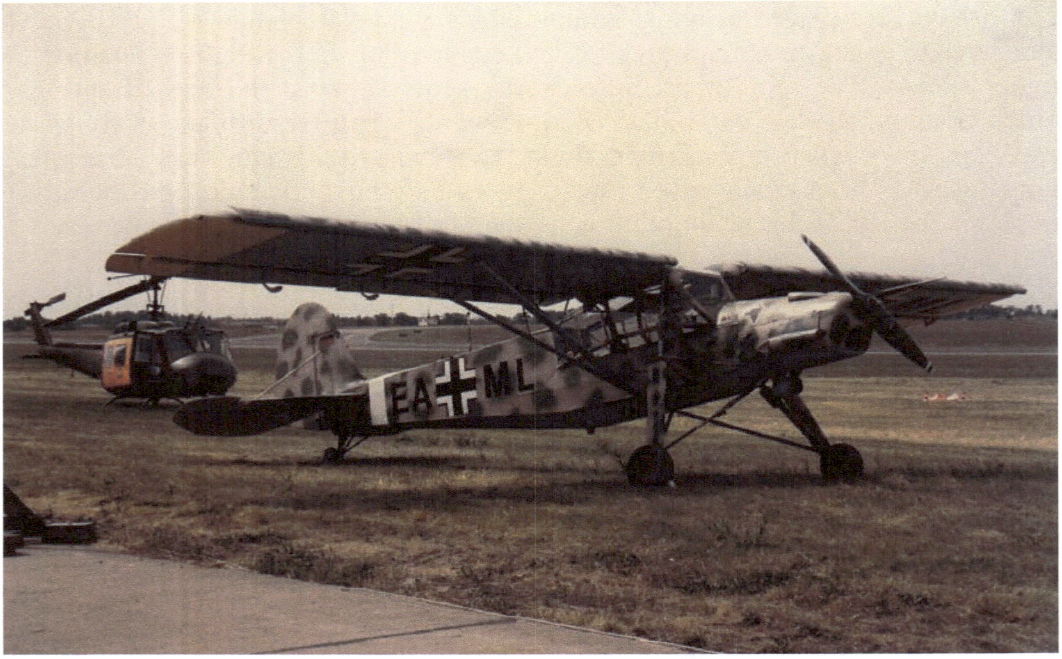

Fig. (2.18). Fieseler Storch at ILA 1992, Berlin Schönfeld (Photo: ©1992 Bento Mattos).

The North American F-86 Sabre, a veteran of the Korean War, presents slats along a large part of the wing leading edge (Fig. **2.19**). The design team of the American jet fighter opted for using an automatic slat system, operated independently of pilot control [32]. However, slats were removed in later versions of the fighter in favor of a fixed leading edge, which enabled an increased internal fuel capacity. This is an interesting point of debate because in fact slats feature some drawbacks such as increased wing weight, more expensive maintenance, they impact aircraft dispatch and wing fitted with slats presents a narrower wingbox, which reduces the fuel storage capacity. Some transport airplanes like the Fokker 100 have no slats and despite this they present a reasonable field performance.

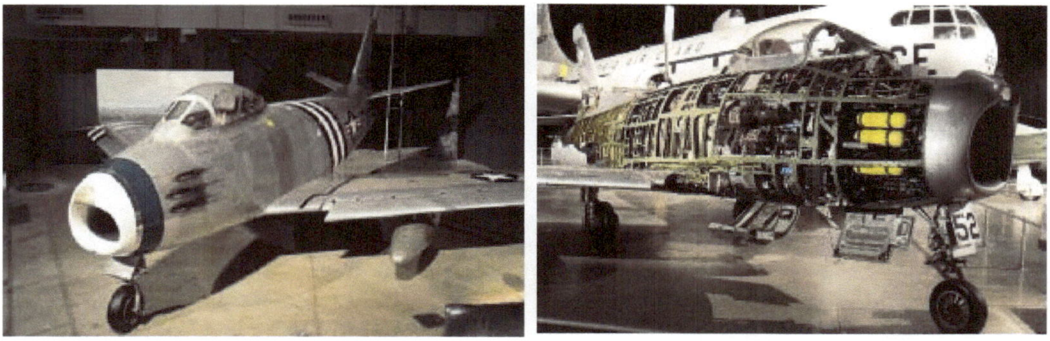

Fig. (2.19). The first versions of North American F-86 Sabre were fitted with slats (Photos: U.S. Air Force National Museum, public domain).

Back to Messerschmitt Bf 109 fighter, which is object of analysis in the present Section, after the fall of France, the Luftwaffe realized that the range of Bf 109E needed to be extended. Thus, Messerschmitt redesigned the airplane, clipped the wing tips, increased its fuel capacity and improved the pilot's shield, among a series of other modifications. The result was the Bf 109F, which entered service in November 1940, and that soon became praised by German pilots thanks to its good maneuverability. The Bf 109F received a redesigned engine cowling, the propeller spinner was enlarged and, in general, several other aerodynamic improvements contributed to a top speed of 650 km/h [33]. A new ejector exhaust arrangement was also incorporated, and on later aircraft a metal shield was fitted over the left-hand banks to deflect exhaust fumes away from the supercharger air-intake. A new three-blade, light-alloy propeller unit with a reduced diameter was used; propeller pitch was changed electrically, and was regulated by a constant-speed unit, though a manual override was still provided. Thanks to the improved aerodynamics and more fuel-efficient engines and all other modifications, the Bf 109F offered an increased maximum range of 650 km compared with the Bf 109E's maximum range of only 560 km on internal fuel [33]. Range could be increased to 1,700 km if external light-alloy drop tanks were used. Several other versions of the Bf 109 were produced each with varying armaments. The Bf 109G series (Fig. **2.20**) was very popular and over 12,000 units were built. In total, over 29,900 Bf 109s were manufactured during the war [33]. Although the Bf 109 was partially replaced by the Focke-Wulf Fw 190 in 1941, it continued to play a major role in the Luftwaffe's fighter operations.

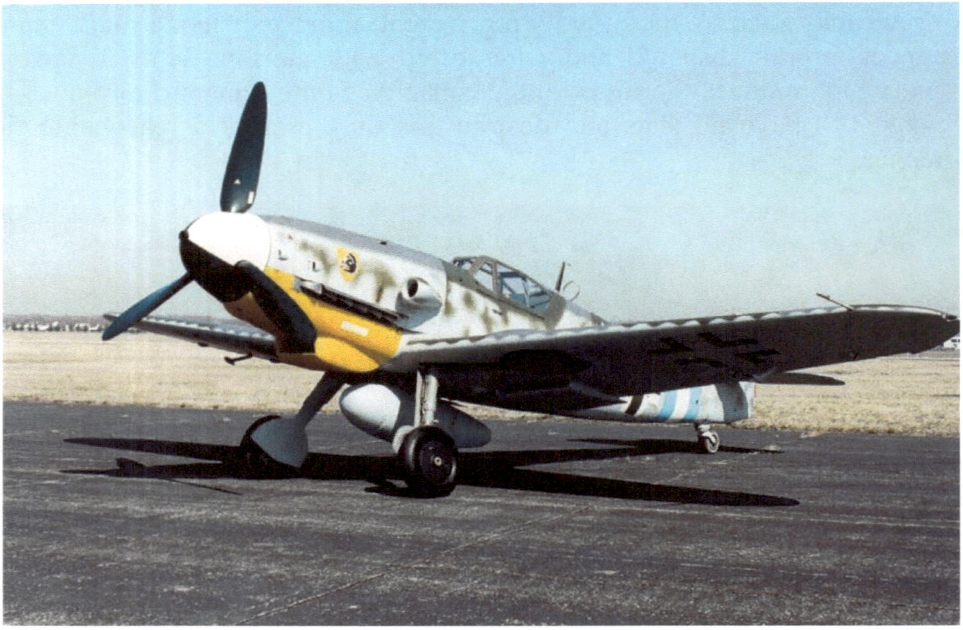

Fig. (2.20). Messerschmitt Bf 109 (Photo: U.S. Air Force, public domain).

Bombers

Bombing of cities, military and industrial facilities were in widespread use during World War II. All types of aircraft were employed for bombing missions: dive bombers like the Junkers Ju 87, medium bombers for tactical operations, the B-25 Mitchell and B-26 Marauder being good representatives of this category, heavy bombers and adapted fighter aircraft for the bombing role. Besides, medium bombers were also modified to attack surface ships and submarines. The Germans used medium bombers for the strategic role, with the twin-engine Heinkel He 111 and Junkers Ju 88 systematically bombing industrial facilities in the beginning of Battle of Britain. Fig. **2.21** shows some Allied and German bombers employed in the conflict.

Germany, England and Italy carried out strategic bombing missions in World War I. Germany utilized airships, besides heavy bombers in such missions. However, these bombing missions were highly inaccurate. Accurate high-altitude bombing was almost impossible before the development of bombsights [34]. To hit the target accurately, airplanes had to fly at lower altitudes, becoming easy targets of anti-aircraft artillery and fighters. The development of the bombsight helped to turn the strategic bomber into an effective weapon [34]. The device compensates for air resistance, which will cause the bomb to trail behind the plane, and cross winds.

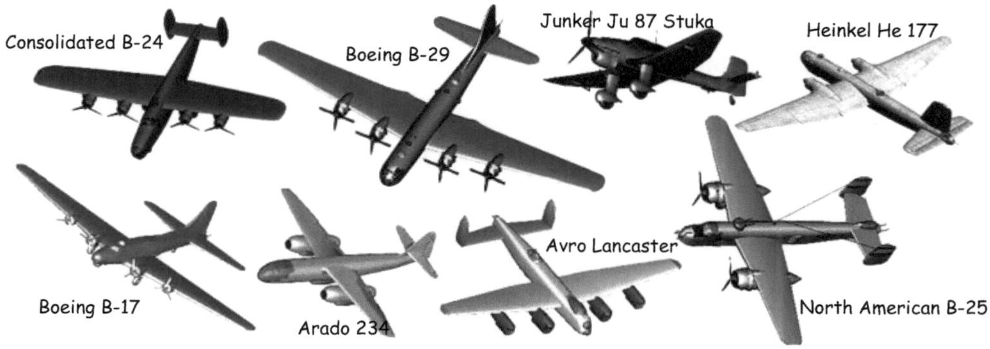

Fig. (2.21). Some allied and German bombers of World War II (Not in same scale).

In the 1930s, mechanical computers with the sufficient performance could solve the equations of motion and they were incorporated in these days into new tachometric bombsights, the most famous being the Norden, the highly secret bombsight from the United States [35]. Later in World War II, tachometric bombsights were often combined with radar systems to allow accurate bombing through clouds or at night.

When post-war studies demonstrated that bomb accuracy was roughly equal when optically or radar guided, optical bombsights were generally removed, and the role passed to dedicated radar bombsights [34].

World War II saw the massive utilization of heavy bombers for strategic operations. Most of them were long-range four-engine airplanes. The United States and England demonstrated their superior utilization of strategic air power during the war. Both countries heavily bombarded Germany: The British with night operations targeting cities and civilians; the Americans in daylight missions for the bombardment of industrials facilities. However, close to the end of war, the Americans switched their strategy and started to bomb German cities, with Berlin being an everyday target.

Against the British night bombing campaign, the Germans developed effective night fighters. The twin-engine Heinkel He 219 Uhu (Eagle owl) was one of them but it was produced in small numbers. The Uhu interceptor airplane incorporated several innovations, including the Lichtenstein SN-2 advanced VHF-band intercept radar, also used on the Ju 88G and Bf 110G night fighters [36]. It was also the first operational military aircraft to be equipped with ejection seats.

Strategic bombing campaigns were part of the United States approach against Japan. The North American air raids on Japan began effectively in October 1944 and escalated into widespread bombing of Japanese Cities with napalm, culminating in the atomic bombings of Hiroshima and Nagasaki on August 6th and 9th, 1945, respectively.

The Boeing B-29 was the airplane that the United States employed for the strategic bombing campaign on Japan (Fig. **2.22**). The type presented a cantilever mid wing with a crew of ten to fourteen men. It was powered by four turbocharged 2,200-hp air-cooled Wright radial engines. Front and aft fuselage of B-29 were pressurized and a small tunnel linked the two regions of the airplane. This allowed for bombing from higher altitudes without the discomfort of unpressurized cabins like that of B-17 and B-24.

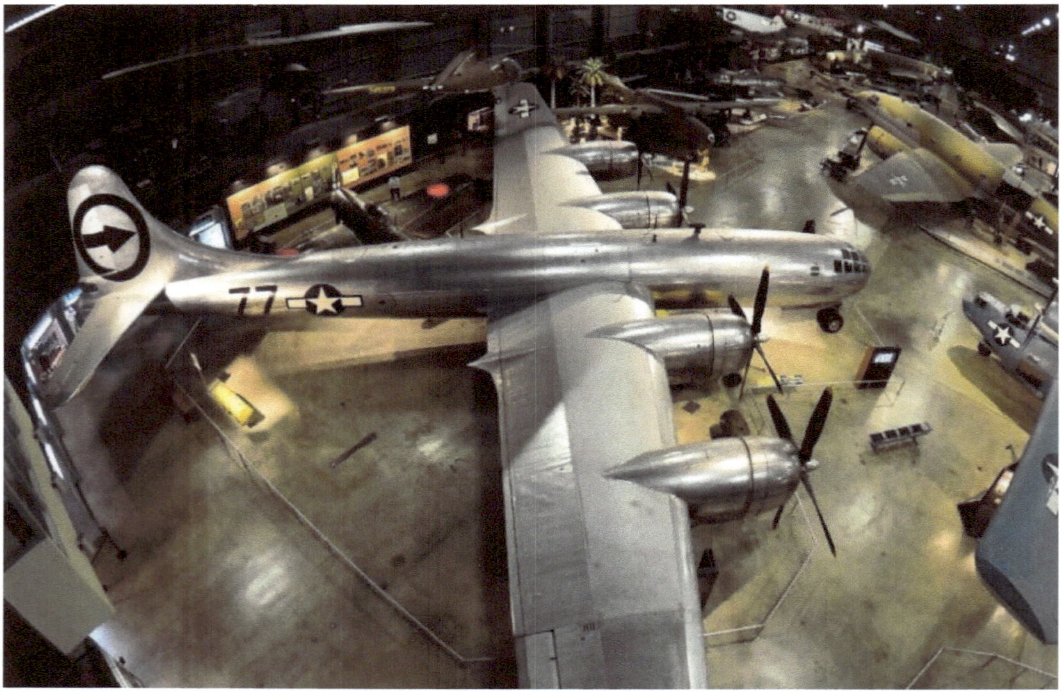

Fig. (2.22). Boeing B-29 in static display at the National Museum of the U.S. Air Force, Dayton, Ohio (Photo: U.S. Air Force, public domain).

It is usually thought that, Germany lacked heavy bombers in World War II. However, the first prototype of its Heinkel He 177 heavy bomber first flew in November, 1939 [37]. Initially the airplane did not see much success. The four-engine Heinkel He 177 Grief (Fig. **2.23**), which had similar range and payload capacity to their American counterparts [37]. The Heinkel He 177 initially possessed two nacelles, with each of them accommodating a pair of DB 601 engines driving a single propeller [37]. The assembly of two 601 engines was designated DB 606. The intention behind this unusual engine configuration was to employ the aircraft in moderate-angle dive bombing to improve accuracy of bombing missions [37]. The coupled-engine arrangement should contribute to a lower aircraft overall drag. After a series of engine failures caused by poor cooling, and ventilation problems, Heinkel conceived an improvement package to avoid the program shutdown by the Reichsluftfahrtministerium (RLM). Luftwaffe staff nicknamed the bomber *Luftwaffenfeuerzeug* ("Luftwaffe's lighter") [37].

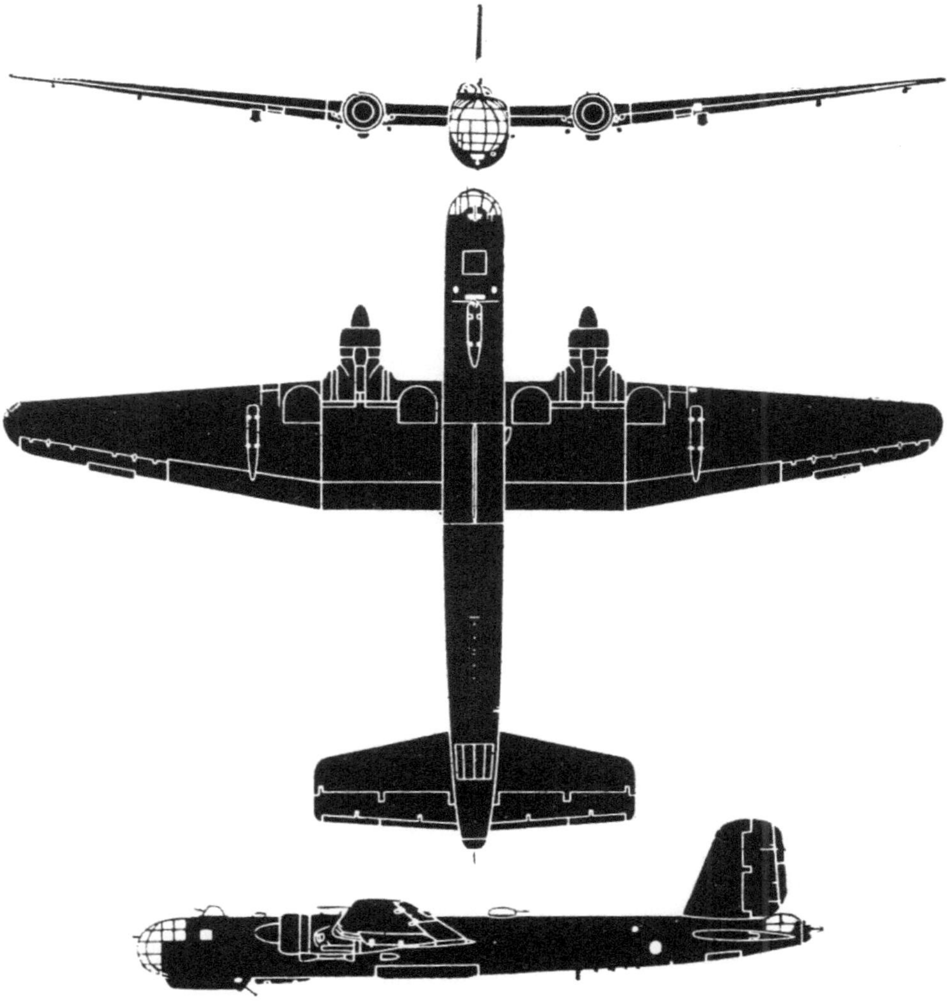

Fig. (2.23). Heinkel He 177 (Source: Wikimedia Commons, public domain).

Due to the continuing problems with the DB 606 engine and its installation into the He 177 bomber, much development work was performed to solve engine troubles. This included a complete redesign of the original He 177, primarily by newer wing designs and layouts to improve the engine installation, in conjunction with the A-3 subtype's lengthened rear fuselage, intended to create a four-engine version of Greif. The first concerns over the proper engine configuration for the He 177 bomber, whether a coupled-engine arrangement or four separate engines should be utilized, emerged in mid-November 1938. By that time, Ernst Heinkel requested that two of the eight He 177 prototypes to be fitted out with four individual engines in place of the coupled-engine arrangements, eventually specifying that the V3 and V4 airframes get four individual Junkers Jumo 211 in a November 17th meeting. Heinkel continue to improve the He 177, starting with the He 177 A-3/R2, which featured a modified engine nacelle with the new Daimler-Benz DB 610, each of which consisting of a Daimler-Benz DB 605 pair. The modification aimed reliability and prevention of engine fires. The introduction of the DB 610 brought some necessary modifications, including the lengthening of the engine mountings by 20 cm, the repositioning of the engine oil tank, the complete redesign of the exhaust system, and the setting of a power limitation on the engines which resulted in greater reliability [38]. These major and minor modifications, were successful in eliminating engine fires, but other minor problems remained, involving the transfer gearbox between the two component engines of each "power system" and their shared propeller.

Cargo Airplanes

Two characteristics cargo airplanes of the pre-war and war period are the Messerschmitt Me 263 Gigant and the Arado Ar 232, both high-wing configurations.

Junkers and Messerschmitt competed in 1940 for the design of a large transport glider, able to carry heavy equipment and soldiers [39, 40]. Junkers proposed the Ju 322 Mammut, which presented a wingspan of incredible 62 m and would have accommodated more than 100 fully equipped troops [39]. However, the type revealed to be unstable and was cancelled by the RLM. Meanwhile, Messerschmit Me 321 was a successful glider of braced high-wing configuration constructed with wood, fabric, and welded-steel tubes [39]. Access to the main cabin was via large clamshell doors in the nose of the aircraft or by doors on each side of the rear fuselage.

The Me 323 was in effect a powered and strengthened variant of Messserschmitt Me 321. French Gnome-Rhône engines were employed for the large cargo transport, four originally and six in subsequent prototypes and production aircraft. The Me 323 was not easy to handle and in certain circumstances they needed rocket to assist their takeoff or simply required a to be towed. Cruise speed of the

E version was 218 km/h [39].

In early 1940, work began on the design of a transport aircraft to replace the venerable three-engine Junkers Ju 52/3m, of which more than 500 had been in service on September 1st, 1939 [40]. Arado proposed a new high-wing transport, which featured an unusual landing gear with an additional set of ten smaller, non-retractable twinned wheels per side, which supported the aircraft when landing on unprepared airfields. This design integrated almost all the features now considered to be standard in modern cargo transport aircraft, including a box-like fuselage slung beneath a high wing; a rear cargo ramp (that had first appeared on the December 1939-flown Junkers Ju 90 V5 fifth prototype four-engined transport); a high tail for easy access to the hold; and various features for operating from rough fields [40]. Although the Luftwaffe was interested in replacing or supplementing its fleet of outdated Junkers Ju 52/3m transports, it had an abundance of types in production at the time and did not purchase large numbers of the Ar 232.

The vertical stabilizers were mounted on the end of a long boom to keep the area behind the doors clear so trucks could drive right up to the ramp, much like the 1944-era American Fairchild C-82 Packet of a differing twin boom fuselage configuration. The high-set tail on its "pod-and-boom" configuration fuselage allowed the Ar 232 to be loaded and unloaded faster than other designs.

Arado also pioneered a boundary-layer control system (BLC). The German company intended to apply the concept to improve the field performance of the Ar 232 transport airplane. The concept is known as Arado BLC system, which increased lift by delaying airfoil stall thanks to a combination of sucking the near separation boundary layer in the inboard wing flap area, and then by blowing energized free stream air over symmetric downward deflected ailerons (actuating therefore as flaperons) and on the outboard flaps. Fig. (**2.24**) displays the effect on boundary layer velocity profiles due to blowing and suction techniques.

Cessna in conjunction with some North American universities conducted some research on Arado boundary-layer control system with a modified Cessna 170 airplane [41]. ITA's Aircraft Design Department also studied theoretically the subject in 1957 (Fig. **2.25**). The impact on maximum lift coefficient due the utilization of the suction techniques on flaps is shown in Fig. (**2.26**).

There is a Japanese company that manufacturers an amphibian airplane with impressive STOL characteristics. The ShinMaywa US-2 (Fig. **2.27**) is capable of takeoff in sea state featuring 3-m height waves [42]. A significant characteristic of the US-2 is the BLC system that provides the aircraft with its outstanding takeoff capabilities. The aircraft has a dedicated an adapted LHTEC T800 helicopter turboshaft that provides flow through a system of pipes and ducts. The momentum that is introduced in the blown flaps and high-lift surfaces keeps the boundary layer attached and diverts the flow downwards thus providing lift in speeds where normally the wing would stall.

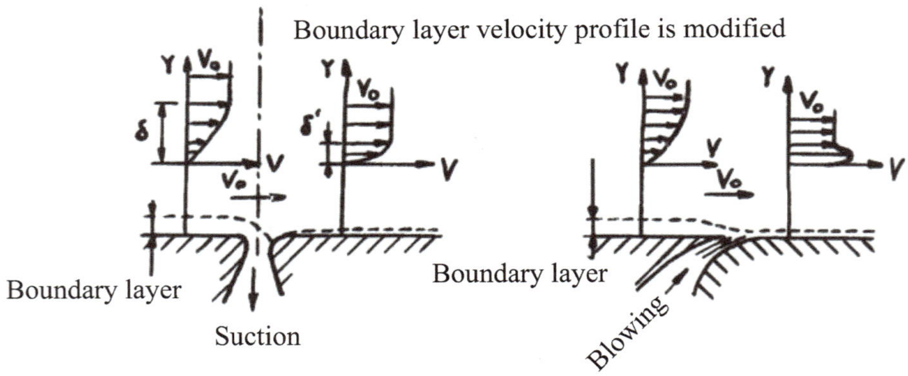

Fig. (2.24). Effect of blowing and suction on the boundary layer velocity profiles.

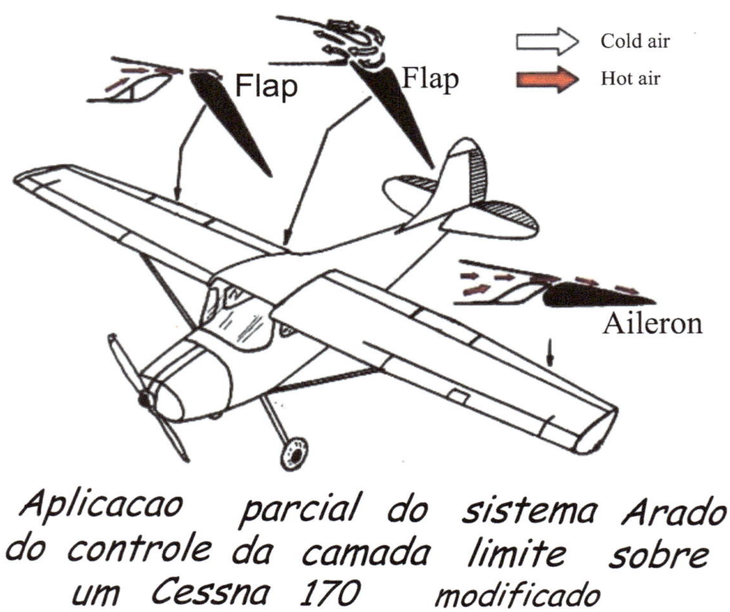

Fig. (2.25). Partial application of Arado's blown system to a modified Cessna 170 (Adapted from ITA, Aircraft Design Department, Drawing no. 727, Fig. II – 87, September 1957).

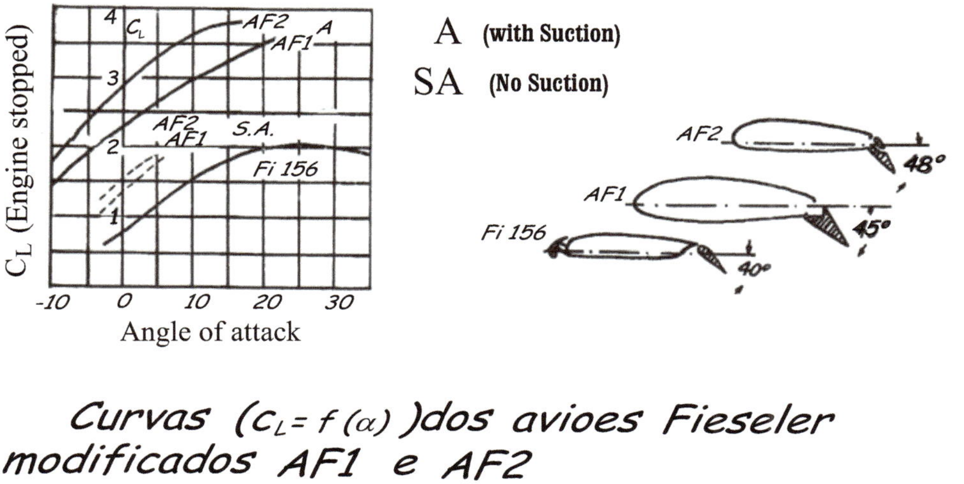

Fig. (2.26). Impact of suction on the lift curve of airfoils. The basic configuration of the Fieseler Fi 156 airplane was used as reference (ITA, Aircraft Design Department, Drawing no. 727, Fig. II – 88, September 1957).

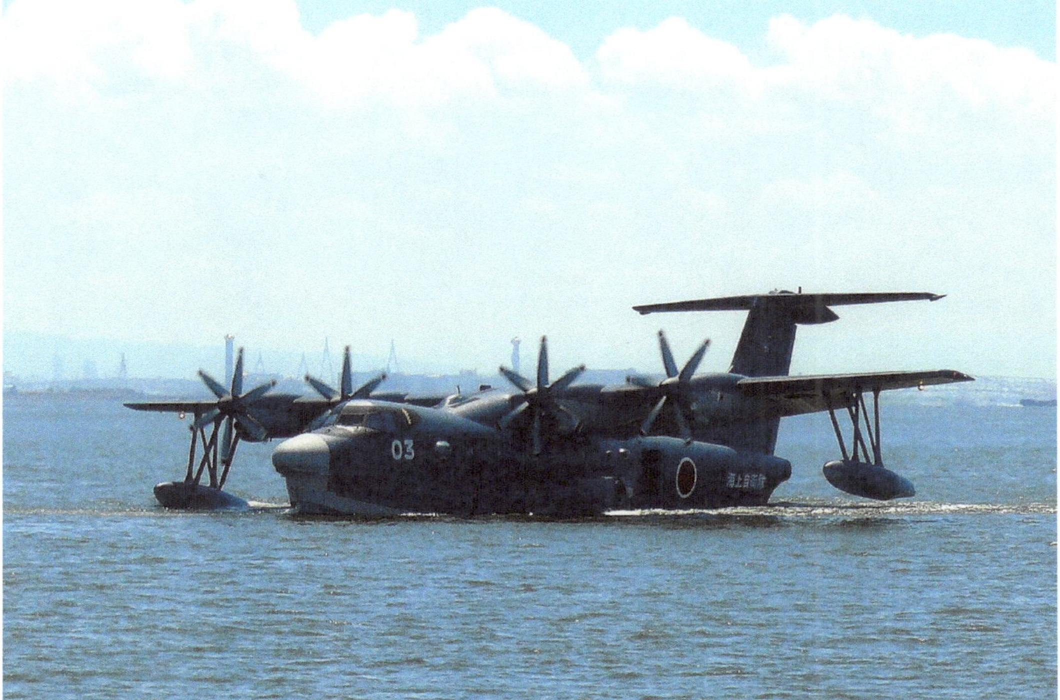

Fig. (2.27). ShinMaywa US-2 (Photo: まも[Mamo], released to public domain. Obtained via Wikimedia Commons).

The Jet Engine

The jet engine rapidly evolved during the World war II. This is one of top technological achievements of that war. It was independently brought to fruition at about the same time in Germany and England [43]. In Great Britain, a Royal Air Force officer, Frank Whittle, invented the gas-turbine engine that powered the first British jet, the Gloster E.28/39, which performed its first flight on May 15, 1941. In Germany, Hans Joachim Pabst von Ohain worked on the problem of gas-turbine engines without any knowledge of Whittle's efforts. Von Ohain found support from the aviation industrialist Ernst Heinkel, who sought an engine-manufacturing capability to complement his aircraft company. Work proceeded swiftly, and on August 27, 1939, von Ohain's He S.3B engine enabled test pilot Erich Warsitz to make the world's first successful turbojet-powered flight in history in the single-engine high-wing Heinkel He 178. The Germans also designed and built some operational jet aircraft during World War II. The Arado Ar 234 reconnaissance and bomber airplane (Fig. **2.28**) and the Messerschmitt Me 262 twinjet are two airplanes that count among successful designs. Prof. Tank from Focke-Wulf was working on a single-engine jet fighter Ta 153. After the war, Prof. Tank helped Argentina to develop the Pulqui II jet airplane, which was based on his Ta 153. Pulqui II performed its first flight in June 1950. Pulqui I, another Argentinian jet fighter, was flown in 1947 and it was designed by the Frenchman Émile Dewoitine.

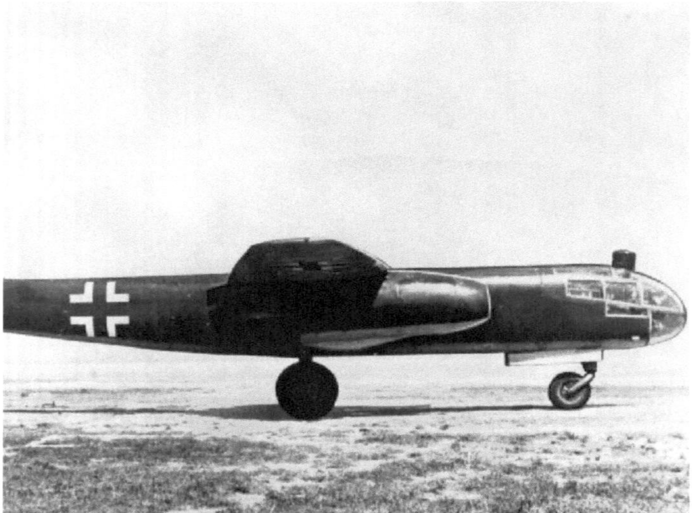

Fig. (2.28). The Arado Ar 234 jet airplane performed reconnaissance and bomber missions during World War II. Above, a twin-engine version fitted with wheeled landing gear. (Photo: Royal Air Force official photographer, public domain, via Wikimedia Commons).

The Arado Ar 234 high-wing airplane was the first jet-powered bomber, also performing strategic reconnaissance missions in from mid to late 1944 [44]. These missions were flown over Western Europe and England, areas which were virtually impenetrable by piston-powered German aircraft. Some of these flights involved calibration sorties for the V-2 (A4) rocket. There were also flights conducted over Northern Italy after findings from the German forces revealed that there was insufficient information about Allied troop movements there. The total number of Ar 234 built amounted to 210 production units [44] and 33 prototypes [44]. Some prototypes and pre-production aircraft were not fitted with pressurized cabins or ejections seats, some of them also tested a three-axis autopilot. They were delivered to the test facilities (*Erprobungsstelle*) of the ReichLuftMinisterium that were in Rechlin. First prototypes received a jettisionable take-off trolley, later replaced by a nose wheel and main landing gear configuration [45], also adopted for operational airplanes.

The Ar 234B-1 was employed as reconnaissance aircraft and the Ar 234B-2 bomber had a maximum payload of 2,000 kg, with bomb racks beneath the engine nacelles. The C-3 was 56 km/h faster than the B-2 version, could climb to 40,000 ft (~ 12,200 m) and offered excellent handling qualities [45]. They were equipped with a three-axes autopilot with overriding control, enabling the pilot to move the control column to a tachometric bombsight be used for the bomber versions. A computer aided bombing system was used in conjunction with a sight periscope for shallow dive-bombing.

The development of Ar 234C employed two prototypes being flown with alternative arrangement for the four engine nacelles, both paired and separate from each other, the former considered to be more efficient. The prototype V19 proved to be the first true Ar 234C series aircraft [45], having four 798-kg thrust BMW 109-003A-1 turbojets in paired nacelles beneath each wing. This prototype was employed for pressurized cabin and icing tests [45].

The Germans designated many advanced aircraft that not became ready for war operations. Plenty of them featured the utilization of jet engines [46, 47]. One of them was the Horten 229 bomber. In 1943, Ministry of Aeronautics (Luftfahrtministerium) issued a request for design proposals to produce a bomber that could carry a 1,000-kg bomb load over 1,000 km, flying at 1,000 km/h. This request was called the 3×1000 project. Conventional German bombers attacking Great Britain were suffering devastating losses by Allied fighters. A high-speed bomber airplane would be then hard to intercept. At the time, there was no way to fulfil the requirements issued by RLM because the high fuel consumption of jet engines, like the Junkers Jumo 004B, compromised the airplane desired range. Thus, Horten intended to employ a low-drag configuration to comply with the range requirement. Per Horten, that would be a low-drag flying wing configuration. In addition, the required high-altitude cruise thrust, also a big issue at that time, could be lowered if the aircraft could present a higher lift-to-drag ratio, something that a flying wing could deliver.

Horten moved forward with a private project, the H.IX, as the basis for the bomber. The RLM approved the Horten proposal, but ordered the incorporation of two 30-mm cannons, as the German officials considered that the aircraft would also be employed as a fighter thanks to its estimated top speed being significantly higher than that of any Allied aircraft. The Horten IX (Fig. **2.29**) was of mixed construction, with the center pod made from welded steel tubing and wing spars built from wood. The wings were made from two thin, carbon-impregnated plywood panels glued together with a charcoal and sawdust mixture [48]. The wing had a single main spar, penetrated by the jet engine inlets, and a secondary spar used for attaching the elevons. It was designed with a 7g load factor and a 1.8× safety rating. The wing airfoils maximum thickness to chord ratio ranged from 15% at the root section to 8% at the wingtip. The aircraft utilized retractable tricycle landing gear, with the nose gear on the first two prototypes taken from a Heinkel He 177's tail-wheel system. The aircraft was originally designed for the BMW 003 jet engine, but that engine was not quite ready, and the Junkers Jumo 004 engine was employed instead. After the war, Reimar Horten said he mixed charcoal dust in with the wood glue to absorb electromagnetic waves (radar), which he believed could shield the aircraft from detection by British early-warning ground-based radar that operated at 20 to 30 MHz (top end of the HF band), known as Chain Home. The only surviving Ho 229 airframe has been restored at the National Air and Space Museum's Garber Restoration Facility.

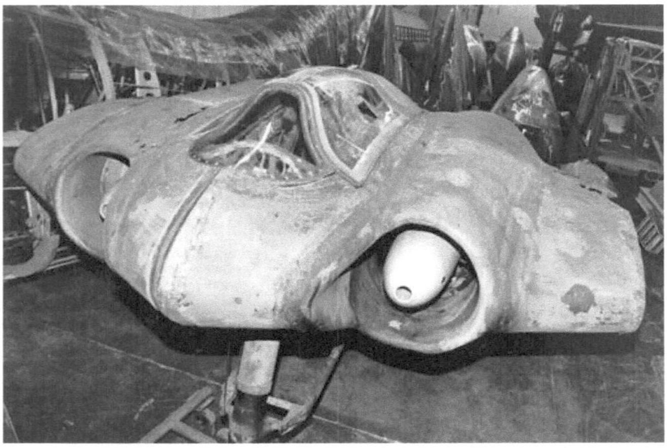

Fig. (2.29). Horten IX (Photo: National Air and Space Museum, Smithsonian Institution, released into the public domain. Via Wikimedia Commons).

High-Speed Flight

The Germans also were at the leading edge of high-speed flight due to research carried out at some universities, noticeably Göttingen University. Research on high speed flow led to study wing sweepback to improve aircraft performance at higher speeds. The Americans gained knowledge on high-speed flight by reading German reports available as war material [32]. The first mention and publication of the concept of wing sweep comes from the aerodynamicist Adolf Busemann in year 1935 [49, 50]. He was then professor at the Technische Hoschule Dresden and gave a lecture entitled *aerodynamic lift at supersonic speeds* at the 5th International Volta Meeting in Rome [49]. Following a recommendation of Albert Betz, a Ludwig Prandtl colleague at Aerodynamic Research Institute in Göttingen, H. Straβl and Hubert Ludwieg conduct systematic wind-tunnel tests with sweep-wing configurations [51]. Upon request from the Messerschmitt aircraft manufacturer experiments with realistic aircraft configurations were also carried out. The results and conclusions of the experimentation, ranging from Mach number 0.5 to 1.2, recommended the utilization of sweep-wing configurations to improve high-speed performance. The researchers communicated their achievements in the meeting High-speed of the General Committee for Fluid Dynamics Research, which took place in 1940 [52]. Fig. **2.30** shows the top view of several sweep-wing combat aircraft conceived until the end of World War II in May 1945.

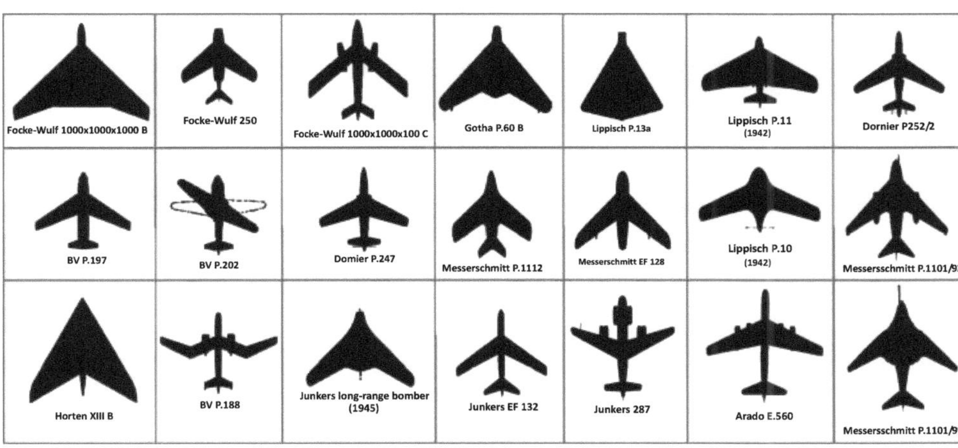

Fig. (2.30). Some German aircraft concepts with sweep wings until 1945.

The area rule is an aerodynamic formulation that addresses the generation of wave drag. The formulation states very simply that the transonic wave drag of an aircraft is essentially the same as the wave drag of an equivalent body of revolution having the same cross-sectional area distribution as the aircraft. This fact, allow the designers to shape the airplane in such way that that it minimizes drag.

The area rule was discovered by Otto Frenzl when comparing a swept wing with a w-wing with extreme high wave drag [49] while working on a transonic wind tunnel at Junkers Flugzeugbau in Germany sometime between 1943 and 1945. He wrote a report on December 17th, 1943 entitled *Arrangement of Displacement Bodies in High-Speed Flight* [53]. This was used in a patent issued by the German office in 1955 but valid from 1944 [54]. The results of this research were widely divulged in March 1944 by Theodor Zobel at the Deutsche Akademie der Luftfahrtforschung in the lecture *Fundamentally New Ways to Increase Performance of High-speed Aircraft* [55].

Some German aircraft design during War World II incorporated the know-how brought by Frenzl, evident in the slender fuselage of aircraft such as:

- Messerschmitt P.1111 Wespe - The Messerschmitt P.1111 was an 8.92-m long tailless airplane with nearly delta-shaped 45°-sweepback wings It was equipped with a pressurized cockpit for a single pilot [56]. Fuselage practically blended with the wings. P.1112 was a further development of P.1111.
- Messerschmitt P.1106 – This concept was intended as an improvement to the Me P.1101. It was redesigned several times. Fuselage section was reduced in the wing-fuselage junction region.
- Focke-Wulf 1000x1000x1000 A long-range bomber that should be powered by a pair of jet HeS 011 engines. The type was conceived to cruise at Mach number of 0.90 at 13,500 m altitude and therefore the fuselage cross-sections in the wing-fuselage junction area was reduced.
- Variable-sweep wings are also a way to apply the area-rule for improve high-speed performance. Several German airplane concepts emerged during World War II: Messerschmitt P.1102, Me P.1109, and Blohm und Voss BV P.202 count among them.

Several other researchers came close to developing a similar theory, notably Dietrich Küchemann who designed a tapered fighter that was dubbed the "Küchemann Coke Bottle" when it was discovered by US forces in 1946. In this case Küchemann arrived at the solution by studying airflow, notably span wise flow, over a swept wing. The swept wing is already an indirect application of the area rule.

Wallace D. Hayes, a pioneer of supersonic flight, developed the transonic area rule in publications beginning in 1947 with his Ph.D. thesis at the California

Institute of Technology. Richard T. Whitcomb, after whom the rule is named, independently discovered this rule in 1952, while working at the NACA.

The area rule was immediately applied to several development efforts in the United States. One of the most famous was Whitcomb's personal work on the re-design of the Convair F-102 Delta Dagger (Fig. **2.31**), a U.S. Air Force jet fighter with disappointing performance [57]. By indenting the fuselage beside the wings, and (paradoxically) adding more volume to the rear of the plane, transonic drag was considerably reduced, and the intended Mach 1.2 design speed was reached. The culminating design of this research was the Convair F-106 Delta Dart, an aircraft which for many years was the USAF's primary all-weather interceptor.

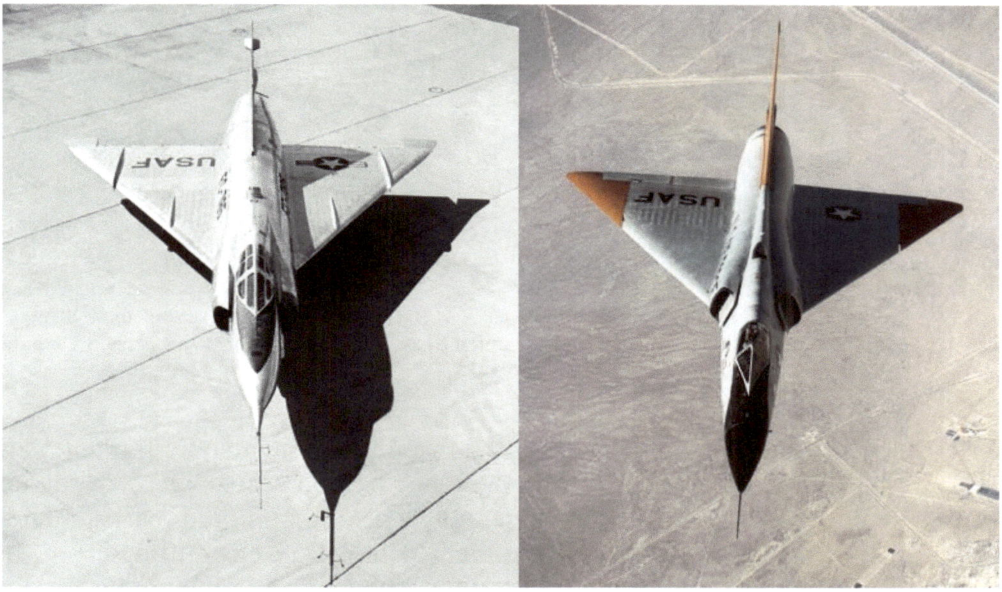

Fig. (2.31). Convair YF-102 before and after modifications (Photos: Courtesy NASA via Wikimedia Commons).

THE JET AGES

From War to Peace II

In the wake of World War II, the aviation experienced an era of experimentation and creativity with fat budgets made available for. No idea or concept seemed impossible to consider, and anything seemed possible. The Korean War signaled the end of the propeller-powered fighter and the World War II B-29 bomber suffered heavy losses. The jet fighter tactics used today were developed during dogfights between North American F-86s and MiG-15s over Korea (Fig. **2.32**).

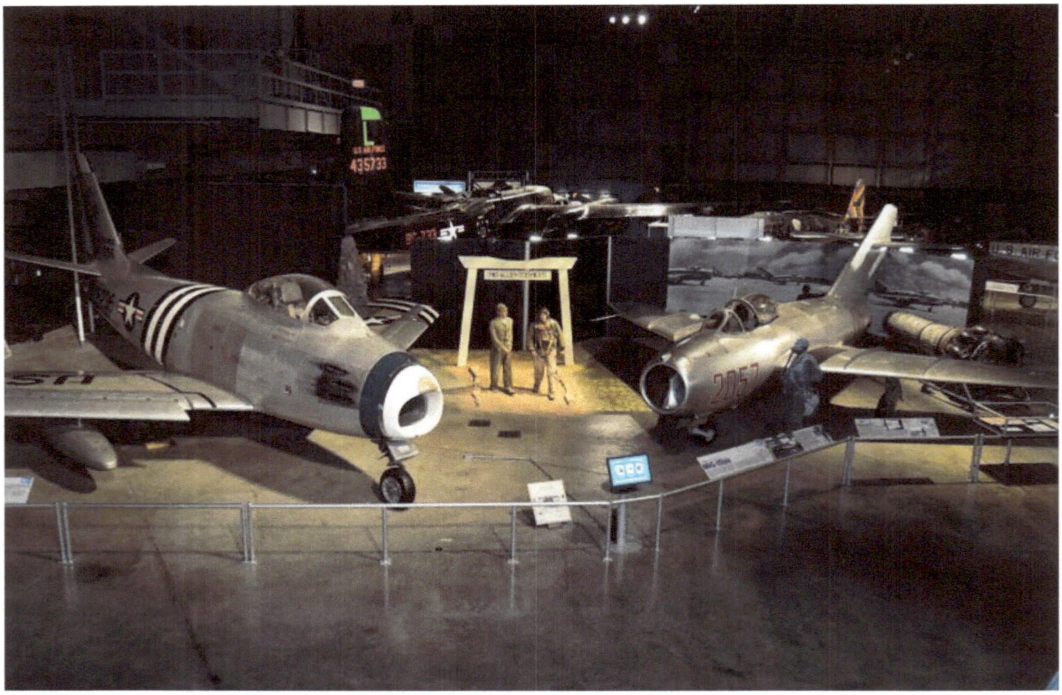

Fig. (2.32). Mikoyan Mig-15 and North American F-86 Sabre, veterans of Korean War in static display at Korean War Gallery at the National Museum of the United States Air Force (Photo: U.S. Air Force, public domain).

A series of new aircraft, consisting of both transonic and supersonic fighters arose (Table **2.2**). Strategic transonic and supersonic bombers also were developed having in mind the need for long-range bombers that could carry nuclear weapons. This first led to the B-47 and then to the B-52 and ultimately to the Convair B-58 Hustler, which was delta-wing supersonic bomber that entered operations in 1960. The idea behind this aircraft was to avoid interception by Soviet fighters flying supersonically at high altitudes.

Table 2.2. Some Cold War fighters from the 1950s and early 1960s (Source: Wikipedia).

Type	Year of Introduction	Max. Level Speed (Mach Number)	Number Built
Lockheed F-94 Starfire	1950	0.84	855
Vought F7U Cutlass	1951	0.92 @ sea level	320
Douglas F3D Skynight	1951	0.80	265
Mikoyan-Gurevich MiG-17	1952	0.97	11,060
Grumman F9F/F-9 Cougar	1952	0.99	1,988

Type	Year of Introduction	Max. Level Speed (Mach Number)	Number Built
Westland Wywern (turboprop)	1953	0.52 @ 3,000 m	127
North American Super Sabre	1954	**1.3**	2,294
North American FJ-2 Fury	1954	0.89	741
Hawker Hunter	1954	0.94 @ sea level	1,972
Republic Thunderstreak	1954	0.91 @ sea level	3,428
Mikoyan-Gurevich MiG-19	1955	**1.35**	2,172
Yakovlev Yak-25	1955	1.0	638
North American FJ-4 Fury	1955	0.89	374
Douglas A-4 Skyhawk	1956	1.0	2,960
Douglas F-4D Skyray	1956	**1.09**	422
Grumman F-11 Tiger	1956	**1.1**	200
Gloster Javelin	1956	0.93 @ sea level	436
SAAB J-32 Lansen	1956	0.91	450
McDonnel F3H Demon	1956	0.97	519
Convair F-102 Delta Dagger	1956	**1.25**	1,000
Chance-Vought Crusader	1957	**1.86**	1,219
McDonnel F-101 Vodooo	1957	**1.72**	807
English Electric Lightning	1957	**2.0**	337
Supermarine Scimitar	1957	0.97 @ sea level	76
Lockheed F-104	1958	**2.0**	2,578
Republic F-105 Thunderchief	1958	**2.08**	833
Convair F-106 Delta Dart	1959	**2.3**	342
Mikoyan Mig-21	1959	**2.0**	11,496
Sukhoi Su-9	1959	**2.0**	1,150
SAAB Draken	1960	**2.2**	651
McDonnel F-4 Phantom II	1960	**2.23**	5,195
Yakovlev Yak-28	1960	**1.73**	1,180
Dassault Mirage III	1961	**2.0**	1,422
		Grand total	**59,507**

New civil concepts and consolidated innovative ideas from the World War II also emerged in the period 1945–1960. Among successful concepts, there was the jet- and turboprop-powered transport. The jet transport was conceived for speed, to shorten time travel of long-distance flights. Boeing and Douglas pioneered the civilian jet age that took place in the late 1950s. Convair arrived late in the dispute with its 880. In 1951, the Boeing B-47 strategic bomber entered service. This bomber featuring wings with high sweep had a spin-off effect on the four-engine Boeing 707 passenger transport.

High-Capacity Turboprop Airliners

After the war, a new generation of passenger transporters began to be developed. Turboprop airliners were on the horizon. As a result of specifications from the British Brarbazon Committee, the turboprop-powered Vickers Viscount first flew in 1948 [58]. The four-engine Vickers Viscount was the first turboprop airliner to enter regular service, which took place in 1953. Initially, the Vickers Vanguard was conceived to fulfil BEA requirements for an airplane with 1600-km range [59]. The airframe also experienced some redesigns: Vanguard fuselage was initially conceived to be the same as that of Viscount, however with the intention to provide a roomier passenger cabin; a new double-bubble layout was introduced to the Vanguard. As a result, Vanguard entered operations only in 1960, facing direct competition with jet airliners. Consequently, only 44 exemplars were produced.

The Bristol Britannia was a medium-range airliner whose development by the Bristol Aeroplane Company began in 1952. Three prototypes were ordered as Mk 1 (piston-engine Centaurus 662), with the second and third prototypes designated Mk 2 (intended to be replaced by Bristol Proteus turboprops, then under development). During the development of Britannia, two prototypes were lost, and the turboprop engines suffered from inlet icing problems, thus delaying entry into service while solutions were sought. The Britannia Model 102 began scheduled service on February 1st, 1957 with BOAC, flying from London to Johannesburg [60].

After a commercial success of the piston-powered Constellation airplane, the North-American aircraft manufacturer Lockheed offered airlines a series of concepts that were successively rejected. Finally, the company attracted interest from Eastern Air Lines for a concept with increased capacity in 1955 [61]. The type became the four-engine Lockheed Electra II turboprop airliner (Fig. **2.33**), which was introduced in 1959 with Eastern Air Lines. Electra II utilized the same Allison 501 engines of the military transport C-130.

Three Electra II airplanes suffered fatal accidents between February 1959 and March 1960, all with the airplanes breaking apart into small pieces [61]. After the third accident, the Federal Administration Agency (FAA) constrained the speed of Electra until the cause that led to the crashes could be determined. According to an extensive investigation, engine mounting was determinant for two of the crashes. They were not strong enough to damp the vibrations that resulted into a whirl flutter at the outboard engine stations. Whirl flutter is a precession type instability that can occur on a flexibly mounted aircraft-engine-propeller combination [62]. When a determined propeller frequency was transmitted to the wings, it was resonant with the vibration modes of the outer wing panels, leading to a catastrophic failure. Lockheed introduced modifications to fix the flutter problem and Electra II returned to civil operations. In 1957, the United States Navy issued a requirement for an advanced maritime patrol aircraft. Lockheed proposed the development of the Electra that was later placed into production as the P-3 Orion (Fig. **2.34**). The Orion has been in continual front-line service for more than 50 years.

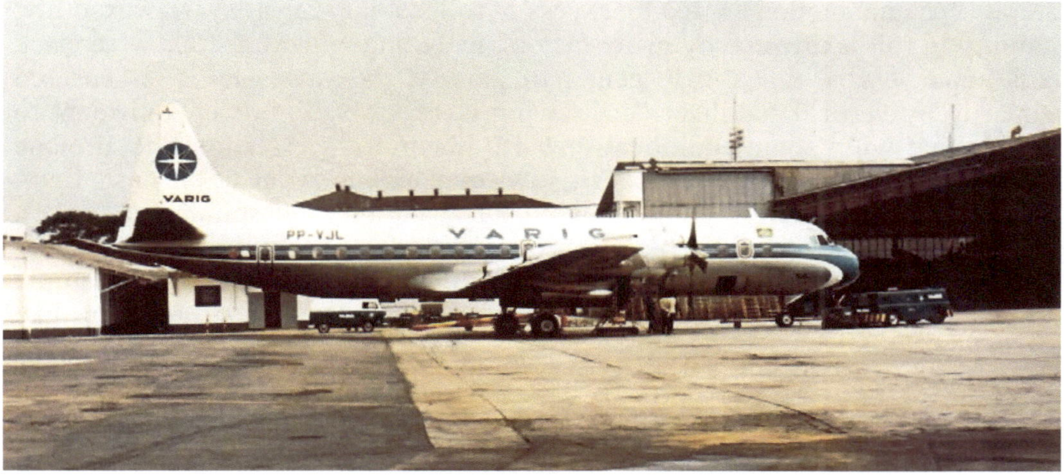

Fig. (2.33). VARIG operated the Lockheed Electra II in the shuttle service between Rio de Janeiro and São Paulo for many years (Photo: ©1985 Bento Mattos).

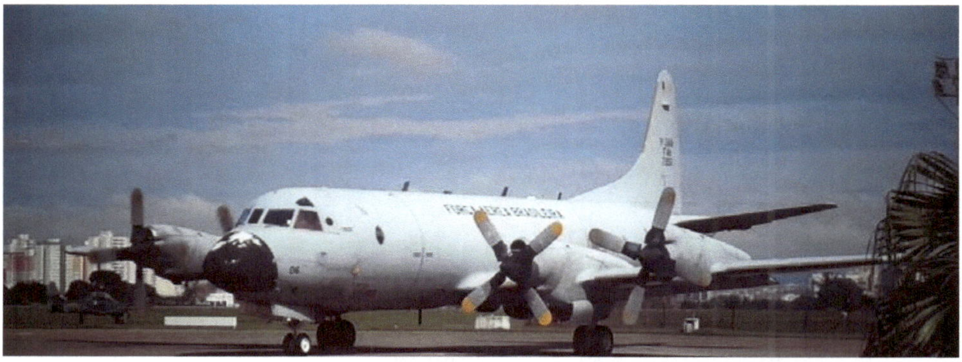

Fig. (2.34). P3 Orion of the Brazilian Air Force (Photo: ©2016 Bento Mattos).

The jetliners replaced the high-capacity turboprops, leaving the market to this kind of airplane for the segment below 80 seats. In the 1990s, the ERJ 145 and Canadair CRJ-100 hit turboprop-powered airplanes again, restricting their market penetration even further.

Inception

The Boeing 707 (Fig. **2.35**) wings were designed with a sweepback of 35 degrees to lower drag at higher speeds and they were inherited in some extent of the B-47 bomber. For this reason, like all swept-wing aircraft, displayed an undesirable Dutch roll flying characteristic that manifested itself as an alternating yawing and rolling motion (the wingtip describes an ellipse) [63]. Dutch roll is a type of aircraft dynamic motion caused by excess of roll stability regarding yaw stability. Stability in roll is affected by many factors, including wing dihedral, sweepback angle, and vertical tail arm to center of gravity; the yaw stability is ensured primarily by vertical stabilizer. If the wing is swept back, this is equivalent to provide that wing some additional upward dihedral angle leading the airplane configuration prone to Ducth roll. This yaw-roll coupling is one of the basic flight dynamic modes (others include phugoid, brief period, and spiral divergence). Boeing already had considerable experience with this phenomenon on the B-47 Stratojet and B-52 bombers, and the company had developed the yaw damper system on the B-47 that would be applied to later swept wing configurations like the 707 [63].

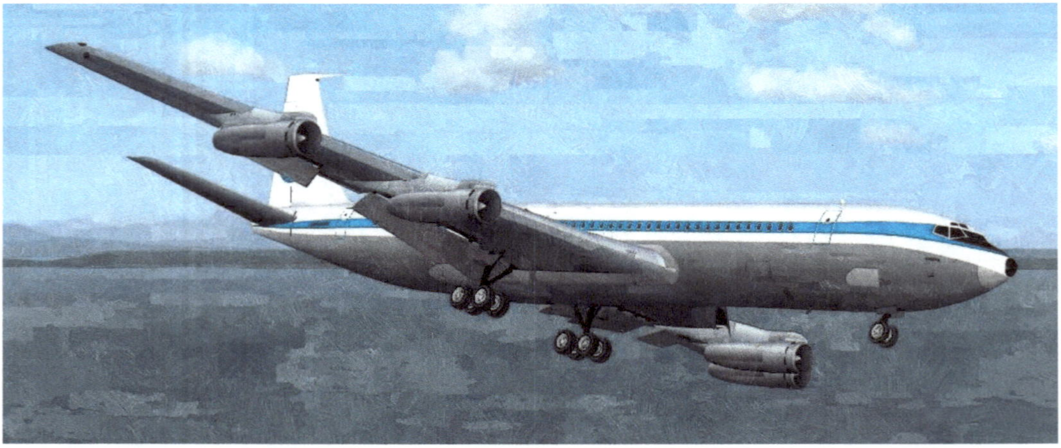

Fig. (2.35). Artistic view of the four-engine Boeing 707 airliner.

Yaw dampers require yaw rate sensors (and, depending on the control adopted, roll rate sensors) and a processor that provides a signal to an actuator connected to the rudder. The use of a yaw damper helps to provide a better ride for passengers, and on some aircraft the yaw damper is a required piece of equipment to ensure that the aircraft stability complains with certification rules. Many new 707 pilots had no experience with the adverse flight behavior caused by Dutch roll, because they were transitioning from straight-wing propeller-driven aircraft such as the Douglas DC-7 and Lockheed Constellation.

On one customer acceptance flight, where the yaw damper was turned off to familiarize the new pilots with flying techniques, a trainee pilot's actions violently exacerbated the Dutch roll motion and caused three of the four engines to be torn from the wings. The plane, a brand new 707-227, N7071, destined for Braniff, crash-landed on a river bed north of Seattle at Arlington, Washington, killing four of the eight occupants [64].

Test pilot Tex Johnston wrote an autobiography where he described a Dutch roll incident experienced by him as a passenger on an early commercial 707 flight [65]. As the aircraft's oscillations did not cease and therefore most of the passengers became uncomfortable and nauseated, he suspected a misrigging of the directional autopilot (yaw damper). He went to the cockpit and found the crew unable to understand and resolve the situation. He introduced himself and replaced the captain who immediately left the cockpit feeling ill. Johnston disconnected the faulty autopilot and manually stabilized the plane "with two slight control movements [65]."

Douglas Aircraft Co. developed a similar airplane to the Boeing 707, the four-engine DC-8. Pan-Am, the airline that will be always associated with the 707, ordered 20 707s and, at the very same time, 25 DC-8s. Boeing was in some disadvantage due the fact that the 707 was narrower and slightly smaller than the DC-8. When William Allen, Boeing's president offered American Airlines an extra half-inch in width over the DC-8, he won an order for fifty 707s [66]. From that moment, the sales success of the Boeing was assured. Boeing built 1,010 707s for commercial airlines between 1958 and 1978, and a further 800 for the military up until 1991, while Douglas assembled 556 DC-8s between 1958 and 1972 [66].

Sud-Aviation Caravelle

The first airliners with turbojet propulsion were experimental conversions of the Avro Lancastrian piston-powered airliner, which were flown with several types of early jet engine, including the De Havilland Ghost and the Rolls-Royce Nene [67]. These, however, retained the two inboard piston engines, the jets being housed in the outboard nacelles, and these aircraft were therefore of "mixed" propulsion. The first airliner with full jet power was the Nene-powered Vickers VC.1 Viking G-AJPH, which first flew on 6 April 1948. The first purpose-built jet airliner was the British De Havilland Comet which first flew in 1949 and entered service in 1952. The Avro Canada Jetliner was also developed in 1949, and although it never reached production, the term jetliner caught on as a generic term for all passenger jet aircraft.

Caravelle 210 (Fig. **2.36**) was the first commercial jet aircraft of short/medium routes. It was designed and manufactured by the French company Sud-Aviation, with production starting in 1955 (when it was still known by the acronym of SNCASE and received an acronym an "SE"). The Caravelle was the first jet to enter service in Brazil, beginning the jet era in that country, Cruzeiro do Sul, VARIG and Panair were the airlines that operated Caravelle in Brazil.

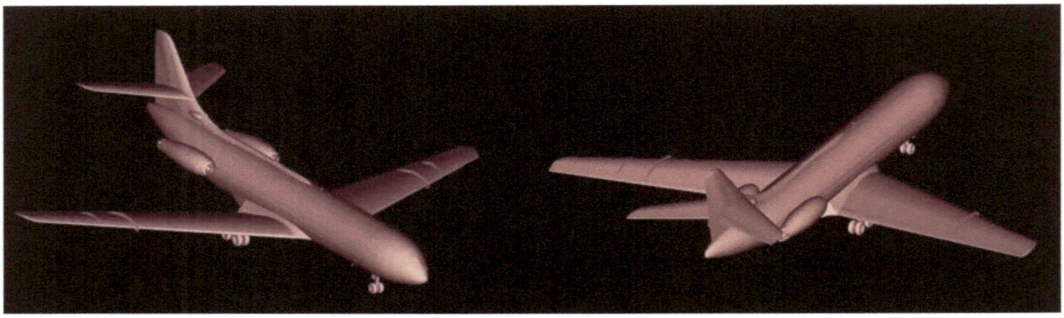

Fig. (2.36). Sud-Aviation Caravelle, the first jetliner with rear-mounted engines.

The Caravelle is generally considered the first commercial jet success since its predecessor, the De Havilland Comet, suffered a series of accidents that forced his premature decommissioning. For several years, the Caravelle was used in Europe and the United States. Historically, the Caravelle was important for being the first aircraft with the engines mounted at rear fuselage, leaving the wing free from disturbances caused by buried engines (buried) as the Comet or underwing configuration like the B-52 bomber and the quadrijet 707. This arrangement of motors was then adopted by many other aircraft, including the DC-9 and BAC 111 airliners.

Because of experience with the construction and operation of the four-engine piston-powered Armagnac, Sud Aviation decided to make use of resistance welding to build the Caravelle twinjet. The Armagnac employed over 150 thousand points and welding although welding machines used were relatively old concept, the results obtained with this type of manufacture have proved to be eminently satisfactory. In at least one accident Armagnac, it was demonstrated that while the rivet lines have failed, the construction spot welding had remained good, demonstrating both the safety and weld strength in aircraft construction.

Sud Aviation examined the welding use the Caravelle and found that [68]:

- The spot welding enables a hermetic structure required for the pressurized fuselage.
- The spot weld quality did not affect the aerodynamics of the aircraft fuselage, i.e. the surface smoothness was not affected by welding.
- Weight Reduction - the spot welding allows higher density of ribs than the riveting due to absence of holes.
- The process of spot welding allows rapid manufacturing, is easy to perform and cheaper than riveting.

As the advantages of spot welding seemed to be very pronounced for Sud-Aviation, the Caravelle was designed to make extensive use of the resistance welding technique. The welding was used throughout the aircraft, except in areas such as the central wing, and all fuselage reinforcements, panels, flooring, the tail end, doors, engine cowling and opening reinforcements are in place welded (Fig. **2.37**). The Caravelle contained over 300,000 points of welding [68].

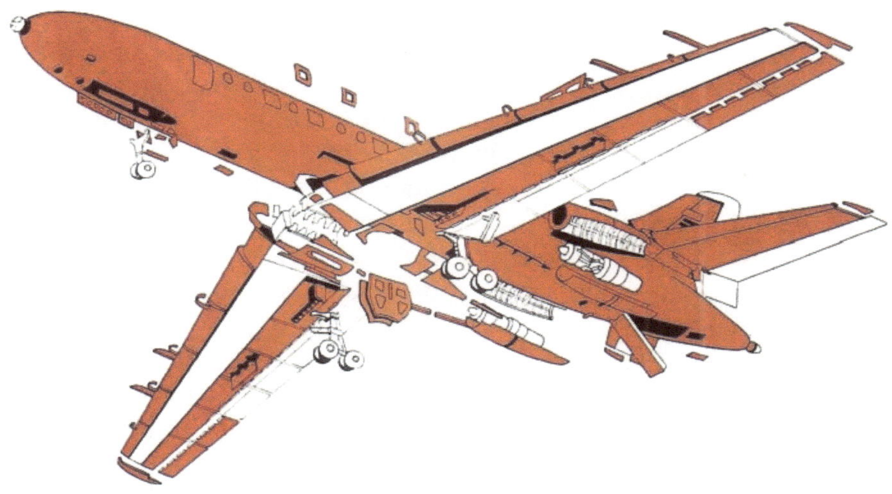

Fig. (2.37). Welded parts of Caravelle (in red).

Several Caravelle versions were produced during the lifetime of its serial production, as the thrust of the engines increased and enabled higher takeoff weights. At a certain time, the Sud Aviation's design bureau turned its efforts to the conceptual design of a supersonic transport with range like that of the Concorde. Sud Aviation named it Super-Caravelle [69]. However, this design endeavor would later be merged with similar work at Britain's Bristol airplane company to produce the Concorde supersonic airliner. In some configurations, Super-Caravelle would have several rearward-facing passenger seats, an uncommon arrangement for civil aircraft [70].

The Super-Caravelle seemed to be a smaller version of Concorde: its wing planform also presented an ogive configuration like Concorde; otherwise it was similar in shape and layout except for the nose area, which was conventional and only the outermost section over the radar featured a droop mechanism for visibility on takeoff and landing. The baseline configuration was conceived to accommodate 70 passengers for a range from 2,000 to 3,000 km [70]. The Super Caravelle should attain a cruise speed of Mach number of 2.

The First Jet Age

With the advent of turbojet, altitude became a critical factor in flight efficiency and performance. Higher cruise altitude was then adopted for better fuel burn and improved performance, basically speed and range. Further cruise altitude increase came with improvements of the turbojet engine. This posed new challenges to designers in regard cabin pressurization because this led to a heavier structure, which, in turn, degrades airplane performance and raises its costs. The Boeing 307 Stratoliner was the first pressurized operational civil airplane. This airliner performed its first flight in 1938. After tests with the Focke-Wulf 190, the Germans introduced a pressurized cabin into a serial produced night fighter, the Heinkel 219 Uhu, which was also fitted with ejection seats. The De Havilland DH 106 Comet was the first production commercial jet. Developed and manufactured by De Havilland, the Comet 1 prototype first flew on July 27, 1949. Fig. **2.38** shows some concepts considered for its configuration. It featured an aerodynamically clean design with four De Havilland Ghost turbojet engines buried in the inboard wing, a pressurized fuselage, and large square windows. For the era, it offered a relatively quiet, comfortable passenger cabin and showed signs of being a commercial success at its 1952 debut. Turbojet engines present higher specific fuel consumption when compared with piston-powered ones that were used in airliners of previous generations. To keep fuel consumption and performance into acceptable levels, jet airplanes fly higher than piston-powered and turboprop ones [71]. This in turn requires a pressurized cabin to keep passengers alive and comfortable. During the descent path, cabin pressure would have to be bled off again. Each cycle causes enormous stress on the airplane's structure; the tubular cabin stretches slightly when pressurized, then contract as pressure is released.

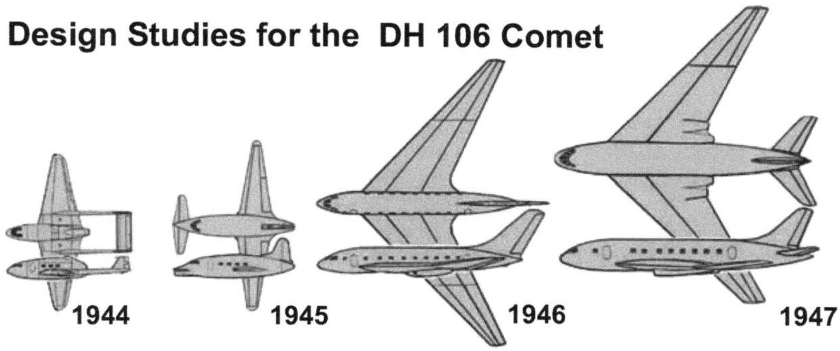

Fig. (2.38). Design studies for the Comet airliner (Author Bzuk, released to the public domain via Wikimedia Commons).

A year after entering commercial service, the Comet airliners started to suffer problems, with three of them breaking up during mid-flight in well-publicized accidents. This was later found to be due to catastrophic airframe metal fatigue. No one had taken into consideration the pressurizing cycles on the fuselage for a given time span, which were faster than the equivalent cycles in the slower, propeller-driven airplanes [71]. Britain authorities lasted to react but later an entire Comet fuselage was placed in a giant water tank, and its sealed interior filled with water to evaluate the effects of pressurization cycles on its structure. To simulate cabin-pressure changes in an aircraft climbing to 10,700 m and then descending again, interior pressure was increased and decreased at three-minute intervals. Around-the-clock testing aged the Comet nearly 40 times faster than it would have performed in actual service. In the meantime, autopsy reports from the Italian pathologist who examined the bodies of victims of one of the crashes indicated they had died by violent movement and explosive decompression. Evidence pointed to the catastrophic failure of the fuselage. The final clue, revealing the weakness in the Comet's structure, turned up on June 24 in the tank at Farnborough, where the immersed test Comet had been subjected to the equivalent of 9,000 flying hours. Instruments showed a sudden drop in cabin pressure, indicating that something had happened in the tank. Although sales never fully recovered, the improved Comet 2 and the prototype Comet 3 culminated in the redesigned Comet 4 series which debuted in 1958 and had a productive career of over 30 years [72]. The Comet was adapted for a variety of military roles such as VIP, medical and passenger transport, as well as surveillance [72]. The most extensive modification resulted in a specialized maritime patrol aircraft variant, the Hawker Siddeley Nimrod.

France succeeded with its first effort at a jet airliner, creating the Sud-Est (later Aérospatiale) SE 210 Caravelle, a medium-range turbojet intended primarily for the continental European market. First flown on May 27, 1955, the Caravelle achieved sales of 282 aircraft, and a turbofan-powered variant was used for domestic routes by airlines in the United States. The Caravelle was the world's first airliner to have rear-mounted engines, a design feature that was adopted for some uses by all other major manufacturers. The type was operated by the Brazilian airline VARIG. Some year later, the Boeing 707 design proved successful and has been adopted for jetliners almost universally since the 1960s [73]. Later, in the 1990s, EMBRAER and Canadair brought the jet revolution to the regional market, with the ERJ 145 (Fig. **2.39**) and CRJ-100 twinjets, respectively.

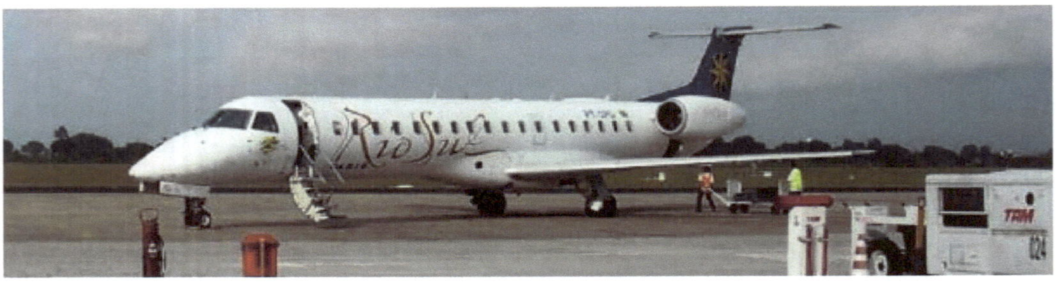

Fig. (2.39). *Top* - EMBRAER ERJ 145LR at São José dos Campos Airport (Photo: ©2002 Bento Mattos).

The Second Jet Age

The Canadair Challenger 600 business jet entered in operation in 1980. Its configuration featured a wider fuselage cross-section than previous business jets in its category. The Challenger was also one of the first bizjets designed with a supercritical wing and powered by turbofan engines. This technological combination gave him a true competitive leap. Canadair considered that a regional jet could be developed from the Challenger 610E seating 24 passengers. This idea did not move forward but studies for a 50-seat regional jet emerged in 1987. Canadair formally launched the CRJ program in 1989. The CL-600 design was stretched 5.92 meters to create the CRJ-100, with fuselage plugs fore and aft of the wing, two more emergency exit doors, plus a reinforced and modified wing. The CRJ high-speed advantage regarding turboprop airplanes of similar capacity should translate in a higher daily utilization rate and offering competitive direct operating costs. The concept of a stretched airliner derivative of the Challenger is not new, Canadair (purchased by Bombardier Aerospace) originally studied a 24-seat stretched development of the CL-600 up to 1981.

Design studies for a stretched airliner based on the 601 however were first undertaken in 1987, leading Canadair to launch the Regional Jet program on

March 31, 1989. The first prototype, of a total of three aircraft, took to the skies for the first time on May 10, 1991. Transport Canada certification was awarded on July 31, 1992, allowing the first customer delivery to Lufthansa that October.

Major changes over the Challenger apart from the stretched fuselage include a new advanced wing optimized for airline operations, higher design weights, EFIS flight deck with Collins Pro-Line 4 avionics suite, new undercarriage, additional fuel capacity and slightly more powerful CF-34 engines. The original CRJ-100 series - the 100, 100ER and 100LR - was augmented by the 200 series (with more efficient engines) in 1995. The Series 200 is available in standard 200, long range 200LR with optional greater fuel capacity, and the extended range Series 200LR (all three are offered in B form with CF34-3B1s for improved hot and high performance).

In the late 1980s, the regional aviation market was dominated by turboprop airplanes. Some airlines were analyzing whether the introduction of small jet airplane into regular service would be viable or not. Favoring the jets, their higher speeds allow for higher utilization rate by airlines; jet aircraft also provide greater passenger comfort because they are quieter, faster, and present lower vibration levels in flight. Despite the market signals and marketing difficulties that EMBRAER was experiencing with the twin-turboprop CBA-123, which should offer 350 kts cruise speed and a quieter cabin, the Swedish company SAAB still bet on the high-performance turboprop airplane after the commercial success of its SAAB 340 for 34 passengers. SAAB began development of the twin-engine 50-seater SAAB 2000 in December 1988. To attach a 400 kts promised cruise speed, the type was equipped with two 4,152 shp Allision AE 2100A engines. To reduce the discomfort caused by noise originated from propellers, the SAAB 2000 incorporated an active noise reduction system in the passenger cabin, which included 72 microphones and 36 speakers. The SAAB 2000 twin turboprop began operation with the launch customer Crossair in 1994 and its commercial failure led SAAB to leave the civil aviation market. A total of 63 exemplars were sold the last aircraft was delivered to Crossair in April 1999. Unlike SAAB, EMBRAER began development of a regional jet 45 seats (later, the capacity was increased to 50 seats) after suggestion made by the president of the airline American Airlines, Mr. Robert Crandall in 1989. The unusual first configuration of the called EMB 145 was characterized by an overwing engine configuration, aiming to reduce costs by taking advantage of the EMB 120 Brasilia wing and the fuselage. This configuration was abandoned because it was unable to deliver any reasonable performance. EMBRAER then considered an underwing configuration (Fig. **2.40**) for the EMB-145 but it demanded evacuation slides and was also abandoned.

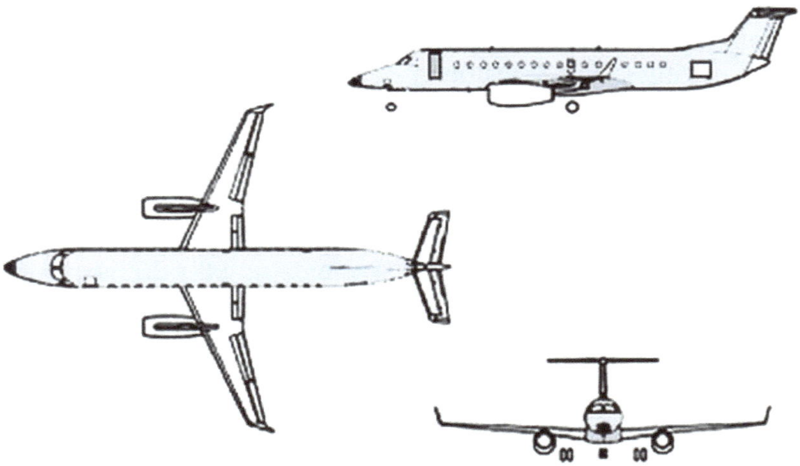

Fig. (2.40). Second configuration considered for the EMB-145 twinjet Note the winglets, which were removed from the ERJ 145 ER and LR versions (only the XR features winglets in its configuration).

In the first half of the 1990s, a crisis caused by the First Gulf War plagued the aviation industry. In addition, EMBRAER was experiencing another crisis because the of the ill-fated CBA-123 twin turboprop program. Thus, the EMB-145 program was substantially delayed.

The EMB-145 finally was redesigned and the engines were placed at the rear fuselage. The type entered operation in early 1997 with Continental Express. Later, EMBRAER renamed its 50-seat twinjet ERJ 145.

In the 2000s, EMBRAER portfolio grew significantly. Its commercial aviation arm experienced a large expansion with the introduction of the successful EMBRAER 170/175/190/195 airliners, known as E-Jets which present a high degree of communality among the airplanes. The first product of the family was the E170, which entered service in 2004 with LOT, a Polish airline. EMBRAER E175 (Fig. **2.41**) is a stretch of the E170 and it can accommodate 88 passengers in a single class with a seat pitch of 29 inches.

However, both EMBRAER ERJ 145 and CRJ-100/200 were not the first in their class. They were preceded by the Yak-40 (Fig. **2.42**) and VFW-614. The Yakovlev Yak-40, a small, three-engine airliner, is the world's first commuter jet airplane. Maiden flight of Yak-40 was performed in 1966. Introduced in September 1968, the Yak-40 was exported since 1970. By the time production ended in November 1981, the factory at Saratov had produced over one thousand aircraft.

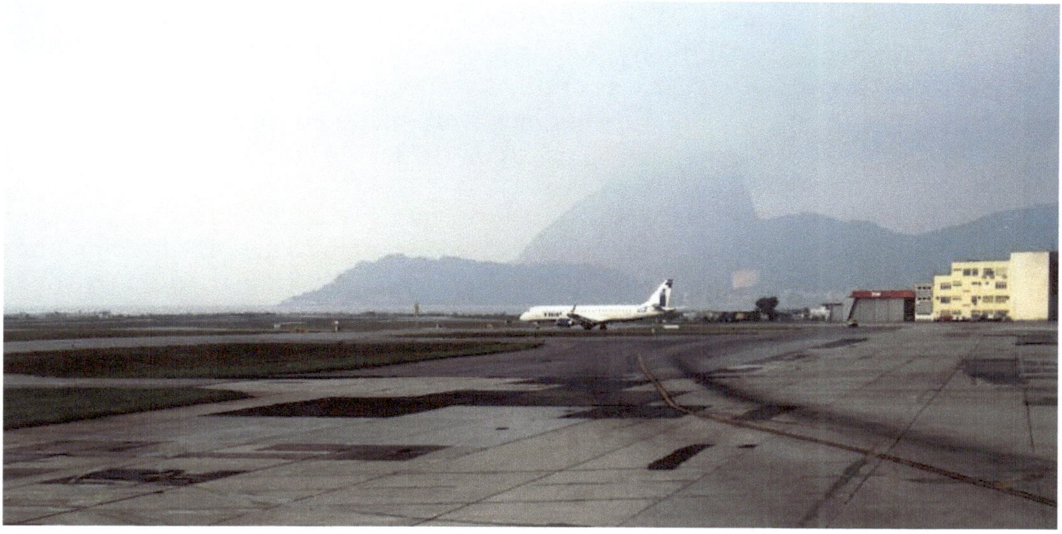

Fig. (2.41). EMBRAER E175 at Santos Dumont Airport in Rio de Janeiro (Photo: ©2013 Bento Mattos).

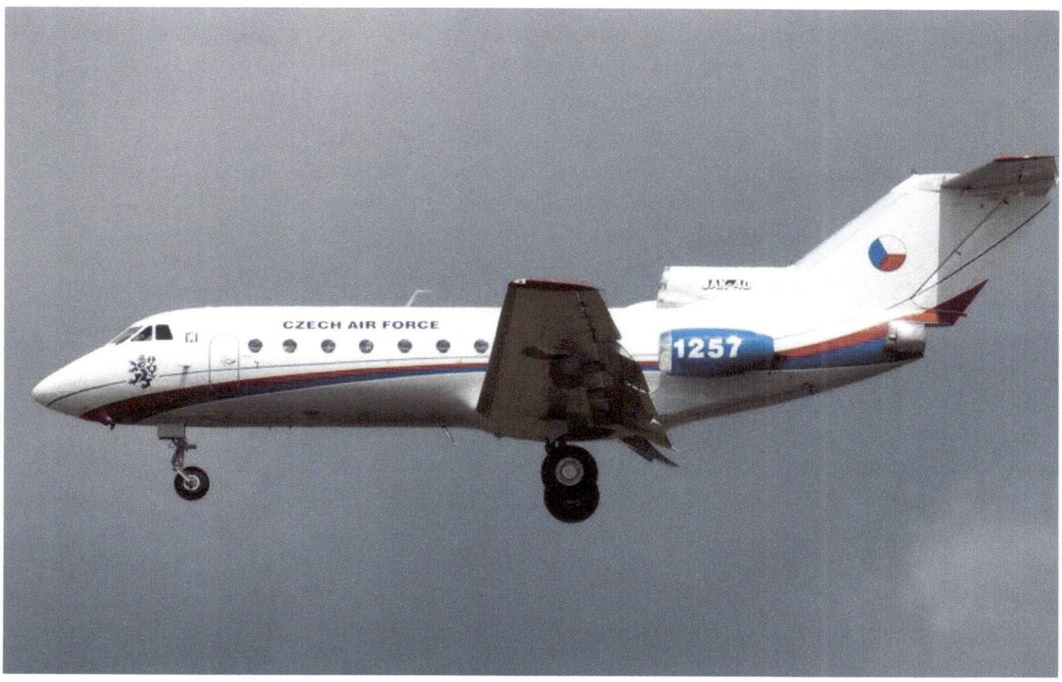

Fig. (2.42). Yak-40 (Photo: Arpingstone, released to the public domain).

The VFW-Fokker 614 (also VFW 614) was a twin-engine jet airliner designed and built in former West Germany. It was produced in small numbers by VFW-Fokker in early- to mid-1970s. It was originally intended as DC-3 replacement. Its most distinctive feature was that its engines were mounted on pylons above the wing. The type was eclipsed by the oil crises of 1973.

Although the Yak-40 was successful in the former Soviet Union, this airplane would be not successful in a market-oriented economy due its three-engine configuration that does not enable a profitable operation. Thanks to the Airline Deregulation Act, which boosted regional aviation, the EMBRAER and Bombardier planes modified the aviation landscape. Airplanes such as Douglas DC-8 and EMBRAER E-Jets also performed a key role in first and second jet revolution, respectively.

Need for Speed

The jet transport boosted the air travel because people felt stimulated by one-day travels. Since large jetliners could also carry more passengers than piston-powered airliners, airfares also declined.

The price to fly in the high transonic regime or at supersonic speeds is the need to burn more fuel because, among other reasons, the required thrust increases if speed goes up. Aircraft structure becomes heavier due to need to resist higher loads as well, which in turn requires engines that are more powerful. To keep fuel consumption within reasonable figures, speedier aircraft cruises at higher altitudes. The quest for even faster airplanes is motivated to provide passengers shorter travels and airlines new business opportunities. However, economics and environmental impacts have hindered the progress towards supersonic airliners.

After World War II, there was a trend to develop faster airliners. Adolph Busemann, a German aerospace engineer, pioneered the concept of swept wings in 1935 [50]. Despite this, Bell X-1, an experimental aircraft with straight wings, performed the first supersonic flight in history in 1947 [74].

In 1958, Convair, a company that was successful manufacturing piston-powered passenger transports, began development of Convair 990 Coronado [75], which was supposed to be faster than the competition. Top speed of improved version Coronado 990A was 621 mph, which translates into Mach number of 0.925 at a cruising altitude of 41,000 ft. The configuration was a faster and elongated version of Convair 600 [75]. The type was later redesignated Convair 990 to avoid the inference that it was an earlier version of Convair 880 [75]. To increase the critical Mach number and reduce transonic drag, Coronado suffered some redesign that incorporated full-span Krüger flaps at wing leading edge,

Küchemann bodies on the upper trailing edge of the wings (Fig. **2.43**), and shorter outboard engine pylons [75]. The aircraft never lived up to its promise of coast-t--coast nonstop capability from JFK to LAX and launch customer American Airlines began to dispose of their 990As in 1967 [76]. Only 37 Coronados were produced, bringing the entire production of commercial jet airliners by Convair to 102 airframes. The airline rejection of Convair 880 and 990 led the Convair Company to suffer what at the time was one of the largest corporate losses in history.

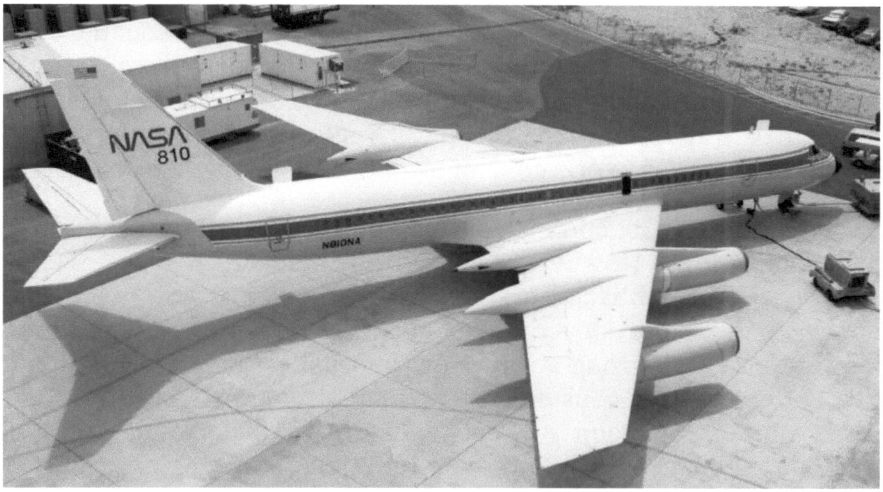

Fig. (2.43). Convair 990A. Note the Küchmann bodies over the wing upper side, which had only aerodynamic function (Photo: Courtesy NASA, public domain).

The Convair 990A is still the fastest non-supersonic commercial transport to have ever been produced. During May of 1961 one of the pre-production 990 prototype aircraft set a record of .97 Mach in level flight at an altitude of 22,500 ft., equivalent to a true airspeed of 675 mph [76].

The Convair Coronado airliner was considerably faster than the competition, but the Europeans intended to fly even faster. The British teamed with the French and founded the Concorde consortium to design and manufacture a supersonic airliner. Both countries had been working on own concepts since a couple of years. A slender-delta-winged configuration emerged from the inter-company discussions. The long- and medium range versions shared the same external dimensions, but they had different internal layouts. The medium-range aircraft could accommodate 100 passengers and it would have a 100-ton maximum takeoff weight; the long-range version had a capacity of 90 passengers and an all up weight of 119 tons.

A review was made of the design, production and research facilities available for the joint project, and general agreement was reached on the allocation of responsibilities between the British Aircraft Corporation and Sud Aviation. At last, on November 29, 1962, an agreement was signed in London by Julian Amery, Minister of Supply, and Geoffroy de Courcel, the French Ambassador to Britain, by which the two governments undertook to finance the development and building of a supersonic airliner [77]. Everything would be shared - costs, work, and proceeds of sales [77]. The airframe work was divided 60-40 in favor of France because the balance of work on the engine was weighted in favor of Britain. By November 1962, the engine selected for the Concorde, the supersonic version of the Bristol-Siddeley Olympus, was already being developed. Engines were in existence and running on the test-bed, and whatever adjustments might be made in the new program to allow joint Anglo-French development of the Olympus 593, the British work content would be greater than the French.

Early considerations for Concorde's configuration envisaged the use of low aspect ratio trapezoidal wings. However, Dietrich Küchemann at the Royal Aircraft Establishment (RAE) published a series of reports on a new wing planform, known as the slender delta concept. Küchemann's team worked with the fact that delta wings can produce strong vortices on their upper surfaces at high angles of attack. The vortex causes a considerably pressure drop, raising the lift coefficient. Küchemann's papers changed the entire nature of supersonic design almost overnight [78 - 80]. Küchemann presented the idea at a meeting where Morien Morgan, director of RAE, was present. Morgan immediately backed the delta wing as the solution to the SST problem and thus Concorde project gained momentum and it was launched in 1962. An ogival delta wing configuration was adopted for Concorde (Fig. **2.44**).

Due to the high speeds at which Concorde travelled, large forces were applied to the aircraft's structure during banks and turns. The resulting stresses twist and distort the aircraft's structure. In addition, there were concerns over maintaining precise control at supersonic speeds. All and other issues were deeply studied. A scaled model of the aircraft structure (Fig. **2.45**) was constructed in France to study structural vibrations. This model was later donated to ISAE (Institut Supérieur de l'Aéronautique et de l'Espace).

The Concorde supersonic transport (SST) airliner never found commercial success in regular flights. Its service entry took place in January 1976. After decades of regular service, a fatal crash near Paris in July 2000 and other factors eventually caused Concorde flights to be discontinued in 2003. This was the only loss of an SST in scheduled flight. There was fierce public opposition to the operation of supersonic airliners, noticeably of Concorde. The Anti-Concorde

Project, founded by Richard Wiggs, challenged the idea of viable supersonic passenger transport, and helped bring about a re-evaluation of Concorde's long-term commercial future [81, 82]. The supersonic airliner was developed based on the assumption that the sonic boom would pose no problem and that population would get used with the noise.

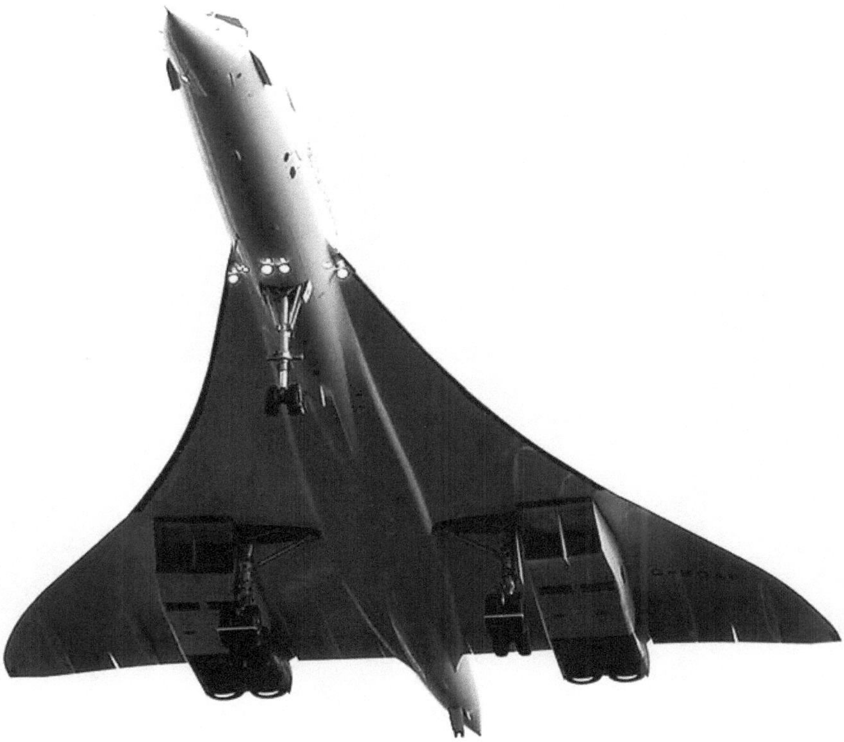

Fig. (2.44). Concorde supersonic airliner (Photo: Adrian Pingstone, released into the public domain. Via Wikimedia Commons).

To better understand the noise effects generated by supersonic airplanes, the United States carried out flight tests with military airplanes. The flights revealed that the sonic boom effects on population are not acceptable [82]. In fact, between 1961 and 1962, 150 flights were performed over St Louis, Missouri; in 1964, Oklahoma City was subjected to 5 months of supersonic over-flights; in 1965, there was further testing over Chicago, Milwaukee, and Pittsburgh; and in 1966–67 at Edwards Air Force Base in California. The flight tests revealed that sonic booms could break windows, crack plaster, tile and brick. There were claims for hundreds of thousands of dollars in damages. In addition, routine exercises flown by USAF (United States Air Force) supersonic jets caused much damage annually: £ 3,800,000 in sonic boom damage claims were presented to the Air Force in a three-month period in 1967. Similarly, there were complaints and compensations for flights close to Oklahoma City in 1964 [83]. In July 1967, the UK Ministry of Technology staged a series of supersonic tests over Southern England (using Lightning fighter aircraft), totaling eleven flights. No official arrangements were made to investigate public reaction, but The Guardian newspaper commissioned a public opinion survey, reporting that population of Bristol was frightened [82]. The Minis try received 12,000 complaints. Between 1970 and 1972, when Concorde no. 2 prototype performed 20 flights over the Irish Sea, there were reports of damage including cracked and broken windows, slates falling from roofs, panicking farm animals and frightened children and adults. The Government had to pay £ 40,000 in damages [82].

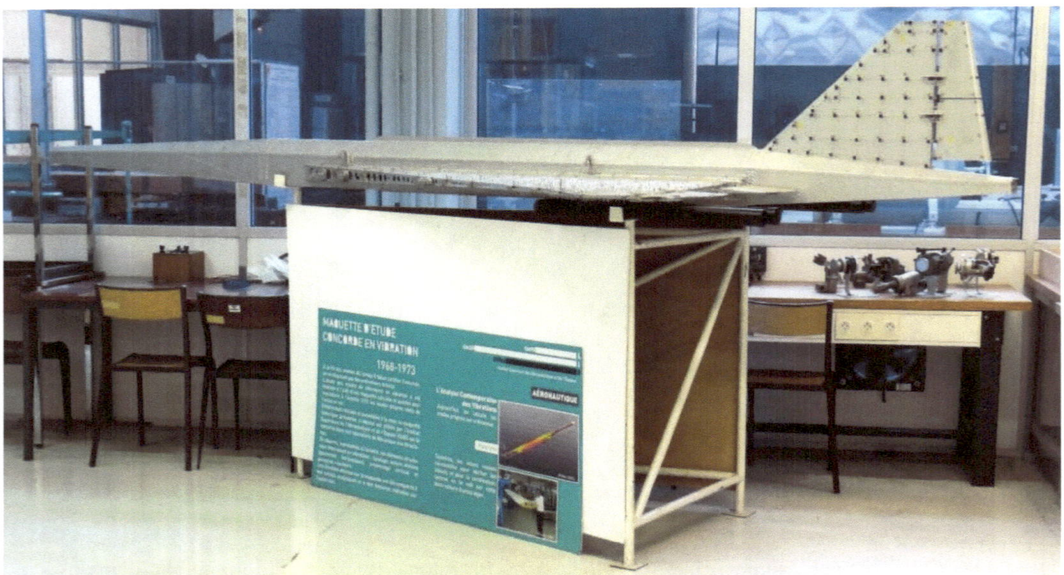

Fig. (2.45). A 250 kg model for vibration studies of Concorde structure (Photo: ©2012 Bento Mattos).

Besides Concorde, the only one supersonic airliner that entered serial production was the Tupolev Tu-144 (Fig. **2.46**). The Soviet SST first flew on December 31, 1968 near Moscow, two months before the first flight of Concorde. The Tu-144 first supersonic flight was performed on June 5, 1969. On May 26, 1970, the type became the first commercial transport to exceed Mach number of 2. The airplane started passenger service on November 1, 1977, almost two years after Concorde. However, the Tu-144 fleet was permanently decommissioned after 55 scheduled flights. The Concorde entered operation in 1976 and was retired in 2003. Air France and British Airways were the only operators of the type.

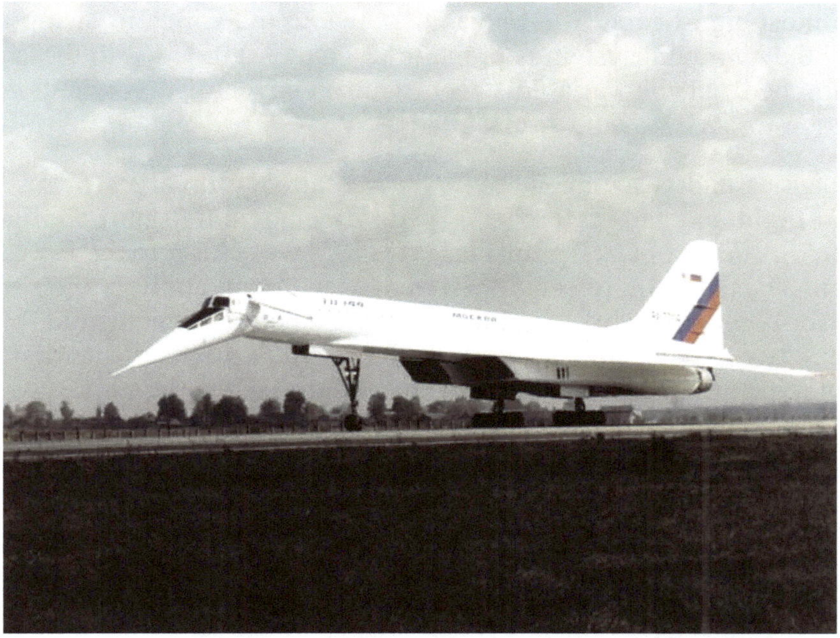

Fig. (2.46). Tupolev Tu-144L (Photo: Courtesy NASA/Jim Ross).

The United States has investigated supersonic technology for civil transport in several waves since the late 1950s. In the early 1960s, various executives of North American aerospace companies publicly affirmed that there were no technical barriers for the introduction of SSTs into service. Pressure on congressional representatives increased when the Concorde project was launched in 1962. Congress then funded a SST program in 1963, which would be conducted by Federal Aviation Administration (FAA). In the first phase, Lockheed L-2000 and Boeing 2707 concepts were selected among proposals from many aircraft manufacturers.

Boeing had started his SSTs design effort with a four-engine configuration featuring a variable-sweep wing, the Boeing 2707-100. By November 1967, this configuration had grown into the Boeing 2707-200. This airplane had a 97 m-long fuselage, able to accommodate 292 passengers.

The swing-wing design attempts to exploit the high-lift characteristics of a primarily straight wing with the low-drag characteristics at high speeds of a sweepback wing. During landing and takeoff, the wing swings into an almost straight position. During cruise, the wing swings into a position that gives it a higher sweep angle. However, there are some drawbacks coming from the utilization of variable-sweep wings, heavier aircraft and higher maintenance cost being the most significant. The hinges that enable the wings to swing are very heavy and the hydraulic system is prone to leakage. Mainly due to these reasons, Boeing dropped out the variable-sweep wing in favor of a conventional delta configuration for its 2707-300 airplane [84].

The aeronautics and space agency NASA was already involved in research on supersonic flight and had researched several supersonic transport configurations already. NASA design SCAT-15F (Fig. **2.47**) [85] was closer to the Boeing 2707-300 design. Thus, NASA selected the fixed-sweep wing configuration from that company for continued work. On May 1, 1967, a contract for the Phase 3 of the SST project was signed with Boeing [86]. The contract stipulated the first flight of a SST prototype in 1970 [86]. When Boeing announced the definitive layout of its SST, two versions were offered with maximum takeoff weight of up to 360,000 kg. A wide-body version presented lower takeoff weight to reduce the sonic boom overpressure for flights in the United States. Later, Boeing discarded the narrow-body version.

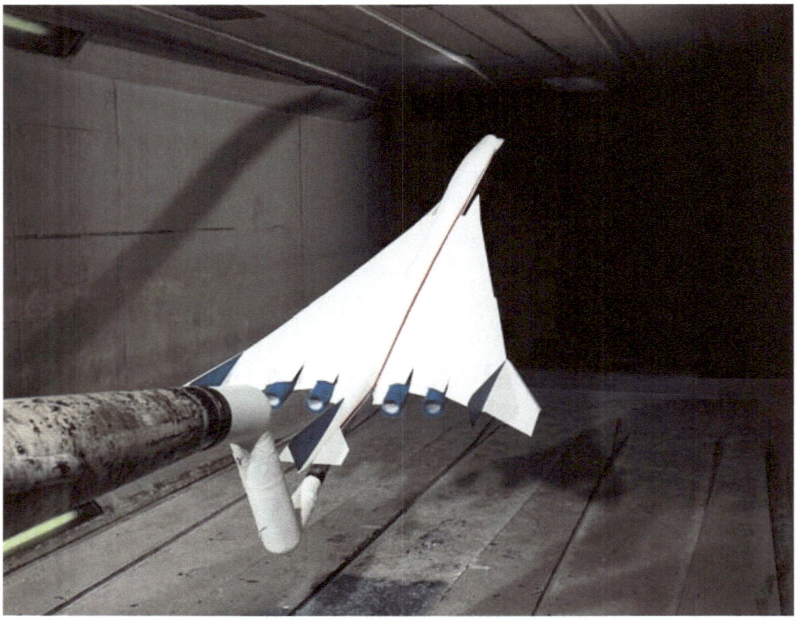

Fig. (2.47). NASA SCAF-25 SST (Photo: Courtesy NASA via Wikimedia Commons).

Although the production issues had not been addressed by 1967, airlines were reserving possible delivery-line positions and backing their orders with refundable deposits of US$ 750,000 (1967 Dollar) [86]. Table **2.3** shows the Boeing SST reservations in November 1967 [86]. Pan Am even promoted supersonic flights to take place in 1969 in one of its advertisements.

Table 2.3. Boeing 2707 orders by November 1967 with refundable deposits [86].

Airline	Units Ordered	Airline	Units Ordered
Aerlinte	2	ElAl	2
Air Canada	6	Iberia	3
Air Fance	6	JAL	8
Air-India	3	KLM	3
Airlift	1	Lufthansa	3
Alitalia	6	Northwest	4
American	6	Pan American	15
Braniff	2	PIA	2
BOAC	6	Qantas	6
CPAL	3	TWA	10
Continental	3	United	6
Delta	3	World	3
Eastern	3		
Total: 115			

Boeing 2707-300 was supposed to accommodate 320 passengers and to present a maximum cruise speed close to Mach number of 3 [84]. Table **2.4** shows a comparison of 2707-300 characteristics with those of Boeing 707 and 747 [87]; Fig. (**2.48**) illustrates the size comparison among the SST concepts from the 1960s.

Table 2.4. Main characteristics of Boeing 707, 747, and 2707-300 [84, 87].

	707	747-200	2707-300
Maximum Operating Mach Number	0.84	0.90	2.70
Trip time New York-Paris (h:min)	6:45	6:20	2:45
Passenger capacity	139-175	366-490	253-321
Cruise altitude (ft)	32,000	35,000	62,000
Length (m)	46..3	70.7	90.8
Wingspan (m)	44.5	59.64	45.6
Wing aspect ratio	7.1	6.96	2.66
Maximum takeoff weight (kg)	151,300	377,840	340,200

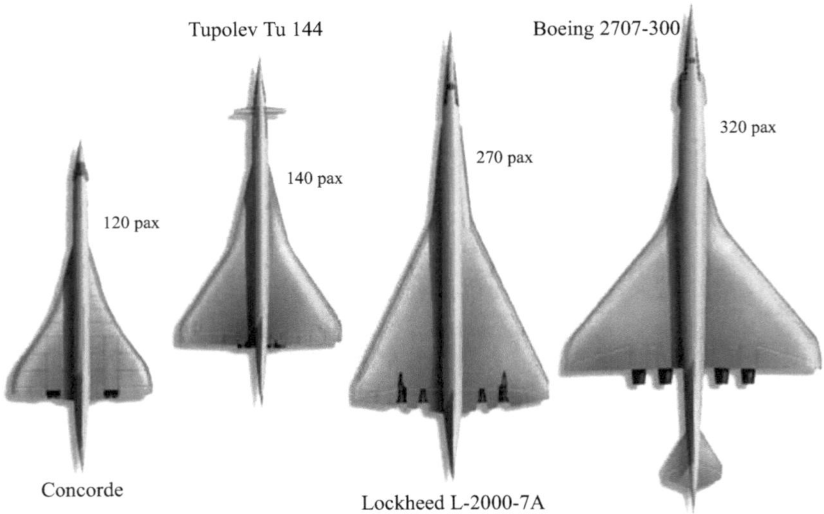

Fig. (2.48). Comparison of SST concepts from the 1960s and its maximum passenger capacity (same scale).

Technological challenges were not overcome, which directly led to the termination of the SST program at the end of 1971. Some of the factors that played a key role in that decision were concerned for:

- high engine noise levels;
- Pollution of upper atmosphere, particularly of ozone layer.
- Flutter characteristics. The sleek fuselage and relatively low payload-to-gross weight ratio made additional structural weight or mass balance particularly difficult to incorporate. The engine's center of gravity is far aft of the main wing box. This is particularly significant in the case of the outboard engines, which are outboard of the wing mid semi-span. This condition may result in unfavorable wing box bending-torsion coupling with attendant adverse flutter characteristics.
- Requirements for stability augmentation systems not available at that time.
- Sonic boom overpressure.
- Low range/payload characteristics caused by excessive structural weight fraction.
- High specific fuel consumption.
- Low lift-to-drag ratio.
- Economics.

In 1972, Boeing continued to study high-speed aircraft. A research on high-transonic airliners was carried out under a NASA contract [88]. The airplane was designated HSCT, which stands for High Speed Civil Transport. In the flight regime studied by Boeing Co., the freestream Mach number is supersonic but airflow in airplane vicinities is characterized for mixed regions, defining the flow pattern as transonic. Certainly, this was an attempt to fly above Mach 1 with a feasible airplane, in terms of economics and environmental impacts. In this study, five distinctive design concepts were elaborated and compared (Fig. **2.49**), which included:

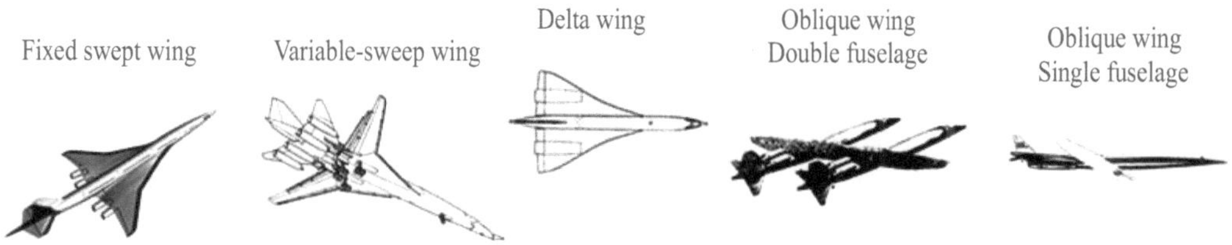

Fig. (2.49). Configurations studied by Boeing for a Mach-1.2 civil transport [88].

- Aircraft fixed swept wing.
- Aircraft with variable-sweep wing.
- A delta-wing airplane.
- Twin-fuselage yawed-wing aircraft.
- Single-fuselage yawed-wing aircraft.

The requirements for the HSCT studied by Boeing were

- Cruise Mach number of 1.2.
- 5560 km (3000 nm) range.
- 15 EPNdB below FAR Part 36 noise levels.
- Passenger payload of 18,143 kg (≡ 195 passengers).

The report issued by the Seattle Company concluded that a configuration that fulfilled the requirements posed by NASA could be achieved by the singe fuselage yawed-wing configuration with a gross weight of 226,796 kg [88]. A configuration with negligible boom effects should feature a gross weight of 211,828 kg [88]. The off-design subsonic range capability for this configuration exceeded the Mach 1.2 design range by more than 20%. Although wing aeroelastic divergence was a primary design consideration for the yawed-wing concepts, the graphite epoxy wings of the study were designed by critical gust and maneuver loads rather than by divergence requirements. The transonic nacelle drag is shown to be very sensitive to the nacelle installation. A six-degree--f-freedom dynamic stability analysis indicated that the control coordination and stability augmentation system would require more development than for a symmetrical airplane, but it would be entirely feasible at that time. A three-phase development plan was recommended by Boeing to establish the full potential of the yawed-wing concept.

To keep on going the supersonic flight technology, the United States started new research programs in the first half of the 1970s, after the failure of the SST commercial airplane. Interest on the subject had also the development of supersonic bombers as motivation. Rockwell variable-sweep B-1 bomber performed its first flight in 1974 but started operation only many years later, in 1986. B-1A could reach speeds above Mach number 2.

The National Aeronautics and Space Administration initiated the Supersonic Cruise Research (SCR) Program in fiscal year 1973 at the direct request of the Executive Office of the President and Congress following termination of the U.S. SST program [89]. Originally, the program was entitled Advanced Supersonic Technology (AST); this was later changed to Supersonic Cruise Aircraft Research (SCAR) and, finally, to SCR [89]. Funding for the SCR Program ended in fiscal year 1981 and its implementation was carried out by contracts and grants with industry and universities and by in-house investigations at the NASA Offices of Aeronautics and Space Technology (NASA/OAST) [89]. The studies included system studies and five disciplines: propulsion, stratospheric emissions impact, materials and structures, aerodynamic performance, and stability and control.

Back to the oblique wing concept it came from studies for the minimization of supersonic drag. NASA Ames Research Center Aeronautical Engineer Robert T. Jones elaborated a simplified expression for minimum supersonic drag [90]:

$$D_{min} \quad \overbrace{qSC_{D0}}^{Zero-lift\ drag} + \overbrace{\frac{W^2}{q\pi b^2}}^{Induced\ drag} + \overbrace{\frac{(M_\infty^2 - 1)W^2}{q\pi l^2}}^{Wave\ drag\ due\ to\ lift} + \overbrace{\frac{128q}{\pi}\frac{Vol^2}{l^4}}^{Wave\ drag\ due\ to\ volume} \tag{2.1}$$

In this expression:

C_{D0} is de zero-lift drag coefficient; q is the dynamic pressure; W is the aircraft weight; M_∞ is the freestream Mach number; b is the wingspan; Vol is the overall volume; S is the wing reference area; and l is the effective length of the aircraft. Fig. **2.50** shows a comparison of drag-due-to-volume of two different wing configurations with same aspect ratio and same maximum relative thickness [90].

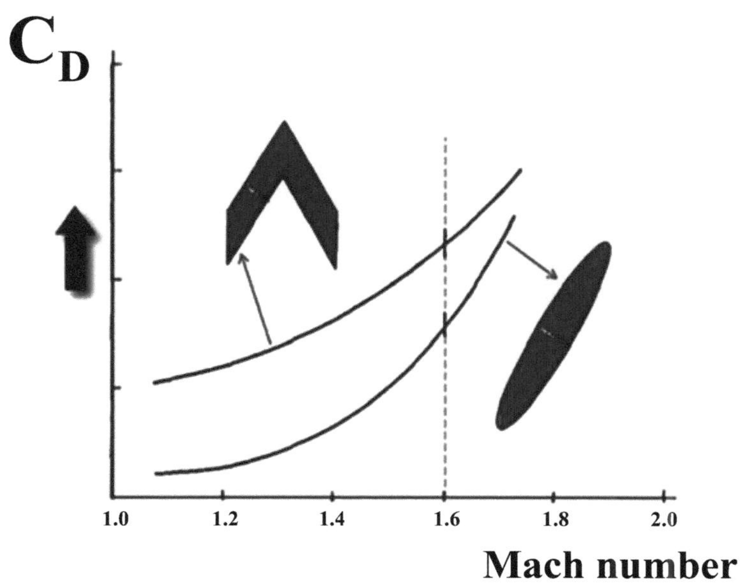

Fig. (2.50). Volume drag for two wing configurations of same aspect ratio and same maximum relative thickness [91].

In the Mach number range of Fig. (**2.50**), the drag coefficient of the oblique wing is considerably lower than that presented by the highly-swept rectangular wing. This drag component is dependent on the fourth power of the effective length. Thus, considering that the oblique-wing configuration presents a longer effective length, this reflects enormously on that drag component [91]. Other basic configuration-related features can be easily derived from the **Eq. 2.**1 [91]. First, the two wave drag terms vary inversely with the length of the vehicle, meaning that a longer supersonic aircraft will lower these two components. Since two of the terms are proportional to q and two are proportional to $1/q$, it is expected that the minimum drag at fixed lift will occur at an altitude that makes the viscous plus volume wave drag terms equal to the lift-dependent terms [91]. Of course, aircraft usually fly lower than this altitude due to Reynolds number effects on $CD0$, propulsion system performance, and structural implications (pressurization loads on the fuselage, for example).

Eq. 2.1 indicated that oblique-wing configurations have a potential for supersonic flight. In addition, wind tunnel studies carried out at NASA Ames confirmed that an oblique wing design on a supersonic transport might achieve twice the fuel economy of an aircraft with conventional wings. Next step was the investigation of an oblique-wing configuration in flight tests. Analyzing in terms of the overall aerodynamics of the configuration, the wave drag reduction of the oblique airplane concept is eclipsed by the dominant volume wave drag of the fuselage [91]. This led to a subsequent focus on oblique flying wings. It is worthy of mention that this conclusion was based on aerodynamic considerations only and it is reasonable that multi-disciplinary aspects should be considered instead. Anyway, NASA designed and built a research airplane fort that purpose, which was designated AD-1, abbreviation of Ames-Dryden-1. The wing could be rotated on its center pivot, so that it could be set at its most efficient angle for the speed at which the aircraft was flying. The oblique wing on the AD-1 pivoted about the fuselage, remaining perpendicular to it during slow flight and rotating to angles of up to 60° as aircraft speed increased. Analytical and wind tunnel studies that Jones conducted at Ames indicated that a transport-sized oblique-wing aircraft flying at speeds of up to Mach number of 1.4 (1.4 times the speed of sound) would have substantially better aerodynamic performance than aircraft with conventional wings [92]. The aircraft was delivered to the Dryden Flight Research Center, Edwards, California, in March 1979 and its first flight was on December 21, 1979. The AD-1 flew a total of 79 times during the research program. The AD-1 program achieved all its technical objectives. However, the vehicle exhibited aeroelastic and pitch-roll-coupling effects that contributed to poor handling at sweep angles above 45 degrees. After completion of the AD-1 project, there was still a need for a transonic oblique-wing research aircraft to assess the effects of compressibility, evaluate a more representative structure, and analyze flight performance at transonic speeds on either side of the sound barrier.

NASA studies carried out in 1995 [93] dealt with the development of a database of aircraft fuel burned and emissions from projected fleets of high-speed civil transports (HSCTs) on a hypothetical universal airline network. The "Universal" HSCT route system is meant to simulate the operation of HSCTs as a mature fleet in a global airline network. The "Universal" system was the sum of several global airlines, although it scheduled as if it is a single airline. Inventories for 500 and 1000 HSCT fleets were considered for this study. Extrapolated inventories for the year 2015 subsonic aircraft fleets in service with these HSCT fleets were also calculated. The objective of the work was to evaluate the changes in geographical distribution of the HSCT emissions as the fleet size grew from 500 to 1000 HSCTs. For this work, flights were projected using a market penetration analysis rather than assuming equal penetration. Emission inventories on this network were calculated for both Mach 2.0 and Mach 2.4 HSCT fleets with NO_x cruise emission indices of approximately 5 and 15 grams NO_x/kilogram fuel. Fuel burned and emissions of nitrogen oxides (NO_x as NO_2), carbon monoxide, and hydrocarbons have been calculated on a 1-degree latitude x 1-degree longitude x 1 kilometer altitude grid.

The NASA study concluded that the geographical distribution of emissions at stratospheric cruise is sensitive to the market penetration assumptions used to distribute projected HSCT passenger demand. An increase in HSCT fleet size from 500 to 1000 units approximately doubled emissions at stratospheric cruise [93]. However, as the fleet grows, emissions in different geographical regions grow at different rates. Consequently, stratospheric emissions in northern mid-latitudes are not projected to double as the fleet size doubles, while emissions in the northern tropics and southern hemisphere mid-latitudes are expected to more than double [93]. For an HSCT combustor with a NO_x emission index of 5, the analyses showed that the total NO_x emissions below 13-kilometer altitude are not very sensitive to the presence or absence of an HSCT fleet [93]. This suggests that to first-order the assessment of the effects of an HSCT fleet are largely decoupled from the assessment of subsonic aircraft effects. Details of the results for different flight segments for the Mach 2.0 HSCT fleets are summarized in Table **2.5**.

Table 2.5. Daily mileage, fuel consumption, NO_x emissions, and NO_X emissions index for the Mach-2 HSCT [93].

Flight Segment	Daily Mileage (nm)	Daily Fuel (1000 lb)	Daily NO_x (1000 lb)	EI (NO_x)
Taxi	0	5,752	40	7.00
Initial climb	87,860	36,689	297	8.10
Supersonic climb	482,933	66,765	541	8.10
Supersonic cruise	6,079,332	367,116	1,925	5.24
Supersonic descent	197,106	1,375	10	6.99
Subsonic cruise	562,131	32,536	214	6.57
Final descent	319,578	11,818	83	6.99
Taxi in	0	2,222	16	6.99
Total	**7,728,940**	**524,273**	**3,125**	**5.96**

MODERN AIRLINERS

Airliners are commonly split down into three categories: long-haul airplanes, wide-body jet airliners, and short-haul civilian passenger airliners. In turn, the short-haul civilian passenger jets are both longer and shorter ranged narrow-body jet and regional jet types. Table **2.6** shows some characteristics of relevant airlines since the introduction of DC-3.

Table 2.6. Evolution of airliner characteristics over time. EIS means Entry into Service.

Aircraft	EIS	Speed (km/h)	Max. Range (full payload, km)	Typical Seating	Wing Loading (kg/m^2)
Douglas DC-3	1936	346	563	21-32	125
Douglas DC-7	1953	555	5,810	64-95	480
Boeing 707-120	1958	917	4,300	110	495
Boeing 727-100	1963	869	5,000	94	503
Boeing 747-100	1970	907	9,800	452	652
McDonnell Douglas DC-10	1971	908	7,415	260	531
Airbus A300	1974	847	3,420	269	635
Boeing 767-200	1982	913	7,130	224	504
Boeing 747-400	1989	912	13,450	524	708
Boeing 777-200LR	1995	905	15,840	317	812
Airbus A340-500	2003	896	16,020	293	847
EMBRAER E170STD	2004	890	2,220	70	500
Airbus A380	2007	945	15,700	644	680
Boeing 787-8	2011	913	13,620	242	701

Fig. (**2.51**) shows a photo taken at a Daimler-Benz Aerospace AG (DASA) stand during the Internationale Luftfhartaustellung (ILA) in 1992. This image reveals some interesting airplane concepts:

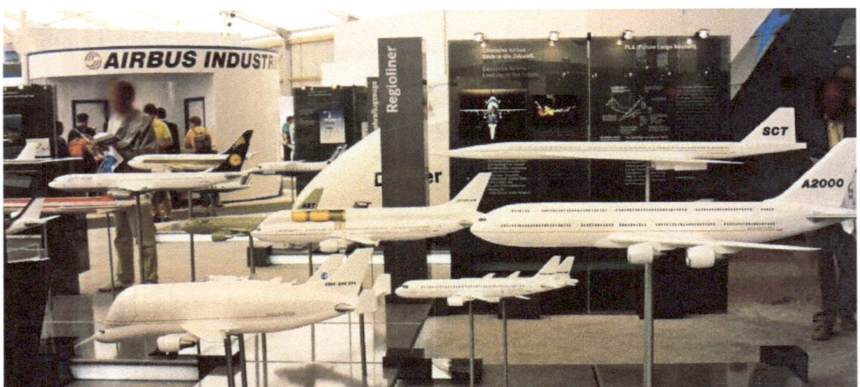

Fig. (2.51). Daimler Benz Aerospace stand at ILA 1992 (Photo: ©1992 Bento Mattos).

- *Supersonic Civil Transport (SCT)*. In early 1990s, British Aerospace, Deutsche Airbus, Boeing, and McDonnel Douglas teamed to investigate the viability of the introduction of a 2nd generation supersonic civil transport (SCT). The study for the SCT addressed the size of the market and the technical standards required to produce an environmentally acceptable and commercially viable airplane [94].

- *Regioliner*. It was a company formed in 1992 com majority participation of DASA, the Aerospatiale and Alenia being the remained partners. The intended to develop and market airliners ranging from 30 to 120 seats. At ILA 1992, the two scaled models on display are the R72 and R122, able to accommodate 70 and 120 passengers, respectively. Regioliner tried to establish without success a partnership with Fokker, which was developing 70- and 130-seat airliners at that time. The R72 and R122 programs were then later cancelled and other DASA subsidiary, Dornier Luftfahrt GmBH, started to develop the 70-seat airliner in 1997, which was designated 728Jet. A larger variant of 728Jet should follow, the 928Jet. However, before the first flight of the 728Jet could be performed, Fairchild Dornier filed for insolvency on April 2nd, 2002, and the whole program came to an end. The 728Jet prototypes were scraped.
- *Hydrogen-fueled aircraft*. After the Tupolev Tu-155 technology demonstrator aircraft successfully flew in 1988 powered by turbofans burning liquid hydrogen and liquid natural gas, DASA signed an aeronautical cooperation agreement with Russia. This agreement produced a set of projects on alternative fuels for aircraft [95]:
    1. German/Russia feasibility study about a cryogenic airplane based on the Airbus A321 airframe (1990/1993),
    2. combustion chamber tests (1992/1996),
    3. EU/INTAS tank tests (1994/1999), APU tests,
    4. 1995/98 German/Russian studies for a demonstrator aircraft based on Do 328.
- *A concept for Airbus A380*. DASA A2000 provides an insight of the ovoid cross-section and double-deck configuration that was adopted for the A3XX program. Some ideas of DASA A2000 were merged with others from the Aerospatiale A500/600 and British Aerospace AC14 to create the Airbus 3E configuration. The Airbus A380 resulted from all these considerations [96]. Double-deck concepts were also considered by both Boeing (VLCT) and McDonnel Douglas. (MD-12) in the 1990s [96].

The Airbus A380 concept evolved into a double-deck, wide-body, four-engine jet airliner manufactured by the European aircraft company Airbus (Fig. **2.52**). It is the world's largest passenger airliner, and the airports at which it operates have upgraded facilities to accommodate it. It was initially named Airbus and designed to challenge Boeing's monopoly in the large-aircraft market. The A380 made its first flight on 27 April 2005 and entered commercial service in October 2007 with Singapore Airlines.

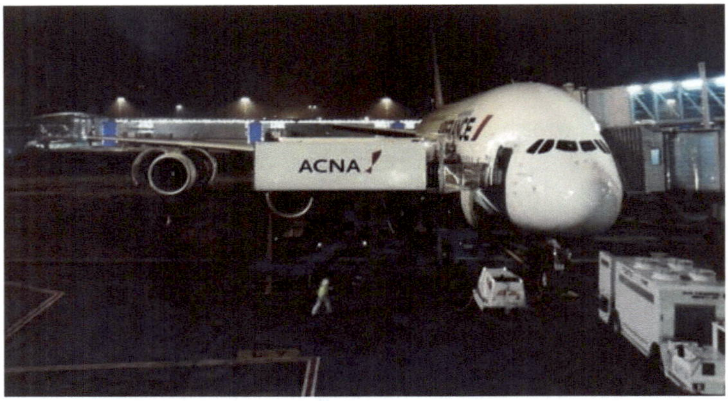

Fig. (2.52). Airbus A380 at Charles de Gaulle Airport (Photo: ©2012 Bento Mattos).

According to Airbus, the A380's main instrument panel incorporates eight identical and interchangeable liquid crystal display Units, providing a primary flight display, navigation display, two multi-function displays, an engine warning display and a system display [97]. Their increased display size provides improved situational awareness for pilots, and allows for such enhanced presentation modes as a vertical situation awareness function that presents a "vertical cut" of the aircraft trajectory integrating flight path, terrain and weather information [97]. A key A380 innovation is the use of an electronic library to avoid paper documentation to be used by pilots. This library allows flight and maintenance crews to easily locate operational information in the various flight manuals, lists and logbooks, while enabling an optimization of performance and weight-an--balance computations [97]. Table **2.7** lists some technological advances in flight physics. Some of the structural technologies employed in A380 are:

Glare® for part of upper fuselage; laser beam welding for lower fuselage; CFRP for wing ribs; CFRP wingbox; flap track fairings in CFRP (Resin transfer molding); CFRP for the horizontal tailplane; CFRP rear pressure bulkhead; finite element analysis with global load behavior.

The Boeing 787 airliner is a long-range, twin-aisle commercial transport developed by Boeing Commercial Airplanes (Fig. **2.53**). Its variants seat 242 to 335 passengers in typical three-class seating configurations [98]. This airplane is the most fuel-efficient airliner that Boeing ever produced. It is a pioneering airliner with the use of composite materials as the primary material in the construction of its airframe. The 787 was designed to be 20% more fuel efficient than the Boeing 767, which it was intended to replace. Boeing 787 was fitted with bleed-less engines and therefore air supply to its interior is provided by a power station that compresses external air. The Boeing 787 distinguishing features include mostly electrical flight systems, raked wingtips for drag reduction, composite fuselage and wings, and noise-reducing chevrons on its engine nacelles. It shares a common type rating with the larger Boeing 777 to allow pilots to be certified in operating both models [98].

Table 2.7. A380 innovative technologies in flight physics (Source: Airbus).

Integrated wing design	Inboard wing with higher loads provided 4-ton weight saving for a slight increase in induced drag
Wake-vortex prediction	Methodology for wake-vortex prediction was validated. It enabled the Airbus airplane to present the same signature of that generated by Boeing 747
Advanced load control	Wing weight reduction of 2.2 t thanks to additional improvements in load control (fatigue/maneuver/turbulence wing load alleviation)
Advanced engine nacelle	Significant (100 kg) weight reduction for the anti-ice system; reduced maintenance
Optimal tailplanes	Variable thickness distribution for the horizontal and vertical saved 350 kg and provided slight drag reduction
Drooped airfoils	Higher lift-to-drag ratio at takeoff
High-Reynolds number performance estimation from wind-tunnel data	Better performance prediction and therefore lower margins for performance guarantee

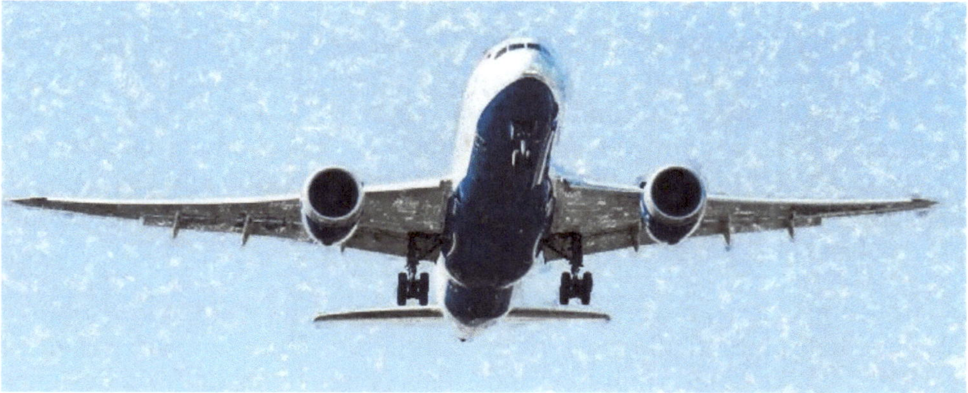

Fig. (2.53). Artistic view of Boeing 787.

GROUND EFFECT AERIAL VEHICLES

Many attempts have been made to build aerial vehicles based on wing in ground effect (WIG). Boeing released a concept in the 1990s, called Pelican Ultra Large Transport Aircraft. In the Soviet Union era, it was designed the so-called

Ekranoplan. The A-90 Orlyonok is one of them and it uses ground effect to fly a coupled of meters above the surface, water or land. Russian categorize Orlyonok as an Ekranoplan Class B - it can achieve an altitude of 3,000 m, placing between Class A - which is limited to ground effect, and Class C, which exploits the ground effect only during take-offs and landings [99].

The layout of the engines on the Orlyonok was unusual and a testament of the special needs of such an unconventional aircraft. Mounted in the top of the tail, it featured a massive Kuznetsov NK-12 turboprop, the most powerful turboprop to find service. This engine provides the required cruise power. Two turbofan engines are in the aircraft nose, with the intakes on top of the nose to prevent water ingestion. Their exhausts are placed sideways along the forward fuselage and the thrust produced by the jet engines are vectored over the wings to produce increased lift and the required propulsion at takeoff. Under cruise conditions and in ground effect, the front engines could be shut off since their power was unnecessary to keep the aircraft lifted, this also minimized intake of water, salt and ingestion of low flying birds.

South Korea developed the Aron M50, capable of an 800-km range in ground effect. The machine presents a top speed of 200 km/h and is employed in coastal patrol by South Korea. Equipped with Optronics systems and a small naval radar, an armed Aron M50 can fire small anti-ship missiles or guided rockets to attack larger ships.

The Wing Ship Technology Corporation, a South Korean company, developed a turboprop vehicle can transport 50 passengers, which was designated WSH-500. It has a catamaran-style hull and a reverse-delta wing. Cruising at 180 km/h, makes it faster than a jetfoil, its principal rival, and the production version will have a range of 1,000 km. Table **2.8** compares the WSH-500 and Orlyonok with big airliners [100]. The WSH-500 has a very small range with full payload but the vehicle reaches 1,000 km with a payload of 22 passengers [101].

The South Korean company believes that the reverse-delta wing is key solution to turn WIG vehicles into viable mean of transportation. This approach was devised in the 1960s by Alexander Lippisch and Hanno Fischer, the latter a designer of Fanliner, an experimental German light aircraft of the 1970s, propelled by a piston engine driving a ducted fan. However, their single-seater Aerofoilboot, as they dubbed it, was not a commercial success. However, Wing Ship Technology believes the idea of a delta wing is revolutionary. The delta wing's geometry amplifies the ground effect, allowing the vehicle to cruise five meters above the water's surface. That means it is less likely to be confined to harbor by rough seas, which was one of the problems encountered by previous designs. It also launches itself by directing some of the airflow from the turbo props downwards, to create a temporary hovercraft effect until it is travelling forwards at full tilt. The difficulty of getting airborne was another bugbear of previous designs. It remains to be seen whether Wing Ship Technology's craft will be the breakthrough that enthusiasts of ground-effect vehicles are hoping for.

Table 2.8. Wing in ground effect vehicles compared with big airliners [100].

	Orlyonok	WSH-500	Boeing 747-400ER	Airbus A380
Length (m)	58	29	70.6	73.0
Wingspan (m)	31.5	28	64.4	79.8
MTOW (tones)	140	17.1	412.8	575
Cruise altitude (m)	0.5-5	2-5	13,747	13,136
Cruise speed (km/h)	370	175	900	946
Payload (tones)	20	4.3	112.7	150
Range with max. payload (km)	1,000	50	14,205	15,200
Wing aspect ratio	3.0	2.5	7.4	7.5
Installed power or thrust	2 x 10 t 1 x 15000 hp	2 x 1,400 hp	4 x 282 kN	4 x 311 kN

Wing Ship Technology advocates that their vehicle presents more advantages in regard fuel consumption and CO_2 emissions (Table **2.9**).

Table 2.9. Fuel burn and CO_2 emissions of several means of transportation [101].

Mean of Transportation	Cruise Speed [km/h]	CO_2 Emission [g/(pax.km)]	Fuel Efficiency [g/(pax.km)]
Ferry	46	396	124
75-seat airliner	800	106	33
WSH-500 WIG vehicle	180	94	29

The Be-2500 super-heavy transport seaplane (Fig. **2.54**) is a concept aircraft of Russian Beriev target to perform specialized service transportation on transoceanic routes [102]. The design concept of super-heavy seaplane allows operate the aircraft both in ground effect mode above the ocean and usual airplane operation. The Be-2500 may also be used for landing operations, search and rescue missions, as well as the vehicle for prospecting and extraction operations at shelves and archipelagos areas [102]. The facilities of existing major ports may provide sufficient support for operation and anchorage of the seaplane. Table **2.10** presents some data for Be-2500.

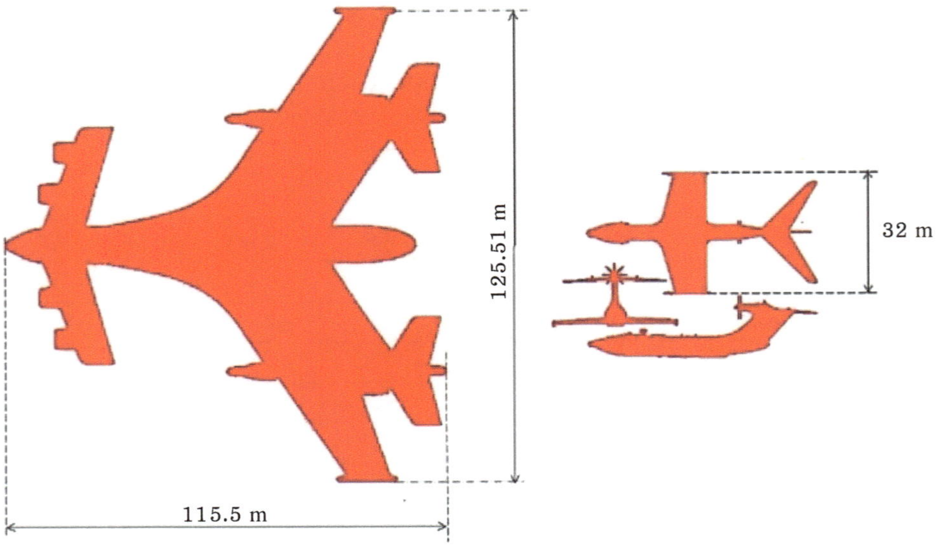

Fig. (2.54). Beriev 2500 concept compared to the Orlyonok ekranoplan.

Table 2.10. Beriev Be-2500 specifications (Source: Beriev Aircraft Company Website).

Wing span	125.51 m
Wing area	3,184 m^2
Aircraft length	115.5 m
Aircraft height	29.12 m
Maximum take-off weight	2,500 t
Maximum payload	up to 1,000 t
Cruise speed: **- high-altitude flight mode** **- WIG flight mode**	770 km/h 450 km/h
Maximum range	16,000 km

ALTERNATIVE FUEL AND POWER

Before airplanes became technologically advanced for a non-stopping intercontinental crossing, airships performed this role. The Graf Zeppelin (Fig. **2.55**), an airship designed by the German company Zeppelin Luftschiffbau, made the very first commercial passenger flight across the Atlantic. The aircraft departed from Friedrichshafen in Germany on October 11, 1928, and landed at Lakehurst, New Jersey, on October 15, 1928, after a flight of 111 hours and 44 minutes [103]. Graf Zeppelin had performed its first flight some time earlier, on September 18, 1928. By the time of Graf Zeppelin's last flight, nine years later, the airship had flown over a million miles, on 590 flights, carrying thousands of passengers and hundreds of thousands of pounds of freight and mail, with an excellent safety record. Graf Zeppelin circled the globe with a stop-over in Japan and it was very famous throughout the world.

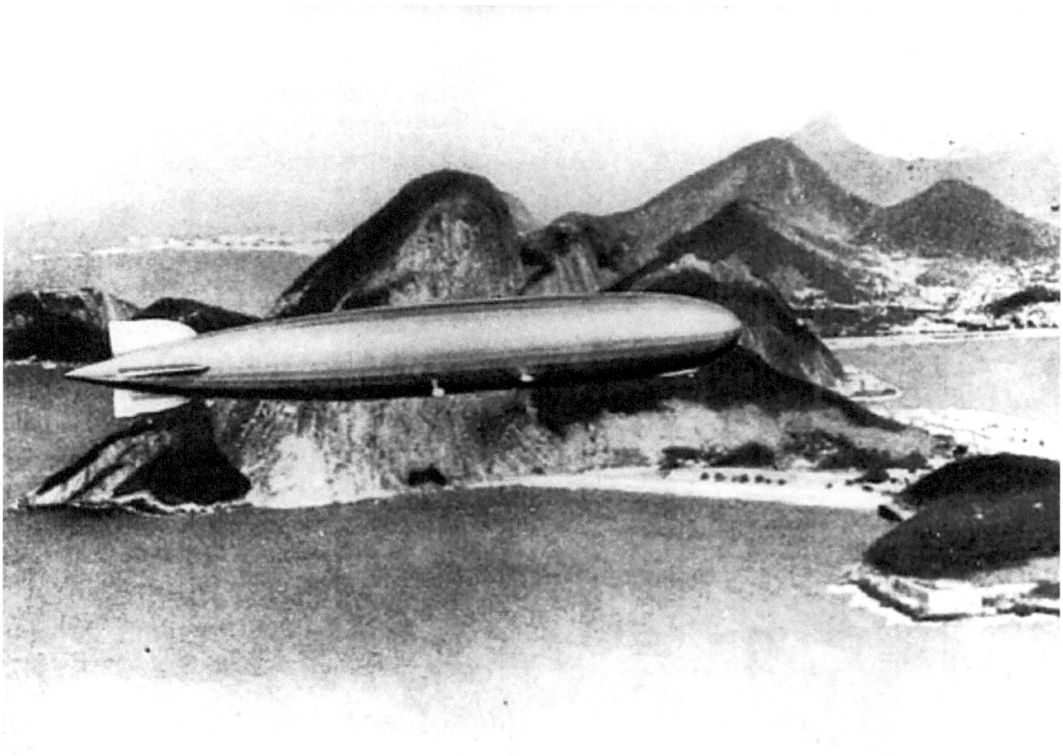

Fig. (2.55). LZ 127 Graf Zeppelin over Rio de Janeiro (Photo: Brazilian Air Force Archive, public domain via Wikimedia Commons).

The Graf Zeppelin airship incorporated an outstanding innovation: the use of the so-called blaugas fuel for its five engines [104]. One of the challenges of lighter-than-air powered flight has been the need to account for the loss of weight as fuel is burned. As gasoline or diesel fuel is consumed during flight, the airship becomes lighter and expensive lifting gas must be released to maintain the aircraft balance. The Zeppelin Company's innovative solution to this issue with the Graf Zeppelin was the use of a gaseous fuel, like propane, named blaugas after its inventor, Hermann Blau [104]. Since blaugas has similar density to air, its consumption during flight did not significantly change the aerostatic balance of the airship, and so it is not necessary to release hydrogen to compensate for blaugas burned by the engines. Blaugas was also more efficient to carry than gasoline, and extended the endurance of the Graf Zeppelin by over 30 hours [105]. The approximately one million cubic feet of blaugas carried by the Graf Zeppelin could power the airship for over one hundred hours, but if that million cubic feet of blaugas had been replaced by hydrogen, the additional hydrogen could have lifted only enough gasoline to power the ship for 70 hours or less.

In early 1930s, ignition systems made life difficult to radio operators, because they created interference that often hindered the communication's understanding. Diesel engines need no ignition and no fire risk was associated with diesel fuel. Diesel engines became therefore highly desirable at that time. Indeed, there were diesel engines as aircraft engines, but offering a weight-to-power ratio of 3 kg/hp, they were practically unusable.

In 1929, after 20 years of development, Hugo Junkers developed a diesel engine for airplane that was comparable with the usual water-cooled petrol engines [106]. Junkers had then developed a large diesel engine, which required no spark plug and could start at low temperatures [106]. A Focke-Wulf A17 Möve airplane was employed to flight test the Junkers engine in May 1933. A 500-hp Junkers Jumo 205B was installed into a Fw A17C airplane and a flight test campaign then began. Due to noise caused by many flights, population resident in the area complained and the tests had to be discontinued. Despite this, Junkers move forward with the development of the engine and several versions were brought to the market. The Jumo 205 powered early versions of the Junkers Ju 86 bomber, but was found too unresponsive for combat and liable to failure at maximum power, common setting for combat aircraft [107].

Some airplanes used the Jumo 205 engine at extreme high-altitude conditions, as with the Ju 86P and -R versions for high-altitude reconnaissance over the British Islands. The Jumo 250 was far more successful as a power unit for airships, for which its characteristics were ideal, and for non-combat applications such as the Blohm & Voss Ha 139 airliner. Its more fuel-efficient operation lent itself for use on Germany's few maritime patrol flying boat designs during World War II, such as the BV 138 and six-engine BV 222 flying boat.

The Blohm & Voss BV 138 was a three-engine flying boat conceived for long-range maritime patrol and naval reconnaissance. BV 138 saw combat in World War II and 227 units were produced. Three 868-hp Junkers Jumo 205 D diesel engines powered the first standardized version, BV 138 B-1 [108]. Diesel engines present lower specific fuel consumption than those burning avgas. Thanks to its diesel engines, the BV 138 airplane could fly over 4,300 kilometers and stay airborne for 20 hours [108]. Range could be increased even further by using RATO packs (Rocket Assisted Takeoffs) or when launched from catapults on ships. The diesel engines also enabled the airplane to undertake refueling missions to surfaced U-boats in remote areas in the Atlantic. The BV 138 also had an unusual structural concept. The BV 138 wing spar consisted of a cylindrical steel-made tube, which was used for fuel storage [108].

Interest in diesel engines in the postwar period was fortuitous. Lower power-t--weight ratio is a known drawback of diesel engines, particularly when they are compared to turboprop ones. Due to relative cheaper avgas and kerosene, and considering most financial support to research on turboprops and jets for high-speed airliners, diesel-powered aircraft virtually disappeared. The collapse of the general aviation market in the 1990s recorded a massive decline in the development of any new aircraft engine types. However, more recently, several factors have changed this picture. First, several new manufacturers of general aviation, a nursery of new ideas, emerged. Second, in some places like Europe, avgas has become very expensive. Third, in several remote locations, avgas is harder to obtain than diesel fuel. Finally, technologies for diesel engines have improved greatly in recent years, offering higher power-to-weight ratios, turning them more suitable for aircraft application.

Austrian Diamond Aircraft (www.diamond-air.at) has designed and certified diesel-powered general aviation airplanes. Information available at Diamond's Website states that fuel consumption of its twin-engine DA42 NG is 40.5 liter/h.

Both the Graf Zeppelin and BV 138 employed alternative fuel to improve performance or the balancing of the aircraft. However, there is an experiment with a Russian airplane that was carried out due to concern on oil supply. The Tupolev Tu-155 was a modified Tu-154 trijet and it was used as an alternative fuel testbed. The airplane performed its first flight on April 15, 1988. This was the first experimental aircraft in the world operating on liquid hydrogen. The trijet was fitted with a thermally-insulated 17.5 m^3 fuel tank aft of the passenger cabin which contained liquid hydrogen at a temperature of minus 253°C [109]. This tank provided fuel to a new engine, the Kuznetsov NK-88, mounted in the number three position on the starboard side. Some 30 other systems were installed in the aircraft including pressurization equipment, cryogenic pumps and injection mechanisms, and safety and monitoring systems to protect against leakage and possible explosion [109]. Operating team needed to refuel the aircraft on the ground remotely. Dedicated rigs were built for this purpose. Although liquid hydrogen was used for the first few flights, the focus quickly shifted to liquid natural gas, in line with the Soviet energy strategy at the time.

The Brazilian national ethanol program was triggered by the 1973 oil crisis. It has been supported by the Brazilian government since the 1970s. Today, Brazil is the world's largest single producer of first generation biofuels, namely ethanol. The Brazilian government has supported private industry in the development of alcohol-based fuels by subsidizing research and development [110]. The program for distributing these subsidies is known as PróÁlcool (National Alcohol Program). Since the 1980, the supply of gasoline versus ethanol has varied, as prices. Today, most vehicles in Brazil are flex-fuel vehicles, which can run on gasoline or 100% ethanol or any combination of the two fuel types. Neiva, an EMBRAER subsidiary, considered alcohol a viable option to the crop-duster market because the fuel is environmentally friendly and research data indicates it can extend the engine maintenance cycle. Neiva modified and certified an alcohol-fueled variant of the agricultural airplane Ipanema EMB-201A (Fig. **2.56**). The modifications basically incorporated a larger injection nozzle and a corrosion protected fuel pump able to deliver a higher mass flow. The newest version of Ipanema is EMB-203, which presents a larger wingspan than that of EMB-201A.

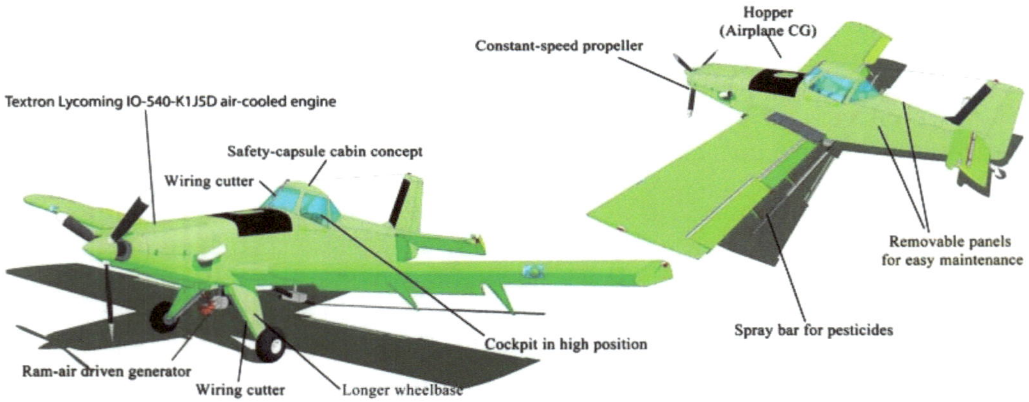

Fig. (2.56). Some characteristics of EMB 201A Ipanema.

The alcohol-powered Ipanema project involved the participation and technical support of Lycoming, Precision and Hartzell, manufacturers of the aircraft's engine, the fuel injection system and the propeller group, respectively. Alcohol-powered Ipanema (Fig. **2.56**) received Brazilian General Command for Aerospace Technology (CTA) certification on October 19, 2004. Produced without interruption for more than 40 years, Ipanema has already surpassed 1,300 delivered units in 2014.

Airbus Group developed an electric aircraft with French Aero Composite Saintonge. The aircraft is equipped with on-board lithium batteries, which supply power for two electric engines. Two occupants find place in the cabin. A test flight was performed in April 2014 at Mérignac Airport, France. Two production variants are planned, a two-seater E-Fan 2.0 for use as a trainer, and the E-Fan 4.0 four-seater. To increase autonomy, the E-Fan 4.0 will have a hybrid-electric system that will have a small engine to charge the battery, which will increase duration from nearly an hour to 3.5 hours [111]. Per information posted at Airbus Website on February 2015, Airbus Group is involved in many technological programs whose breakthroughs could eventually also be applied to an all-electric helicopter and a 90-seat-passenger regional airliner with fully electric or hybrid propulsion.

The E-Aircraft System House is located at Airbus Group Innovations facilities in Munich and its duty is to contribute to the development of electric-powered aircraft at Airbus. The E-Aircraft System House resulted from collaboration between Airbus Group and Siemens, which signed a Memorandum of Understanding signed with company Diamond Aircraft in 2013. These three partners already successfully flew a second-generation prototype of the DA36 E-Star 2 hybrid aircraft in Vienna in June 2011. Inside this aircraft, there is a small Wankel engine which supplies the electricity by driving a generator. The aircraft, which was based on HK36 Super Dimona, relies on a battery to provide the extra power needed for takeoff and climb, and recharges it during cruise. Because of the airplane's low engine output, Diamond states that DA-36 E-Star presents fuel consumption and carbon emissions by 25 percent lower when compared to conventional aircraft.

CONCLUDING REMARKS

Santos-Dumont designed the first operational airplane, the Demoiselle, which influenced up to a certain extent the Blériot XI design, the first flying machine that crossed the English Channel. Blériot delivered military airplanes to the French armed forces, which already were obsolete when World War I began.

World War I recorded an impressive increase in engine power and airplane speed. Top speed of the Blériot XI was 75 km/h. Fokker D.VII, an outstanding fighter that saw combat in the last years of war, could reach 200 km/h. Engine power of Blériot XI was a mere 25 hp while that of Fokker D.VII was 185 hp. Zeppelin Staaken R.XVI was a German heavy bomber powered by four engines in a push-pull configuration. Two of these engines could deliver 530 hp each, a twenty-fold rate when compared with the power provided by the Blériot XI engine.

Between the great wars, airships were the sole flying machines able to perform non-stop transoceanic flights and they also offered a unique level of comfort. Apart from the Hindenburg disaster in 1937, the successful non-stop flight of the Focke-Wulf 200C airliner from Berlin to New York represented the end of the airship era. Flying boats followed suit, being then replaced by land-based airplanes after World War II. Aviation also killed ocean liners, ships designed for regular transport service of passengers from a port of origin to an established destination. They became obsolete and the maritime passenger transport is nowadays exclusively restricted to transatlantic ships, which transport people for leisure.

The Graf Zeppelin airship burned an original fuel, which was called Blaugas, an artificial illuminating gas. This fuel has the same density of air, avoiding the release of expensive hydrogen gas by the airship crew to maintain its course. Blaugas (Blau is the German word for blue) is not blue, but has a rather water-like color [112]. It can be stored in steel cylinders for shipment and its advantage relies on the fact that it possesses the highest specific energy of all artificially produced gases. However, unlike coal gas, Blaugas is free of carbon monoxide. Blaugas was also more efficient to store than gasoline, and extended the Graf Zeppelin's autonomy by over 30 hours of flying time.

For the No. 3 airship, Santos-Dumont employed illuminating gas as lifting medium instead of hydrogen, which is expensive to produce, as previously mentioned. His intent was to build a low-cost airship that would be affordable for many people, an attempt to turn aviation popular at his time. Dumont returned to hydrogen with his No.4 airship.

The introduction of the first jet transport in the 1950s marked the beginning of a revolution in transportation. The technology of the jet engine developed in World War II took some time to establish itself in the commercial aviation sector. The pioneer introduction of the De Havilland Comet of the early 1950's, unfortunately marred by a sad history, led to the highly efficient, safe, reliable, and economical transport aircraft of today. The modern jet transport has altered forever the travel concepts and habits of people all over the world. This includes the second jet age that was triggered by EMBRAER and Canadair aircraft manufacturers with their regional jets in the early 1990s in the wake of the 1978 North-American Deregulation Act. This was a breakthrough in air transportation, which this time was not caused by technological advance but by a political-economical move. The Deregulation changed aviation profoundly, making it possible for airlines to offer jet and turboprop transport to small and medium cities, which in turn resulted in economic development for those communities.

The present Chapter also describes several attempts to design and manufacture civil supersonic airliners. The British-French Concorde was the only airplane to enter service on a regular basis; its Russian competitor, the Tu-144, was retired prematurely from service after an accident over Paris. Concorde was not economically viable to operate, but it remained in regular service thanks to heavy subsidies from France and Great Britain. Research will continue in the following decades to enable commercial supersonic passenger service at a reasonable cost.

The Convair 990 was not capable to fly supersonically, but was able to cruise at Mach number of 0.92. Its immense fuel consumption caused one of the largest corporate losses in history at the time. In 1994, the General Dynamics Corporation split and sold the original Convair Division, along with other General Dynamics aerospace units that had been incorporated over the decades.

Environmental concerns about a fleet of supersonic commercial airplanes pose a great barrier to the widespread use of such airplanes, even in a short-to-medium timeframe. A 5000-nm range 8-passenger capable supersonic business jet will probably present a maximum takeoff weight of 55 tons, burning 30 tons of fuel. The EMBRAER 195AR airliner has a maximum takeoff weight like that, 52,450 kg, but can transport 124 passengers for a 2000-nm journey. The emission levels per seat are far from acceptable for the supersonic business jet.

Despite environmental concerns, a supersonic small business jet (SSBJ) has nevertheless some appeal. A SSBJ able to cruise a Mach number 2 will cut the time from Los Angeles to Tokyo to 3.5 h and on longer trips it could reduce travel time by half including ground refueling. For this kind of airplane, ground refueling is a big issue because it takes considerable time due to the large amount of fuel needed. A SSBJ able to accommodate 8 passengers and capable to cruise at Mach number 2 SSBJ would probably cost US$75 million or more, depending on the units that could be put on the market. Certainly, there are some categories of people and corporations that can afford to pay that price in benefit of time travel saving. However, this market size lacks a more accurate estimation and the environment hazard poses a great barrier to commercial operations on a large scale.

Early in 2001, the Boeing Company announced the development of a completely new 250-passenger high-speed aircraft, which was designated Sonic Cruiser. The most impressive features of this new concept were a range of up to 10,000 nm, a cruise Mach number of 0.98 and the claim of a large reduction in flight time. Martin Epperle from the German Research Institute DLR carried out a feasibility study about the sonic cruiser and concluded [113]:

"Combining the aerodynamic data, the structure/fuel mass ratio, the tank volume and taking the fuel consumption into account, a range of 6,500 nautical miles is just reachable when flying at Mach number of 0.98. To extend the range to 7,500 miles, the TSFC of the engines must be reduced from 0.67 to about 0.55 in cruise, which seems to be possible. A further extension of the range to 9,000 miles would require engines operating with a TSFC of less than 0.55, which seems not to be feasible, at least not with a BPR below 8."

Mr. Epperle did not address the potential operating cost of the Sonic Cruiser, especially regarding other existing transport airplanes of similar capacity. In fact, the benefit of shorter flight time was overshadowed by higher operating costs. By any means, airlines lost interest in the concept and Boeing cancelled the Sonic Cruiser program in 2002. Afterwards, the 787 program started.

Many airplanes flying in 2016 were developed with the technology level from the 1980s, as, for example, the Airbus A320, EMBRAER ERJ 145, and Boeing 737-300. Transport aircraft currently in production, among them the Boeing 787 and Airbus A350, will continue to leave assembly line for many years to come. They will incorporate improvements, modifications, and adaptations to new routes and markets and will continue to operate as technologies evolve.

The concept of the Be-2500 ekranoplan started envisaging military applications, but it could also provide an interesting mean of civil transportation. A lot of "energy" is necessary to put an airplane flying at 12,000 m cruise altitude, special efforts must be made to keep passengers safe and sound and well taken care of. Be-2500 can fly at 400 meters above the ground or sea, taking advantage of the ground effect. In this flight mode, its speed is only a little bit more than 400 km/h. It would be more efficient in terms of design, if an unpressurized vehicle were designed instead, preventing the structure from being too heavy. A fleet of such flying vehicles would cause such an impact on aviation that it could suffer a total recall. Unfortunately, the investment needed for that change is huge, both for the vehicle and for changing and establishing a new airport infrastructure.

Alongside upgraded airplane designs, new transport aircraft will certainly be developed in the next two or three decades and innovative technologies in aerodynamics, structures, guidance and control, and propulsion will be incorporated. Laminar flow, unusual configurations such as truss-braced wing, composite structures, active controls, and engines of improved efficiency and reduced noise are only a few of the new key technical developments. Fuel-efficient airplanes are important to reduce emission levels. Technological improvements play a key role for the mitigation of the aviation impact on the environment. New products must be continuously developed and regularly introduced into the airline fleets everywhere to properly reduce the environmental impact of aviation. However, significant global improvement is a lengthy process. While the current and future generation of commercial transport aircraft will eventually burn less than 3 liters of fuel per passenger, per 100 kilometers, achieving this average fuel consumption for the worldwide fleet will take approximately 20 years.

In addition to advances in disciplinary technologies, improved methods for integrating discipline-based design into a better system are being developed. The field of multi-disciplinary design optimization permits detailed analyses and design methods in several disciplines to be combined to the best advantage for the overall system. It is a key methodology to design green airplanes with satisfactory performance tradeoffs.

Apart from evolutionary improvements in conventional aircraft, revolutionary changes are possible when the "rules" are changed. This is possible when the configuration concept itself is changed and when new roles or requirements are introduced.

SOME MILESTONES IN AIRCRAFT TECHNOLOGY

Aircraft	Year	Major Innovations
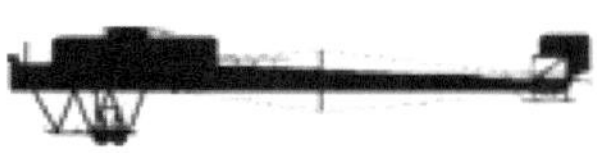 **Sikorsky Russky Vityaz**	1913	• World's first multi-engine airplane • Storage room • Passengers could walk during flight causing no stability problem to the airplane • Dual control column
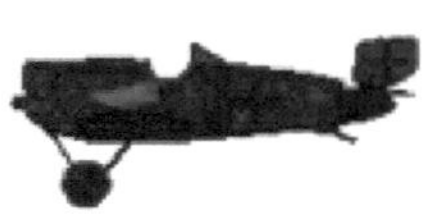 **Junkers D-I**	1919	• First all-metal airplane • Cantilevered low-wing design • Corrugated duralumin skin • Variable-incidence horizontal empennage • Advanced engine radiator design layout: the radiator was placed in a ventral belly position under the forward fuselage
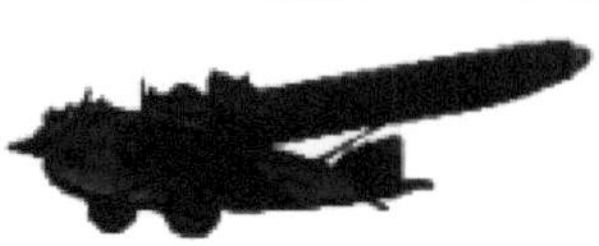 **Zeppelin-Staaken E4/20**	1920	• Stressed skin • Torsion-box spar • Wing leading-edge mounted engines with most part at wing lower side for low drag
 **Dornier Wal**	1923	• Transatlantic cargo and passenger flights became possible • Semi-cantilever wing • Duralumin construction • Stabilizing sponsons

Aircraft	Year	Major Innovations
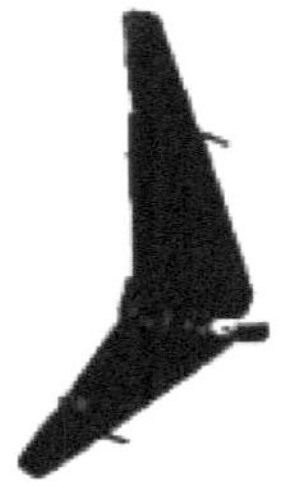 **Westland-Hill Pterodactyl I**	1928	• Tailless airplane • Wing tips pivoted to act as slab elevons providing control in pitch and roll • The wing was "washed out", having a slight twist which reduced the angle of incidence progressively towards the tips, providing a near-stationary overall center of pressure and ensuring that the aircraft was stable in pitch.
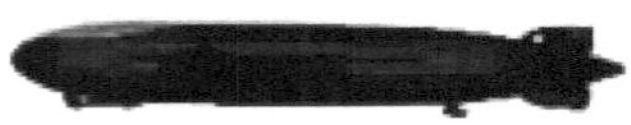 **Graf Zeppelin**	1928	• First around-the-world flight by an aircraft in 1929 • Non-stop Atlantic regular crossings • Innovative fuel bauhaus, which has the same density as the air
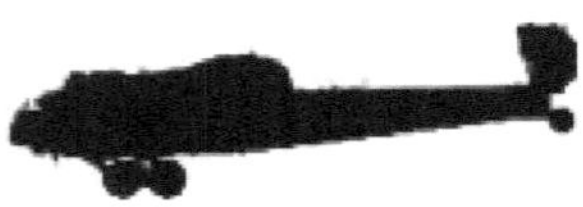 **Junkers G38**	1929	• Part of passengers seated in the wings • Diesel engines (Later version) • All-metal construction • Blend wing-body configuration • Flaperons
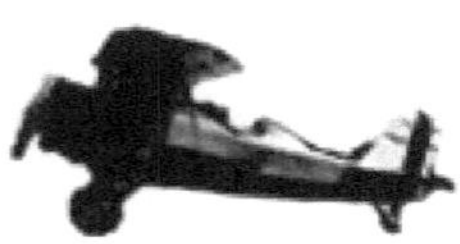 **Hall XFH**	1929	• Hall Aluminum, a U.S. Company, built the XFH, which was the first aircraft with a riveted metal fuselage - a watertight aluminum skin over steel tubing. Hall also pioneered flush rivets and butt joints between skin panels in the PH flying boat, which first flew in 1929
 **Polikarpov I-16**	1933	• First low-wing monoplane with a retractable undercarriage • Cantilever wing construction • Variable-pitch propeller • Enclosed cockpit (some versions) • Ailerons acting as flaps (flaperons)
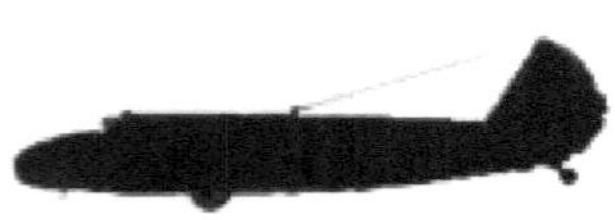 **Boeing 247**	1933	• First autopilot in civil aircraft • First civil aircraft with de-icing boots • Variable-pitch propellers • All-metal semi-monocoque construction • Cantilever wing • NACA cowlings • Air conditioning
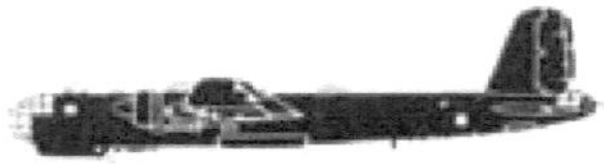 **Heinkel He 177**	1939	• Evaporative cooling system to avoid the utilization of drag-producing radiators.

Aircraft	Year	Major Innovations
 **Boeing 307**	1940	• First pressurized airliner. Work on this field began with Hugo Junkers, who built and flew the experimental airplane Ju 49 • First airplane to include a flight engineer station
 **Messerschmitt Me 262**	1942	• First production aircraft with jet engines • Swept wings • Tricycle landing gear
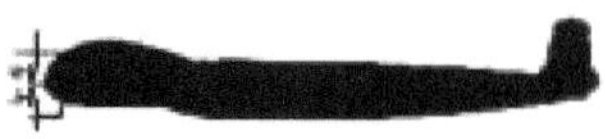 **Heinkel He 219**	1943	• First aircraft with ejection seats • Pressurized cabin • First steerable nose wheel of a German aircraft
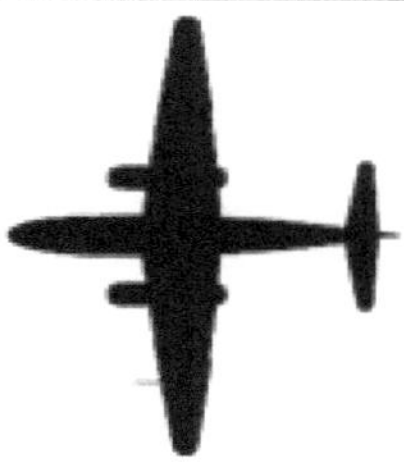 **Arado Ar 234**	1943	• Rocket-assisted takeoff • Integration of several new technologies: • Pressurized cabin • Autopilot • Jet engine • Ejection seat • Bombing computers
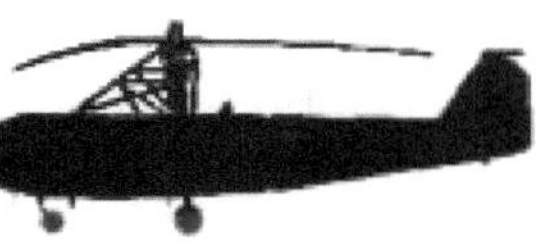 **Focke-Achgelis Fa 223**	1944	• Thanks to its rotor design it was the first Helicopter able to externally transport outsized cargo even at higher altitudes. • Some cabin equipment could be throw out for crew evacuation in an emergency event
 **Vickers Viscount**	1950	• First turboprop aircraft in regular service • Pressurization
 **Chance-Vought Cutlass**	1951	• First swept-wing naval aircraft • First production aircraft with afterburner • First fighter to carry radar-guided missiles • High-pressure hydraulic system (3000 psi) • Tailless configuration
 **De Havilland Comet**	1952	• First production jetliner • Pressurized cabin • Four-wheel bogie main landing gear • Integral fuel tanks • Redundant hydraulic systems • Irreversible powered flight controls • New alloys, both riveted and chemically bonded

Aircraft	Year	Major Innovations
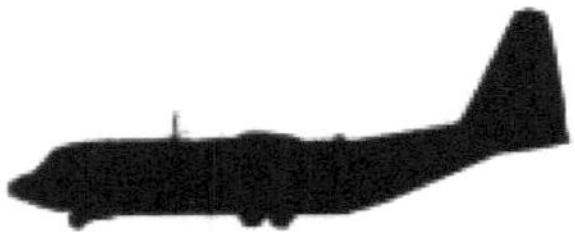 **Hercules C-130**	1954	• First airplane fitted with ice detectors
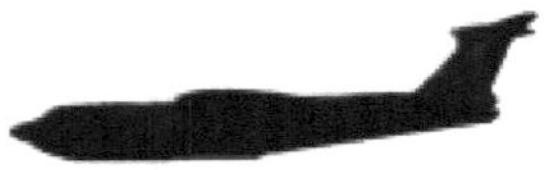 **Martin P6A Seamaster**	1955	• First amphibious airplane to reach Mach 0.90 in level flight
 **Sud-Aviation Caravelle**	1959	• Rear-mounted engines configuration • Jet transport for short-range operations • Welding for structural components. • Engine electric start
 **Convair B-58 Hustler**	1960	• First supersonic bomber • Ejection capsule • One of the first extensive applications of aluminum honeycomb panels, which bonded outer and inner aluminum skins to a honeycomb of aluminum and fiberglass.
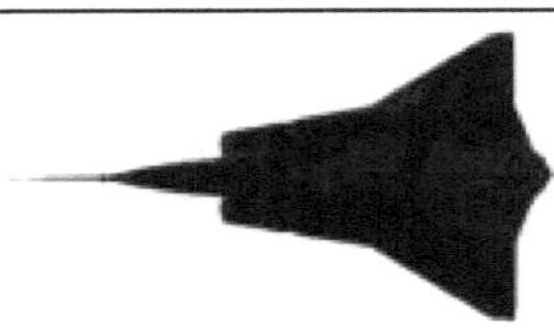 **Saab Draken**	1960	• Double-delta wing configuration • Capable of operating from public roads • Ram air turbine providing emergency power
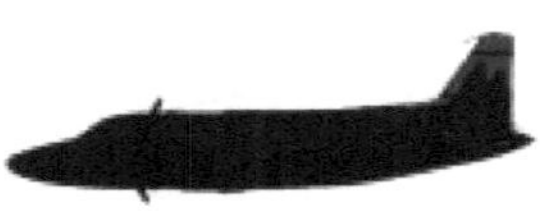 **Rockwell Sabreliner**	1962	• First business jet fitted with turbofans engines. First turbofan saw some development in WWII by the Germans. However, due to lack of technology at that time development stopped • First serial airplane whose wings were fitted with supercritical airfoils (Series 65)
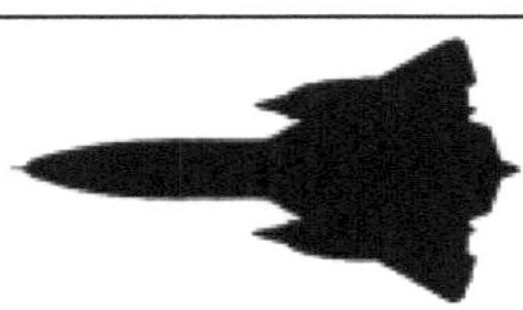 **Lockheed SR-71**	1964	• First jet aircraft to reach Mach 3.4 • Astro-inertial navigation system • First airplane designed with stealth capabilities • Titanium construction • Cooling of structure by cycling fuel
 **Vickers_armstrong VC-10**	1964	• Autopilot enabled fully-automatic landings • Quadruplicated systems

Aircraft	Year	Major Innovations
 **BAC-111**	1965	• Equipped with stick shaker and pusher systems
 **General Dynamics F-111**	1967	• Variable-sweep wing • Afterburner for a turbofan engine • Automated terrain-following radar for low-level, high-speed flight
 **Windecker Eagle**	1969	• The Windecker Eagle became the first all-composite aircraft to receive FAA certification, using a flexible, non-woven glass fiber material, "Fibaloy," developed by Dow Chemical. Carbon replaced glass as the reinforcing fiber in subsequent designs. The Eagle also was the first aircraft certified under the Part 23 FAA regulations, new at that time.
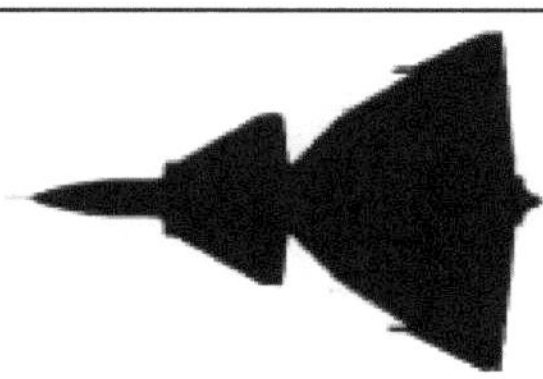 **SAAB Viggen**	1972	• Canard surfaces • Engine fitted with afterburner and thrust reverser
 **Boeing 747**	1970	• First wide-body airliner • Redundant structural components and hydraulic systems for improved safety • Variable camber flaps at leading edge of honeycomb construction
 **Airbus A300**	1974	• First medium-range wide-body airliner • Supercritical airfoils • Structures made of metal billets, reducing weight • First airliner fitted with wind shear protection • Advanced autopilots capable of flying the aircraft from climb-out to landing • Electrically controlled braking system • Two-man crew by automating the flight engineer's functions, an industry first • Glass cockpit flight instruments • Extensive use of composites for an aircraft of its era • Center-of-gravity control by shifting around fuel • The first airliner to use wingtip fences for increasing flutter margins • Manufacturing employed just-in-time concept, an industry first • First ETOPS compliant aircraft

Aircraft	Year	Major Innovations
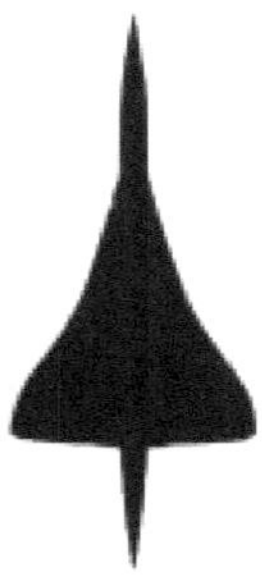 **Concorde**	1976	• Ogee/Ogival- shaped delta wing • Supercruise capability • Variable inlet ramps • Thrust-by-wire engines, predecessor of today's FADEC-controlled engines • Droop-nose section for improved visibility at landing • Mach 2.04 cruising speed • Full-regime autopilot and auto throttle allowing “hands off” control of the aircraft from climb out to landing • Fully electrically controlled analogue fly-by-wire flight controls systems • Multifunction flight control surfaces • High-pressure hydraulic system of 28 MPa (4,000 lbf/in^2) for lighter hydraulic systems components • Fully electrically controlled analogue brake-by-wire system • Pitch trim by shifting fuel around the fuselage for center-o--gravity control Parts milled from single alloy billet reducing the part-number count
 **General Dynamics F-16**	1978	• Relaxed static stability/fly-by-wire flight control system • Side-mounted control stick • Variable camber wing • Reclined seat to reduce g-forces • Blended wing body configuration
 **Boeing 767**	1982	• First twinjet to receive regulatory approval for extended overseas flights • One the first airliners to eliminate the flight engineer station • The first twinjet wide-body type to reach 1,000 aircraft delivered
 **Airbus A310**	1982	• The first carbon-fiber primary structure in a production commercial aircraft was the vertical stabilizer of the Airbus A310-300. It marked the beginning of increasing composite use in the European manufacturer’s airliners that added the horizontal stabilizer with the A320 in 1987 and A330/A340 in 1994 and the center wing-box and aft fuselage of the A380 in 2005.
 **Airbus A320**	1988	• First civil aircraft fitted with digital fly-by-wire control system • Side-stick control • Full glass cockpit
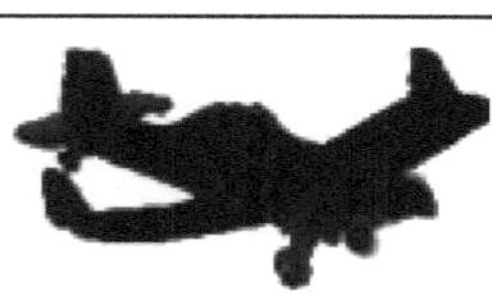 **EMB 202 Ipanema**	2004	• First serial-produced aircraft powered by an engine burning ethanol

Aircraft	Year	Major Innovations
 **ShinMaywa US-2**	2007	• Short takeoff and landing amphibian airplane • Land on rough seas with waves height of 3 m • Internal engine to blown flaps elevator and rudder (maximum lift coefficient approx. 7)
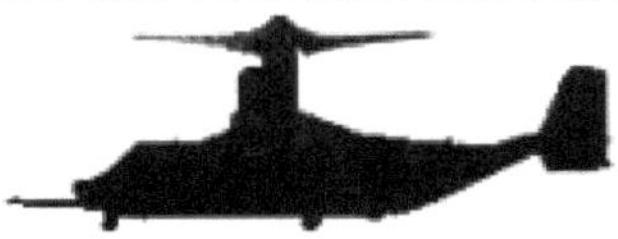 **Bell/Boeing V-22 Osprey**	2007	• First production VTOL aircraft
 **Airbus A380**	2007	• Skin to stringer welding • Center wingbox in CFRP • Variable-frequency power generation • GLARE utilization. GLARE is a composite laminate construction of alternating layers of thin aluminum and layers of fiber glass and plastic matrix material. The fiber orientation of the fiberglass can be tailored to produce desired strength and stiffness.
 **Boeing 787**	2011	• Composite fuselage and wings • Electric wing anti-ice system • Bleed-less engine • Electronic circuit breakers

REFERENCES

[1] B.S. Mattos, "Open Source Philosophy and the Dawn of Aviation", *J. Aerosp. Technol. Manag.,* vol. 4, no. 3, 2012.
[http://dx.doi.org/10.5028/jatm.2012.04030812]

[2] "Progress in Mechanical Flight", In: *Flight Magazine*, 1909, pp. 12-13.

[3] "M. Santos Dumont's New Achievements", In: *Flight Magazine*, 1909, p. 561.

[4] G. Schmitt, "Fliegende Kisten - von Kitty Hawk bis Kiew", Berlin: Verlag für Verkehrswesen, 1990.

[5] Wikipedia, the Free Encyclopedia, "Sikorsky Ilia Muromets", Wikipedia, 08 2017. [Online]. Available: https://en.wikipedia.org/wiki/Sikorsky_Ilya_Muromets

[6] I. Sikorsky, *Story of the Winged-S: An Autobiography by Igor Sikorsky.* Dodd, Mead & Company: New York, 1938.

[7] E. Angelucci, *Flugzeuge - 1000 Maschinen aus aller Welt mit sämtlichen Technischen Daten - von Ersten Fluggerät bis zum Überschalljet.* Falken Verlag und Motor Buch Verlag: Stuttgart, 1974.

[8] K. Iatrou, *100 Years of Commercial Aviation 1914-2014.* Hermes Air Transport Club, 2014.

[9] Wikipedia, The Free Encyclopedia, "Farman F.60 Goliath", Wikipedia, August 2017. [Online]. Available: https://en. wikipedia.org/ wiki/ Farman_ F.60_ Goliath

[10] J.A. Watkins, *A History of Commercial Airliners,* 2011. https://hubpages.com/technology/A-Histor--of-Commercial-Airliners

[11] H. Wings, *The First Midair Airline Disaster,* 2013. http://fly. historicwings.com/ 2013/04/ the-firs--midair-airline-disaster/

[12] L. Prandtl, *Über Flüssigkeitsbewegung bei sehr kleiner Reibung," in III Internationaler Math. Krongress.* Heildelberg, 1904.

[13] Wikipedia, The Free Encyclopedia, "Ludwig Prandtl," Wikipedia, https://en. wikipedia.org/ wiki/ Ludwig_Prandtl

[14] Wikipedia, the Free Encyclopedia, "Mixing Length Theory," Wikipedia, https:// en.wikipedia.org/ wiki/ Mixing_length_model

[15] R.M. Doshi, and N.W. Gill, "A Note on Mixing Length Theory of Turbulent Flow", In: *AIChE*, 1970, pp. 885-888.

[16] Wikipedia, The Free Wikipedia, "Junkers D.I," Wikipedia, https:// en.wikipedia.org/ wiki/ Junkers_D.I

[17] Wikipedia, The Free Wikipedia, "Junkers F.13," Wikipedia, https://en. wikipedia.org/ wiki/ Junkers_F.13

[18] RIMOWA FLUGZEUWERKE AG, "A Legend grows new Wings", RIMOWA, 2017 http://www. rimowa-f13. com/ en/#home

[19] Northtrop grumman, "History of Sperry Marine", Northtrop Grumman, 2017. [Online]. Available: http://www.sperrymarine.com/corporate-history/sperry-marine. [Accessed 24 August 2017].

[20] Wikipedia, The Free Encyclopedia, "In-flight entertainment," Wikipedia, September 1 2017. [Online]. Available: https://en.wikipedia.org/wiki/In-flight_entertainment. [Accessed 4 September 2017].

[21] Wikipedia, The Free Wikipedia, "Curtiss T-32 Condor II," Wikipedia, 2016. [Online]. Available: https://en.wikipedia.org/wiki/Curtiss_T-32_Condor_II. [Accessed 08 April 2016].

[22] P.L. Jakab, "Wood to Metal: The structural origins of modern airplane", *Journal of Aircraft, November-December,* 1999.
[http://dx.doi.org/10.2514/2.2551]

[23] "Rotachute, Rotabuggy and Rotatank", *Flying Review International,* vol. 19, no. 3, p. 45, 1963.

[24] J. Forsgren, *The Junkers Ju 52 Story.* Fonthill Media, 2017.

[25] Wikipedia, The Free Encyclopedia, "Boeing 247," Wikipedia, 28 August 2017. [Online]. Available: https://en.wikipedia.org/wiki/Boeing_247. [Accessed 2017 September 2017].

[26] Wikipedia, The Free Encyclopedia, "Boeing 307 Stratoliner," Wikipedia, 22 July 2017. [Online]. Available: https://en.wikipedia.org/wiki?curid=1882449. [Accessed 5 September 2017].

[27] Wikipedia, The Free Encyclopedia, "Focke-Wulf Fw 200 Condor," Wikipedia, 22 August 2017. [Online]. Available: https://en.wikipedia.org/wiki/Focke-Wulf_Fw_200_Condor. [Accessed 29 August 2017].

[28] J.R. Smith, *Focke-Wulf Fw 200.* Profile Books Ltda, 1982.

[29] Wikipedia, The Free Encyclopedia, "Messerschmitt Bf 109," Wikipedia, 24 August 2017. [Online]. Available: https://en.wikipedia.org/wiki/Messerschmitt_Bf_109. [Accessed 5 August 2017].

[30] Wikipedia, the Free Encyclopedia, "Leading-edge slats," Wikipedia, The Free Encyclopedia, 8 December 2015. [Online]. Available: https://en.wikipedia.org/wiki/Leading-edge_slats. [Accessed 17 April 2016].

[31] Wikipedia, The Free Encyclopedia, "Fieseler Fi 156," Wikipedia, 13 August 2017. [Online]. Available: https://en.wikipedia.org/wiki?curid=176773. [Accessed 6 September 2017].

[32] E.R. McDowell, and R. Ward, North American F-86A-L Sabre.*USAF & Foreign Service.* vol. Vol. 17. Osprey Publications Ltda: Canterbury, Kent, 1970.

[33] H.J. Nowarra, *Messerschmitt Bf 109 1936-1945.* Schiffer Publishing Ltd.: West Chester, 1991.

[34] F. Sean, "World War II Technology that Changed Warfare - Radar and Bombsights", *Academic Symposium of Undergraduate Johnson,* 2011 Wales

[35] Wikipedia The Free Encyclopedia, "Bombsight," Wikipedia, 30 May 2017. [Online]. Available: https://en.wikipedia.org/wiki/Bombsight. [Accessed 5 September 2017].

[36] Wikipedia The Free Encyclopedia, "Heinkel He 219," Wikipedia, 16 August 2017. [Online]. Available: https://en.wikipedia.org/wiki/Heinkel_He_219. [Accessed 6 September 2017].

[37] M. Griehl, and J. Dressel, *Heinkel 177, 277, 274.* Airlife Publishing Ltd: Shrewsbury, 1998.

[38] Wikipedia, The Free Wikipedia, "Heinkel He 177," Wikipedia, 22 august 2017. [Online]. Available: https://en.wikipedia.org/wiki?curid=455366. [Accessed 29 August 2017].

[39] B. Gunston, A.J. Jackson, D. Mondey, M. Passingham, J. Stroud, M.J. Taylor, and S.H. Young, *Jane's Encyclopedia of Aviation.* Crescent Books: New York, 1996.

[40] Wikipedia, The Free Encyclopedia, "Arado Ar 232," Wikipedia, 19 July 2017. [Online]. Available: https://en.wikipedia.org/wiki?curid=646085. [Accessed 23 July 2017].

[41] H. Clements, "Leading Edge Aeronautical Research on the Plains," Air Facts - The Journal for Personal Air Travel, February 2013. [Online]. Available: http://airfactsjournal.com/2013/02/leading-edge-aeronautical-research-on-the-plains/. [Accessed 24 April 2016].

[42] ShinMaywa Industries, "By Land, Sea, or Air US-2," ShinMaywa Industries, 2017. [Online]. Available: https://www.shinmaywa.co.jp/aircraft/english/us2/index.html. [Accessed 2017].

[43] Encyclopaedia Britannica, Inc. , "The Jet Age," Encyclopaedia Britannica, 2017. [Online]. Available: https://www.britannica.com/technology/history-of-flight/The-jet-age. [Accessed 4 September 2017].

[44] J.R. Smith, and E.J. Creek, *Arado 234B.* Monogram Aviation Publications, 1983.

[45] R.P. Bateson, *Arado Ar 234 Blitz, Profile 215.* Profile Publications, 1972.

[46] D. Herwig, and H. Rode, *Luftwaffe Secret Projects - Strategic Bombers 1935-1945.* Midlan Publishing: Leicester, 2000.

[47] W. Schick, and I. Meyer, *Luftwaffe Secret Projects - Fighters 1939-1945.* Midland Publishing: Leicester, 1997.

[48] Wikipedia, the free encyclopedia, "Horten Ho 229," Wikipedia, the free encyclopedia, 13 April 2016. [Online]. Available: https://en.wikipedia.org/wiki/Horten_Ho_229. [Accessed 24 April 2016].

[49] W. Heinzerling, "Flügelpfeilung und Flächenregel, zwei grundlegende deutsche Patente der Flugzeugaerodynamik," In: *Beiträge des 9. Kolloquiums Luftverkehr und der neunten August Euler-Preisverleihung,* Darmstadt, 2002.

[50] R. L. Benson, Quieting the Boom: The Shaped Sonic Boom Demonstrator and the Quest for Supersonic Flight, NASA eBook Series, 2013.

[51] H. Straßl, and H. Ludwieg, *Verringerung des Wiederstandes von Tragflügeln bei hohen Geschwinigkeiten durch Pfeilform.* Aerodynamischen Versuchsanstalt Göttingen, 1939.

[52] H. Ludwieg, *Pfeilflügel bei hohen Geschwindigkeiten (Versuchs Ergebinisse)*, 1940.

[53] Wikipedia, The Free Encyclopedia, "Area Rule," Wikipedia, 24 August 2017. [Online]. Available: https://en.wikipedia.org/wiki?curid=34036. [Accessed 5 September 2017].

[54] H. Hertel, A. Berre, O. Frenztl, W. Hempel, and D. Ziebigk, "Patentschrift zur Flächenregel". Germany Patent 932419, 1955.

[55] H-U. Meier, *Die Pfeilflügelentwicklung in Deutschland bis 1945.* Bernard & Graefe, 2005.

[56] Wikipedia, The Free Encyclopedia, "Messerschmitt P.1111," Wikipedia, 24 June 2017. [Online]. Available: https://en.wikipedia.org/wiki?curid=39592726. [Accessed 6 September 2017].

[57] D. Baals, "Wind Tunnels of NASA," NASA, 1981. [Online]. Available: http://history.nasa.gov/SP-440/contents.htm. [Accessed 17 March 2016].

[58] P. Mike, *The Brabazon Committee and British airliners, 1945-1960.* Tempus: Stroud, 2007.

[59] M.L. Hill, *Vickers Viscount and Vanguard, Ramsbury.* Crowood Press Ltd: Malborough, Wiltshire, 2004.

[60] Wikipedia, The Free Encyclopedia, "Bristol Britannia," Wikipedia, 2017. [Online]. Available: https://en.wikipedia.org/wiki/Bristol_Britannia#cite_note-BAhis-40. [Accessed October 2017].

[61] Wikipedia, The Free Encyclopedia, "Lockheed L-188 Electra," Wikipedia, 2017. [Online]. Available: https://en.wikipedia.org/wiki/Lockheed_L-188_Electra. [Accessed October 2017].

[62] W. Reed, *Review of Propeller-Rotor Whirl Flutter.* NASA Langley: Hampton, VA, 1967.

[63] Wikipedia, the Free Encyclopedia, "Boeing 707," Wikipedia, 22 August 2017. [Online]. Available: https://en.wikipedia.org/wiki/Boeing_707. [Accessed 22 August 2017].

[64] Flight Safety Foundation, "Boeing 707 N7071 Accident," Aviation Safety Network, 2015. [Online]. Available: http://aviation-safety.net/database/record.php?id=19591019-0. [Accessed 12 March 2015].

[65] A.M. Johnston, *Jet-Age Test Pilot.* Smithsonian Books: Washington, 2000.

[66] J. Glancey, *Boeing 707: The Airplane that Changed the Way We Fly,* 2014. http://www.bbc.co.uk/ culture/ story/ 20141020-the-plane-that-changed-air-travel

[67] PediaView.com, "Jet Airliner," PediaView.com, 2017. [Online]. Available: https://pediaview.com/openpedia/Jet_airliner. [Accessed 2017].

[68] E. Backfiles, "Resistance Spot Welding in the Caravelle", *Aircr. Eng. Aerosp. Technol.,* pp. 86-87, 1962.

[69] Wikipedia, The Free Encyclopedia, "Sud Aviation Caravelle," Wikipedia, September 2017. [Online]. Available: https://en.wikipedia.org/wiki/Sud_Aviation_Caravelle. [Accessed September 2017].

[70] L. Ortega, *Reactores Comerciales 1948-1994.* Agualarga: Madrid, 1994.

[71] R. G. Pushkar, "Comet's Tale," Smithsonian Magazine, June 2002. [Online]. Available: http://www.smithsonianmag.com/history/comets-tale-63573615/?no-ist=&page=2. [Accessed August 2017].

[72] World Heritage Encyclopedia, "De Havilland Comet," World Library, 2017. [Online]. Available: http://www.worldlibrary.org/article/whebn0000182728/de. [Accessed 4 September 2017].

[73] E. Torenbeek, *Advanced Aircraft Design.* John Wiley & Sons, 2013. [http://dx.doi.org/10.1002/9781118568101]

[74] R. P. Hallion, Supersonic Flight: Breaking the Sound Barrier and Beyond - The Story of Bell X-1 and Douglas D-558, The Macmillian Co. in association with the Smithsonian National Air and Space Museum, 1972.

[75] K. Muson, *Airliners Since 1946.* 2nd ed. Blandford Press, 1975, pp. 167-168.

[76] Wikipedia, The Free Encyclopedia, "Convair 990 Coronado," Wikpedia, 17 August 2017. [Online]. Available: https://en.wikipedia.org/wiki/Convair_990_Coronado. [Accessed 5 September 2017].

[77] Gordon, "Concorde History: Early History," June 2001. [Online]. Available: http://concordesst.com/history/eh1.html. [Accessed 5 September 2017].

[78] D. Küchemann, "A Brief Survey of the Work Done in Aerodynamics Department on Swept and Slender Wings," RAE Tech. emo Aero, 1958.

[79] D. Küchemann, *Some Considerations of Aircraft Shapes and their Aerodynamics for Flights at Supersonic Speeds.* RAE Tech. Memo Aero, 1959.

[80] D. Küchemann, *A Brief Outline of some of the Present Aerodynamic Work on Supersonic Transport Aircraft.* RAE Tech. Memo Aero, 1961.

[81] R. Wiggs, *Concorde: The Case against Supersonic Transport.* Ballantine Books/Friends of the Earth, 1970.

[82] Wikipedia, "Anti-Concorde Project," Wikipedia, [Online]. Available: https://en. wikipedia.org/ wiki/ Anti-Concorde_ Project. [Accessed 17 February 2015].

[83] M. Novak, "When the FAA Blasted Oklahoma City with Sonic Booms For 6 Months," GIZMODO, April 2015. [Online]. Available: https://paleofuture.gizmodo.com/when-the-faa-blasted-okla-oma-city-with-sonic-booms-for-1649589210. [Accessed September 2017].

[84] *General Descripton Boeing 2707-300 Supersonic Transport.* Boeing Co.: Seattle, 1969.

[85] *NASA SCAT 15 15-F Feasibility Study.* Boeing Co.: Seattle, 1965.

[86] Flight Magazine, "Commercial Aircraft Survey," Flight Magazine, 23 November 1967. [Online]. Available: http://www.flightglobal.com/pdfarchive/view/1967/1967-2245.html . [Accessed 17 03 2015].

[87] The Boeing Company, "747 Airplane Characteristics - Airport Planning," May 1984. [Online]. Available: http://www.boeing.com/assets/pdf/commercial/airports/acaps/747_8.pdf. [Accessed January 2015].

[88] M. R. Kulfen, "High Transonic Speed Transonic Aircraft Study - Final Report," NASA, CR-114658, 1973.

[89] S. Hoffman, "Bibliography of Supersonic Cruise Research (SCR) Program from 1980-1983," NASA RP-1117, 1984.

[90] R.T. Jones, "Theoretical Determination of the Minimum Drag of Airfoils at Supersonic Speeds", *J. Aeronaut. Sci.,* 1952.

[91] I. Kroo, "Unconventional Configurations for Efficient Supersonic Flight," in VKI Lectures Series on Innovative Configurations and Advanced Concepts for Future Civil Aircraft, 2005.

[92] Y. Gibbs, "Past Projects: AD-1 Oblique Wing," NASA, 4 August 2017. [Online]. Available: https://www.nasa.gov/centers/dryden/history/pastprojects/AD1/index.html. [Accessed 6 September 2017].

[93] S. Baughcum and C. S. Henderson, "Aircraft Emission Inventories Projected in year 2015 for a High Speed Civil Transport (HSCT) Airline Network," NASA CR-4659, 1995.

[94] G.B. Feilden, A.H. Wickens, and I. Yates, *Passenger Aircraft After 2000 AD.* E & FN Spon: London, 1995.

[95] R. Faaß, "Cryoplane - Flugzeuge mit Wasserstoffantrieb," 06 December 2001. [Online]. Available: http://www.fzt.haw-hamburg.de/pers/Scholz/dglr/hh/text_2001_12_06_Cryoplane.pdf. [Accessed 25 April 2016].

[96] G. Norris, and M. Wagner, *Airbus A380 - Superjumbo of the 21st Century.* Zenith Press: St. Paul, USA, 2005.

[97] Airbus, "A380 on The Sky," Airbus, 2017. [Online]. Available: http://www.aircraft. airbus. com/ aircraftfamilies/ passengeraircraft/ a380family/innovation/. [Accessed 5 September 2017].

[98] Wikipedia, The Free Encyclopedia, "Boeing 787 Dreamliner," Wikipedia, 18 August 2017. [Online]. Available: https://en.wikipedia.org/wiki/Boeing_787_Dreamliner. [Accessed 22 August 2017].

[99] Wikipedia, The Free Encyclopedia, "A-90 Orlyonok," Wikipedia, 10 August 2017. [Online]. Available: https://en.wikipedia.org/wiki/A-90_Orlyonok. [Accessed 209 August 2017].

[100] L. Yun, and J. Doo, *WIG craft and Ekranoplan.* Springer, 2010. [http://dx.doi.org/10.1007/978-1-4419-0042-5]

[101] Wingship Technology, "WSH-500 Product Brochure," Wingship Technology, Seul, 2014.

[102] Beriev Aircraft Company, "Beriev 2500," Beriev Aircraft Company, 2017. [Online]. Available: http://www.beriev.com/eng/Be-2500_e/Be-2500_e.html. [Accessed 5 September 2017].

[103] D. Grossman, "Graf Zeppelin History," Airship.Net, 2010. [Online]. Available: http://www.airships.net/lz127-graf-zeppelin/history/. [Accessed 5 September 2017].

[104] P.L. Teed, "Gas Fuels for Airships: The Manufacture of Blau Gas, with Details of some Possible Alternatives", *Aircr. Eng. Aerosp. Technol.,* vol. 3, pp. 41-42, 1931. [http://dx.doi.org/10.1108/eb029368]

[105] D. Grossman, "Graf Zeppelin Design and Technology," Airships.net, October 2016. [Online]. Available: http://www.airships.net/lz127-graf-zeppelin/graf-zeppelin-design-technology/. [Accessed 29 August 2017].

[106] E. Springmann, Flugzeug und Hubschrauber von Heinrich Focke 1912-1961, Oberhaching: Aviatic Verlag, 1997.

[107] Wikipedia, The Free Encyclopedia, "Junkers Jumo 205," Wikipedia, 19 June 2017. [Online]. Available: https://en.wikipedia.org/wiki?curid=638303. [Accessed 5 September 2017].

[108] F. Kober, BV 138 Der Fliegende Holzschuh, Friedberg: Podzun-Pallas Verlag, 1973.

[109] F. Magazine, *Soviet Designer Tupolev Describes Hydrogen Fuel Safety Measures.* Flight Magazine, 1989, p. 16.

[110] BioFuel.org.uk, "National Fuel Alcohol Program (Proalcool)," Biofuel.org.uk, 2010. [Online]. Available: http://biofuel.org.uk/National-Fuel-Alcohol-Program.html. [Accessed 5 September 2017].

[111] Airbus, "Airbus E-Fan," Airbus, 2017. [Online]. Available: http://company.airbus.com/responsibility/airbus-e-fan-the-future-of-electric-aircraft.html. [Accessed 5 September 2017].

[112] Wikipedia, The Free Encyclopedia, "Blau gas," Wikipedia, 21 July 2017. [Online]. Available: https://en.wikipedia.org/wiki?curid=6474209. [Accessed 6 September 2017].

[113] M. Epperle, "The Sonic Cruiser – A Concept Analysis," International Symposium Aviation Technologies of the XXI Century: New Aircraft Concepts and Flight Simulation, 2002. [Online]. Available: http://www.mh-aerotools.de/company/paper_7/astec_2002.htm. [Accessed September 2017].

CHAPTER 3

Entropy Statistics and Cluster Analysis Applied to Jet Airliner and Fighter Aircraft Classification

Abstract: The present work describes the entropy statistics theory and its application to analyze the commercial aviation market and fighter aircraft. Airliners are designed to comply with certification requirements and to provide operational profitability to airlines. They need to be more economical, lighter, faster and better than its predecessors. Understanding the technological evolution of aviation is extremely useful when one is designing new aircraft. Saviotti (1984) and later, Frenken (1997) proposed a method of analysis of aircraft technological evolution. This method, based on information theory developed by Shannon (1948), specially the concept of entropy statistics, has proved to be very effective for product classification. Thus, a methodology based on entropy statistics was employed to analyze the jet airliners since the 1950s and fighter aircraft since World War I. The results show the impact of notable events such as the 1978 Airline Deregulation Act on the airplane designs and naturally, the world wars. The airplanes can be classified into four groups: niche, fuzzy, scaled trajectories and breakthrough designs. Some airplanes were chosen for a deeper analysis and the entropy statistics methodology could correct label some airplanes like the ERJ 145 family, the Boeing 777-300, and Airbus 340-500. Fighter airplanes like the Vought Cutlass, Westland Wyvern, and IA-54 Pucará also could be adequately categorized and rated.

Keywords: Aircraft design, Airliner, Airplane evolution, Entropy statistics, Fighter aircraft, Information theory.

INTRODUCTION

Objectives

In the present work, elements of information theory are described to evaluate key airliners designs, *i.e.,* airplane configurations that played decisive role in commercial aviation and for fighter aircraft, either by successfully integrating previous technologies or transmitting their characteristics to airplanes that succeeded them.

Indeed, aeronautical evolution is deeply related to technological evolution. As such, like any other form of evolution, it follows certain rules or heuristics. These

Bento S. de Mattos, José A. T. G. Fregnani & Paulo Eduardo C. S. Magalhães

rules can vary in complexity; from the relatively simple arithmetical progression to the more intricate biological evolution. Technology fits closely to the complex end of that spectrum. This form of evolution can potentially be lucrative if well understood, especially at a corporate level. By employing the entropy statistics methodology, analyses concerning airplane evolution were carried out and aircraft could be categorized regarding their importance in terms of aviation contribution [1]. However, the entropy statistics tool does not just consider technology involved in product evolution. Technology is of major importance for improving aircraft performance as it is widely known, but sometimes aviation evolves thanks to discoveries of new business models. For instance, this is the case of the business aviation, which had a considerable boost in the 2000s thanks to the shared ownership concept. This in turn led to an increase in new business aircraft configurations. The entropy statistics dealing with the information and distance between the designs can easily map such kind of evolution. This is also valid for the effects that the 1978 Deregulation Act exerted on airliner design.

The work presented here is an improved and extended effort regarding the one performed by Frenken and Leydesdorff [2]. Here, more suitable variables adequately represent the aircraft configuration and its embedded technology. The variables were carefully selected after an extensive study. Both works also differ in range of application. Two analyses were performed to evaluate the applicability of the methodology. One is concerned with the evolution of civil aviation transportation in the jet age (1955-2015) and the other with the evolution of fighter aircraft (from 1914 to 2009). After the creation of the databank containing aircraft characteristics, a numerical tool that was developed takes the variables as input to evaluate two important evolutionary indexes: convergence and diffusion. Studies analyzing the combination of the diffusion and the convergence indexes, as well as the critical transition of the airplanes were carried out here. Based on this approach, other computer tools can be elaborated to assist decision-making process in the aircraft conceptual design phase.

In addition to the entropy statistics classification of the aircraft, cluster analysis for commercial jet airliners made it possible to accommodate them into 11 groups. Dendrogram plots were also obtained for the jet airliners and fighter aircraft and this tool proved to combine the airplanes very efficiently and very reasonably.

An extended utilization of entropy statistics and cluster analysis can enable design teams to conceive niche airplanes or to discover what characteristics of certain aircraft must be changed to turn it from failure to a niche aircraft or even a breakthrough design, for example.

How Products Evolve

It can be easily observed that the tools and instruments devised by human beings undergo an evolution themselves that is strangely analogous to ordinary evolution, almost as if these artifacts propagated themselves as animals do. Aircraft began as birdlike objects but evolved into fishlike objects for much the same hydrodynamic reasons as those which caused fish to evolve into fishlike objects. Bicycles have evolved and so did motor cars [1].

The challenge of understanding the dynamics of technological development has long been a concern of every branch of manufacturing enterprises. Two approaches dominate the scene: one suggests that the external requirements of the market [3], while the other views the activities and internal capabilities of firms as primary drivers of innovation [4]. Taken separately, each approach highlights key aspects of technological development but, as many have argued, the greatest insight derives from their joint consideration [5].

Convergence contends that products evolve into unified devices through linear evolutions; whereas with divergence innovation is spurred through disruptive revolutions. The Internet was a disruptive technology and the same will certainly occur to the air transportation. Another way of moving in the atmosphere will not be called "airplane" anymore. Convergence captures the imagination, but divergence is tuned to the market.

Today, many types of aircraft, jet aircraft, propeller-driven airplanes, and helicopters, and many types of automobiles, sedans, convertibles, station wagons, minivans, sport-utility vehicles, are available by manufacturers. However, no flying car really succeeded, although many attempts have been made to bring them into life. Ries [6] asks the question "Why divergence and not convergence?" Per them, that is because convergence requires compromise and divergence satisfies the evolving needs of different market segments. An automobile needs to be heavy enough to stay on the highway; an airplane needs to be light enough to take off from a runway and perform its mission providing profit to its operator.

No flying car will ever be as drivable as an automobile or as well flyable as an airplane. The auto boat, another convergence concept that has been floating around for decades, suffers from the same flaws.

The codification of design principles associated with the emergence of a dominant design also implies a convergence of design principles that have been developed in the past. Thus, the coming into existence of a scaling trajectory at the industry level is essentially a two-sided phenomenon. It refers both to the diffusion of design principles, and to the convergence of design principles. These phenomena are different: the diffusion of design principles does not necessarily imply convergence of design principles, since a design can be scaled in various and potentially divergent directions. For example, some aircraft firms may scale a dominant design with respect to maximum take-off weight, others with respect to speed, and still others with respect to range. Hence, to test the dominant design hypothesis, one needs to distinguish between the diffusion of design principles through time and the convergence of design principles that can be observed in retrospect.

At this point, it is worthy of mention the different meanings of divergence and diffusion. Considering the computer as example, it can be easily perceived that there are supercomputers, network computers, personal computers, laptop computers, tablet computers and handheld computers. That is a typical divergence case, a family of products having the same *common ancestral*. Diffusion is related to various products sharing *common technologies or features*. The fly-by-wire flight and control system appeared in a Western commercial plane in the supersonic Concorde airliner. Since those days, this technology has spread her legs to a large variety of airplanes. Even small to medium capacity airliners like the EMBRAER E170 (Fig. **3.1**) have adopted such technology, although in this case is an analogic one and not all control surfaces are electrically controlled and commanded. EMBRAER redesigned its larger E-Jets and provided them with a digital fly-by-wire system. That is a typical example of diffusion.

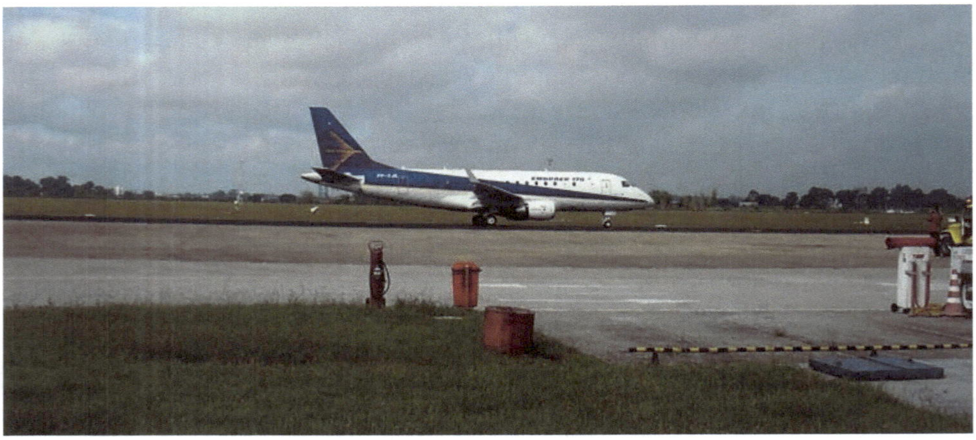

Fig. (3.1). EMBRAER E170 short before its first flight (Photo: ©2002 Bento Mattos).

MODELING TECHNOLOGICAL EVOLUTION

Utterback and Abernathy [7] have proposed the concept of a product life-cycle to describe technological evolution at industry level. A product innovation contains a recent technology or combination of technologies incorporated into it to meet a user or a market need [7]. Similar what happens in process development, a basic idea for product innovation is that products will be developed over time in a predictable manner with initial emphasis on product performance, then emphasis on product variety and later emphasis on product standardization and costs [7]. This concept allows the researcher to distinguish both among the innovative patterns of firms in an industry at a given time and among those of a given firm at various times based on dominant competitive strategy [7]. Thus, innovation concentrates on process and incremental improvement of the product regarding the dominant design. Nelson and Winter [8] and Dosi [4] proposed to describe a series of incremental innovations within a stable design framework as a natural trajectory or technological trajectory, respectively. Along a trajectory, development is guided and constrained by a set of heuristics which make up a technological paradigm. The trajectory concept can be appreciated as the dynamic analogue of the concept of a dominant design.

Nelson and Winter [8] and Sahal [9] highlighted that trajectories do not only concern periods during which the basic technological principles remain unchanged, but also a stage of incremental scaling of designs. A prime example of a series of scaled models in civil aircraft has been the piston propeller Douglas airliner trajectory. The scaling of the engine power, wing span, and fuselage length have led to improvements in speed by a factor of two, and in maximum take-off weight and range by a factor of five from the introduction of the DC-3 in 1936 to that of the DC-7 in 1956.

Information theory was first mentioned by Claude E. Shannon in his 1948 paper entitled *A Mathematical Theory of Communication* [10]. The main purpose of Shannon's work is to deal with the problem of transmitting information over a noisy channel. He could not imagine that a whole new field of mathematics would result from his proposition. Many deep and far reaching mathematical theories were created, such as channel capacity, source-coding and self-information. A great contribution of Shannon was his use of *entropy* playing a vital role in information theory as measures of information, choice and uncertainty [10].

Entropy appeared as *thermodynamic entropy* by Rudolf Clausius in 1850, in his work on Sadi Carnot's 1824 thermodynamic efficiency study. Clausius derived a proportional relationship between entropy and the energy flow by heating (δQ) into a system [11]. In a system, this heat energy can be transformed into work, and work can be transformed into heat through a cyclical process [12].

Clausius writes that [12]: “The algebraic sum of all the transformations occurring in a cyclical process can only be less than zero, or, as an extreme case, equal to nothing.”

The amount of entropy S added to the system during the cycle is defined as

$$\Delta S = \oint \frac{\partial Q}{T} \tag{3.1}$$

However, the more modern definition of entropy as a measure of “disorder” in a system was introduced by Ludwig Boltzmann in 1877. This “disorder” entropy, or *statistic entropy*, then became the cornerstone of the theory of statistical mechanics and was later used by Shannon in his information theory [10]. In this context, some textbooks erroneously employ the “student desk increasing disorder with time” as an example of entropy. This can be misleading since the more precise example would be, “which system has higher entropy: the organized desk or the messy one?” The answer would probably be the messy one, because there are many more ways of arranging the items in a chaotic manner than there are in an organized one. This is basically the definition of entropy elaborated by Shannon, and the one used in this paper.

Many researchers credit Shannon as the actual architect of entropy, since his definition of entropy is broader than the original thermodynamic definition. Those researchers claim that thermodynamic entropy is a category of information entropy. How does this statistical entropy relate to the study of technological evolution? Any system that contains a macroscopic state ruled by many different microscopic systems, such as biological evolution, economic growth, image reconstruction and technological evolution; can be studied using entropy.

If a certain technology has established itself over an extended period without any major breakthroughs, one can conclude that the entropy of that era is very low, since there is a low degree of uncertainty. This means that some breakthrough has occurred in the past and that most of the competitors, if there are any, have borrowed information from that breakthrough. The appearance of a dominant design usually precludes a low entropy era, while an era of experimentation, with high diversity shows no dominant designs, and thus, high entropy. Therefore, one can use these far-reaching theories to study the evolution of technology in a specific sector of industry, such as civil aviation, automobiles, computers, etc.

In the present study, the analysis the evolution of civil transport aviation of the jet age (1950-2017) is carried out. Specific points from information theory and entropy statistics were employed and are discussed in the next section. Although many calculations are performed in this analysis, the results can only be interpreted in a qualitative manner. Entropy statistics is best employed, outside of pure information theory and thermodynamics, as a tool for qualitative analysis of a subject.

METHODOLOGY FOR AIRPLANE CLASSIFICATION

Entropy

Entropy can be also understood as de degree of uncertainty of a transmitted message. Shannon, more specifically described it as the minimum number of bits that must be communicated to as interlocutor for him to know the value of a random variable. Consider, for example, that a transmission of data is composed of a series of ASCII characters. If the characters are random, the entropy of the message is seven times the number of characters (since each ASCII character is composed of seven bits, and entropy is given in bits). If, however, we know in advance that this series is a repetition of the same character, then the entropy is zero, since we, by knowing one of the characters will know all the others. On the other hand, if the message is composed of true text, the entropy is not zero, but is not its maximum value (as was in the random text). The value of the entropy is going to be something in between, since written language allows us to infer the rest of a message by knowing only parts of its content. Written language is, in other words, redundant, which reduces its entropy. English language, for example, has an average entropy of 1 to 1,5 bits per character, instead of the 7 bits per character in a random message.

Shannon [10] proposed that the entropy of a message is given by:

$$H = -\sum_{i=1}^{n} p_i . log_2(p_i) \tag{3.2}$$

In **Eq. 3.2** n is the set of all possible messages, whereas p_i is the probability of occurrence of the *i*-th possible value of the source symbol. Note that by using the logarithmic base 2 the entropy will be measured in bits. H reaches its maximum when all messages have the same probability of occurrence, *i.e.*, $p(x) = 1/n$ and hence $H = log_2 n$.

As it is defined, entropy has a set of properties that are relevant for this work:

- Continuity: The measure of entropy is a continuous function, which allows for easier convergence.
- Symmetry: The measure of entropy is unchanged if the order of probability p is

changed. This allows data for aircraft to be added at will, with no regard for the order in which it is arranged, without change in the entropy values.

- Additivity: Entropy remains the same independently on the way in which the system is divides in subsystems, which in turn allows each aircraft to be compared to others independently.

The work performed by Frenken and Leydesdorff [2] provided a baseline methodology for the present study about aircraft evolution and product characterization. The targeted improvements are the choice of variables for each design, the availability of newer design data and the focus on regional airliners, while conducting firm-level analysis. Another expected conclusion for this work is to ascertain how robust the applied theory and methodology really is in this case.

The most effective way to numerically represent a product is to model its various concepts (trade-offs), which are the expression of years of technical development and engineering hours. To model these trade-offs, it is necessary to create ratios between every characteristic of a product. Arranging these ratios in matrix form, a model for the trade-offs is created. This matrix is a reasonable representation of a product design, but it is not useful in information theory. By dividing all these ratios by their sum, a probabilistic distribution is then obtained, here denoted by $(p_1, p_2, \ldots, p_n)$, where n is the total number of ratios. This way, a probabilistic representation for each product is provided. Every product contains some information from previous designs and provides information to those ones that followed it (Fig. **3.2**). Using information theory, we can calculate how much information is passed among designs using the formula below:

$$I(q \mid p) = \sum_{i=1}^{n} q_i \log_2 \left(\frac{q_i}{p_i} \right)_i \tag{3.3}$$

In **Eq. 3.3**, I is a measure of distance between two product designs, with q chronologically after p. This is the same as the amount of information passed on from p to q. If no information is passed on then parameter I is equal to zero, because every trade-off is the same, even if the characteristics are not the same. This would be a perfectly scaled version of a previous product. Mathematically this means that $q_i/p_i = 1$ and its log is then zero. Interestingly no matter what I is, it will always be positive, this is called probabilistic entropy, and it is because every message that change has occurred is expected to contain information. Lower I means less change occurred from p to q, i. e., the more similar the products are.

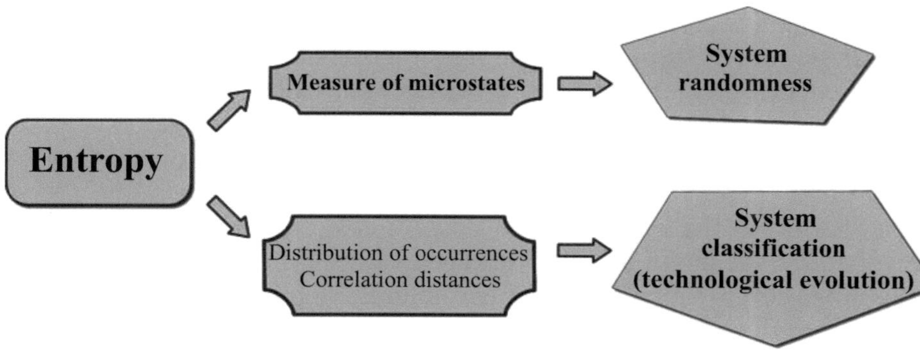

Fig. (3.2). Entropy application to product evolution.

Convergence and Diffusion

For application in product evolution, in Eq. **3.3**, p is a posteriori distribution and q is a priori one. From this, two important parameters can be derived, which are important for product categorization. These parameters are called convergence and diffusion. Convergence is obtained when we consider an individual p and look a certain period past in time and considers the characteristics from another individual q in that timeframe. In the case of diffusion of a design through time, the frame of reference is a product design as the a priori expectation of future designs [2].

The diffusion of a product design can then be measured by its distance I calculated by **Eq. 3.3** to all the members of the technological population as a posteriori events at next moments in time. The average of I-values is then obtained by dividing the sum of I-values by the number of comparisons N during the respective timeframe of observation [2]. Table **3.1** summarizes the definition of these parameters.

Table 3.1. Definition of the convergence and diffusion parameters employed in the present work.

Diffusion	Convergence
Measure the propagation of information contained in each design for its successors	Measure the information contained in each design derived from its predecessors
The diffusion coefficient is calculated by averaging the coefficients obtained considering the airplanes that succeed the reference product in desired time window	The convergence coefficient is calculated by averaging the coefficients that were obtained considering the previous airplanes in a desired time window

According to Frenken [13], industrial products can be classified as follow: innovations; scaled trajectories; niches; and failures. Innovations are introduction of a new, redesigned or substantially improved good or service, well distinguished from its predecessors. Innovative products influence their successors and introduce dominant designs. They are characterized by a low value of diffusion and a high value of convergence. Scaled trajectories are projects that follow patterns defined by previous projects and influence their successors, the scaled trajectories are under the influence of dominant designs, and are characterized by a low diffusion value and a low convergence value. Products that fit into market niches are those complying with standards defined by previous designs and do not exert profound influence on designs that come after it. They are characterized by a high-diffusion and a low-convergence indexes. Failures are concepts that differ from their predecessors and do not influence their successors, being characterized by a high value of its diffusion coefficient and a high value of the convergence index as well. This kind of design classification of industrial products was introduced by Frenken [2]. Table **3.2** provides a compilation of this classification with the "failure" classification replaced by a better one: "fuzzy" configurations.

Products that lie in the Northeast quadrant were classified by Frenken as failures. However, we prefer the cognomen "fuzzy," placing them as an indistinct product. This also considers that must be a gradation among the quadrants for the products that lies close to the boundaries. In addition, the convergence and diffusion indexes are highly dependent on the timeframe selected for their calculation and the normalization employed for the variables that characterize the products.

Table 3.2. product classification according to diffusion and convergence indexes

<table>
<tr><td rowspan="2">Convergence</td><td>High I-values</td><td>Breakthroughs</td><td>Fuzzy</td></tr>
<tr><td>Low I-values</td><td>Dominant Designs</td><td>Niche, Monopolies</td></tr>
<tr><td></td><td></td><td>Low I-values</td><td>High I-values</td></tr>
<tr><td></td><td></td><td colspan="2">Diffusion</td></tr>
</table>

An evaluation of the impact of the timeframe on the convergence and diffusion *I*-values was carried out by Vale [14]. In his work, analysis of the fixed-wing business aviation market was carried out considering timeframes of 5, 10, and 20 years. The smaller value for the timeframe seems to fit better with the airplanes employed in his study. A MATLAB® code was elaborated by the authors to apply the entropy statistics theory for airplane classification, more specifically, jet airliners. A Microsoft Excel® worksheet is needed for running the code and therefore worksheets containing data for 98 jet airliners and 281 fighter aircraft were compiled to feed the code with all data it needs.

Dendrogram and Cophenetic Correlation Coefficient

Cluster analysis is a convenient method for identifying homogenous groups of objects (cases, data) [15]. Besides useful in cluster analysis, a Dendrogram plot is a useful tool to illustrate the arrangement of the clusters produced by hierarchical clustering. A Dendrogram consists of many U-shaped lines that connect data points in a hierarchical tree [15]. The height of each U represents the distance between the two data points being connected. The height of the vertical lines, indicates the degree of difference between branches. The longer the line, the greater the difference. The horizontal orientation of Dendrograms shows the design neighborhood. In statistics, cophenetic correlation coefficient is a measure of how close a dendrogram preserves the pairwise distances between the original unmodeled data points [16].

Considering that Y is the distance matrix and Z is a hierarchical tree, the cophenetic correlation coefficient is then given by:

$$c = \frac{\sum_{i<j}(Y_{ij}-y)(Z_{ij}-z)}{\sqrt{\sum_{i<j}(Z_{ij}-z)^2 \sum_{i<j}(Y_{ij}-y)^2}} \quad \textbf{(3.4)}$$

Y_{ij} is the distance between object *i* and *j*; Z_{ij} is the dendrogrammatic distance between objects *i* and *j*; y and z are the averaged values of Y and Z.

The magnitude of the calculated value of *c* should be very close to 1 for a high-quality solution. This measure can also be used to compare alternative cluster solutions obtained using different algorithms.

RESULTS OF APPLICATION

The methodology outlined before was applied to study the evolution of jet airplanes and fighter aircraft. The jet airliners with entry into service of the period 1950-2018 were considered. The other study involved fighter aircraft from 1914 to 2009. A considerable effort was carried out to consider variables that can deliver a good representation of the aircraft. The jet airplanes are described by 24 variables and the fighter aircraft by just 19 ones.

Jetliners

The first column of the Excel® worksheet was filled with airplane names; the second one contains the year of service entry of the airliners. The remained columns contain the parameters employed for airplane description and they are as follow:

1) Entry into service 2) MTOW [kg] 3) Maximum Zero-Fuel Weight [kg] 4) Operating empty weight [kg] 5) Fuel capacity [kg] 6) Wing reference area [m^2] 7) Wing aspect ratio 8) Wing taper ratio 9) Wing quarter-chord sweepback angle (Degrees) 10) Vertical tail aspect ratio	11) Vertical tail taper ratio 12) Vertical tail quarter-chord sweep angle 13) Horizontal tail aspect ratio 14) Horizontal tail taper ratio 15) Horizontal tail sweepback angle 16) Takeoff thrust-to-MTOW ratio 17) Maximum operating Mach number 18) Maximum range with typical payload (nm) 19) Engine location (1= two underwing; 2= two at rear fuselage; 3=two underwing+one at center fuselage; 4= four underwing; 5= four at rear fuselage) 20) Number of engines 21) Seating abreast 22) Wing position (1= low; 2=high) 23) Tail configuration (1=conventional; 2= "T" tail) 24) Number of corridors in passenger cabin

The earliest design is the Sud-Aviation Caravelle twinjet. The Embraer 190E2, with service entry envisaged for 2018, was also considered in the computations. The Concorde and Tupolev Tu-144 supersonic airliners also compose the databank.

Fig. **3.3** displays the MTOW and wing area of all airplanes in the databank. There is a considerable spread of this variable over the years.

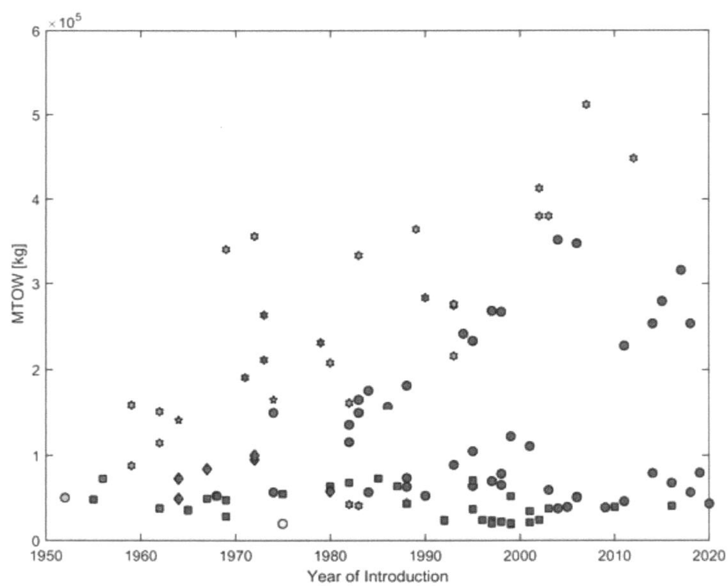

Fig. 3.3 contd.....

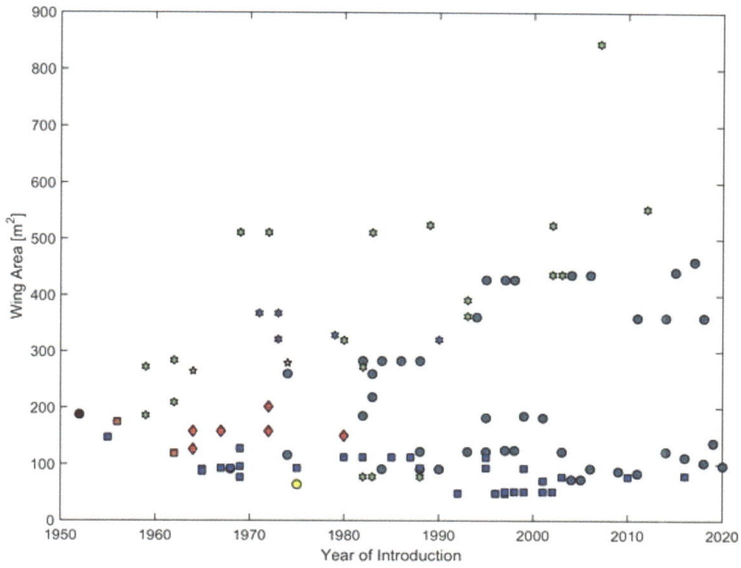

Fig. (3.3). MTOW and wing area of the airplanes in the databank that were employed to entropy statistics calculation.

Featured Aircraft

Canadair (acquired by Bombardier Aerospace) is considered as the creator of the term regional jet because it brought into the aviation market its 50-seat CRJ-100 twinjet in 1992. However, the first regional jet is thought to be the Yakovlev Yak-40 trijet, which was introduced in the Soviet Union, flying for Aeroflot in 1968. In the Western world, there were other important aircraft of slightly larger size such as the Sud Aviation Caravelle and the Fokker F-28 that fit into the acronym regional jet. In addition, the VFW-Fokker 614 (also VFW 614) was a twin-engine jetliner designed and built in West Germany. It offered passenger accommodation between 36-40 seats and had an unusual configuration, with two M45H turbofans mounted on pylons above the wings. VFW 614 was produced in small numbers by VFW-Fokker in the early- to mid-1970s. It was originally intended as a DC-3 replacement. Embraer entered the regional jet market in 1997, after Continental Express started operations with a batch of ERJ 145ER airliners. The ERJ 145ER range was considerable shorter than the competition in the form of Bombardier CRJ-200 airplane and in 1998 Embraer was delivering the 1600-nm LR version. The ERJ 145XR is a later version and more powerful version of the ERJ 145. The ERJ 145XR climbs faster (at 300 kts) and burns less fuel than the ERJ 145ER/LR. Table **3.3** compares some characteristics of the ERJ 145 versions.

Table 3.3. Data for some ERJ 145 versions (Source: EMBRAER).

Version	Maximum Takeoff Weight [kg]	Operational Empty Weight [kg]	Max Usable Fuel [kg]	Takeoff Field Length (MTOW, ISA, Sea Level) [m]	Range (MLW, ISA, Sea Level) [nm]
ER (MK)	19,990	12,038	4,132	1,850	900
LR	22,000	12,114	5,136	2,270	1,550
XR	24,100	12,591	5,973	2,070	2,000

Results

The resulting entropy index variation over time is displayed in Fig. (**3.4**). There are three peaks in entropy, the largest of them recorded in the 1982-1984 period.

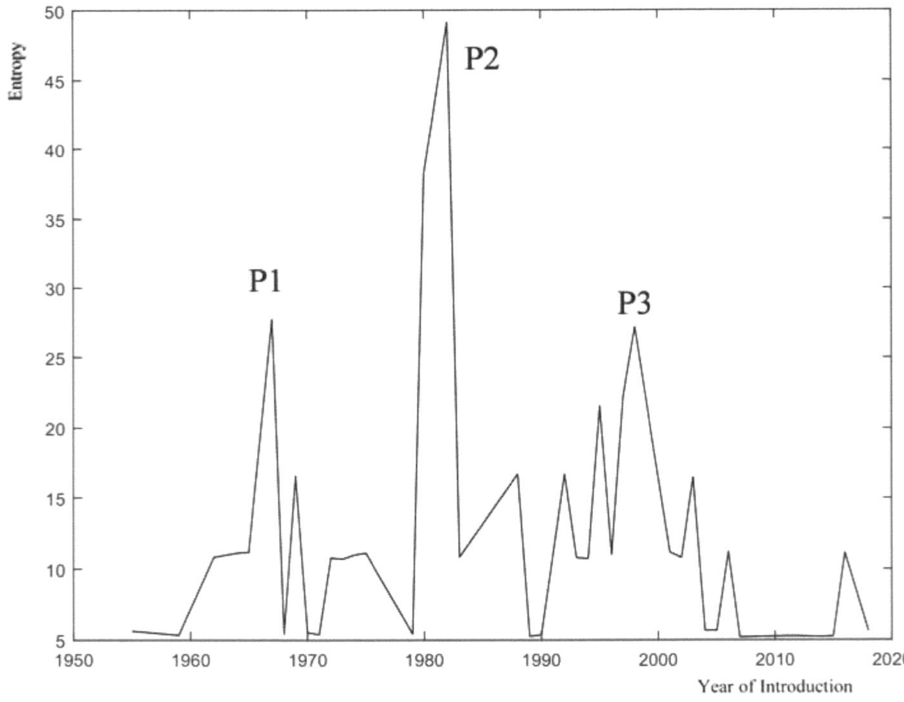

Fig. (3.4). Entropy index variation over time.

The three peaks that are displayed in Fig. (**3.4**) were analyzed and some possible explanations for their appearance have been developed as follows:

P1 – The 1960s are well known for a large diversity of new commercial airplane designs - some of them have never materialized, like the Boeing SST. The Boeing 747-100, Boeing 737-100, DC-9 and many others belong to this creative decade in terms of designs that made history.
P2 – The turbofan engine and supercritical airfoil triggered a new-generation of high-efficiency airplanes that were needed after the 1973 oil crisis. The Boeing 737-200 underwent a deep redesign from which the -300 version with turbofan engines emerged, and consequently sales soared. The 1978 Deregulation Act shook the aviation market and the aircraft manufacturers were agile enough to cope with the new world that appeared thereafter. Thus, the P2 entropy peak is a result of all these factors: technology, the Deregulation, and the oil crisis.
P3 – It took some time after the Deregulation for the introduction of efficient regional jet airplanes. In the 1980s most of them were turboprop airplanes. This peak can be clearly credited to regional jets of the 1990s.

The accumulated entropy over time is shown in Fig. (**3.5**). It seems to be stagnating in recent times. Is that a sign that a new revolution in technology is needed?

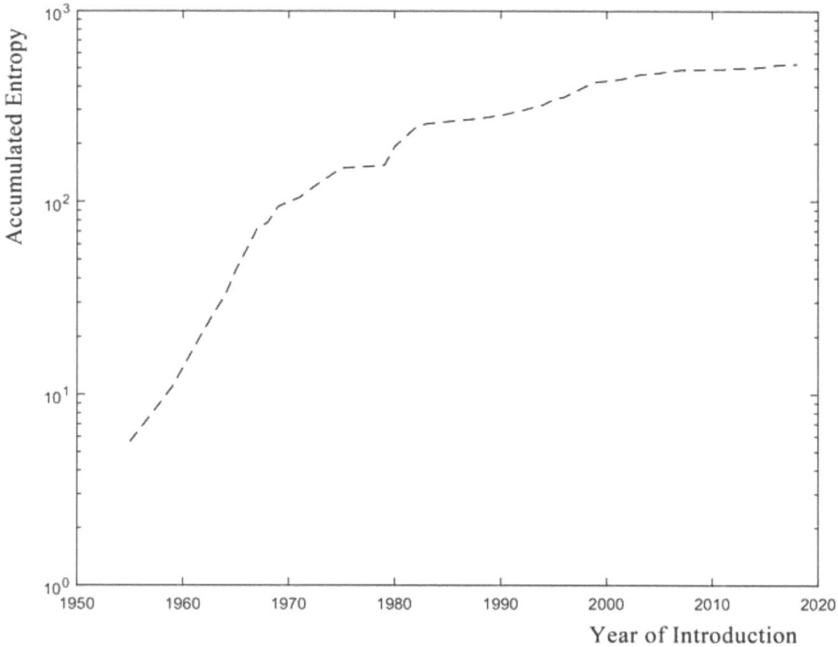

Fig. (3.5). Accumulated entropy over time.

The classification of the designs in the databank according to Frenken's criterium is shown in Fig. (**3.6**). A time window of 5 years was utilized for the calculation of both convergence and diffusion indexes. In fact, instead of defined boundaries between the quadrants a better approach would be to employ a color gradient for the classification.

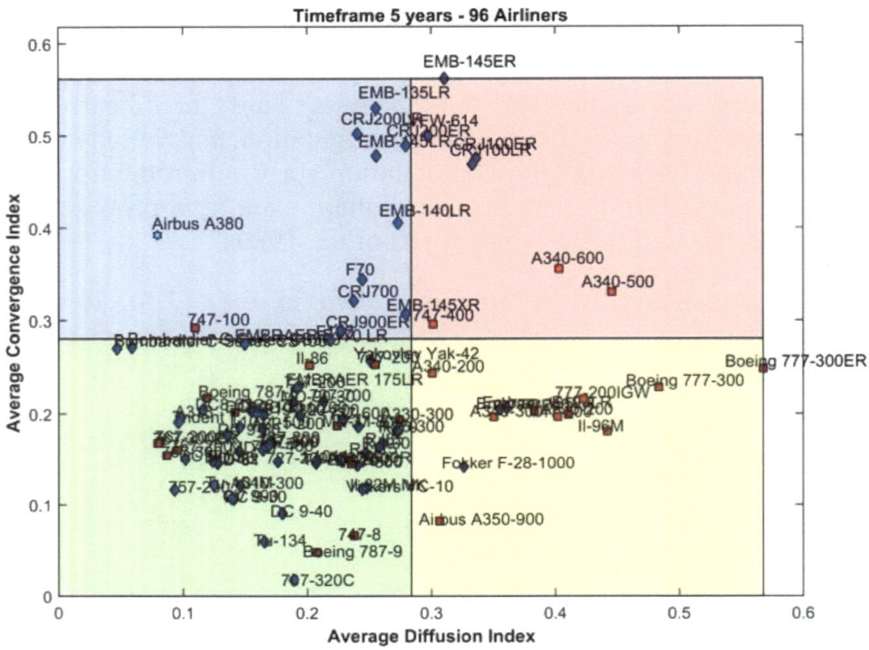

Fig. (3.6). Design classification according to Frenken's criterium.

Based on Fig. (**3.6**), the entropy statistics methodology results for the three ERJ 145 versions are analyzed as follows:

- ERJ 145ER was labeled as "fuzzy" design. Indeed, this seems to be correct due to its short range. The ER was the first ERJ 145 version and entered service in 1997. EMBRAER soon perceived this shortcoming and offered the LR version with greater range already in 1998.
- ERJ 145LR. This version was labeled as a breakthrough design which also seems to be correct. Why then was the CRJ100, which entered service earlier in 1992, not also a breakthrough? This can be possibly credited to its shorter range (1,305 nm) and heavier MTOW (23,133 kg). Probably in this category, the ERJ 145LR seems to present the right characteristics to be classified a breakthrough. Bombardier introduced the CRJ-200LR in 1996 [17], which features an 1,800-

nm range (50 PAX) and better airfield performance when compared to the -100ER version. Alongside with the ERJ-145LR, the CRJ-200LR airliner appears in the classification box as a breakthrough concept.

- ERJ 145XR. This airplane really seems to have been designed to fulfill a market niche. This version of the ERJ 145 presenting improved performance was purchased by ExpressJet only, a subsidiary of Continental Airlines. The Newark airport was the main operational base for the type. Thanks to the better performance when compared to the LR version, the ERJ 145XR enabled ExpressJet to service more distant cities from Newark.

Other airplanes labeled as "fuzzy' designs are the Boeing 747-300 and Airbus A340-500, the first recording 56 aircraft delivered [18]; the four-engine A340-500 of which only 34 were delivered [19]. The poor record sales for both types points to be an indication of product undefinition for the market.

Cluster Analysis

Classification of similar customers and products into groups is a fundamental industrial strategy. Cluster analysis allows segments to be formed that are based on data that are less dependent on subjectivity.

In cluster analysis, the k-means algorithm can be used to partition the input data set into k partitions. A useful plot is that the combine the average distance in regard the number of clusters. Using this plot, a search is performed for distinctive break (elbow).

Using MATLAB® tools a cluster analysis was performed with the database used in the entropy statistics study. Fig. (**3.7**) shows the averaged Euclidian distance in function of the cluster number. Considering that all 99 airplanes can be divided into 11 groups, Fig. (**3.8**) displays the relation between their MTOW and wing area.

Table **3.4** shows the classification of the airliners into 11 groups carried out using the *k*-means cluster analysis. Each group really contains airplanes that presents similarities with each other. The Boeing 777-300 lies isolated in a group. This may indicate that the type is a failure or a niche airplane. In this context, there is a good agreement with the entropy statistics analysis, which placed that Boeing airliner close to the niche-fuzzy boundary (Fig. **3.6**). This seems to agree with the poor sales record of the Boeing 777-300 [20]. Table **3.5** shows deliveries of the various versions of Boeing 777. The extended range version of the 777 registered an excellent sales record instead, what was also well captured by the entropy statistical analysis Fig. (**3.6**).

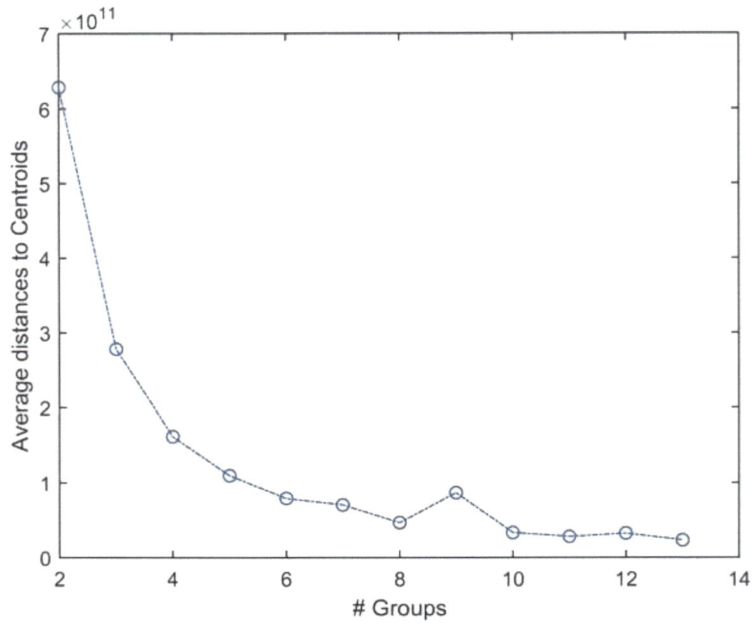

Fig. (3.7). Average distance variation with the number of clusters.

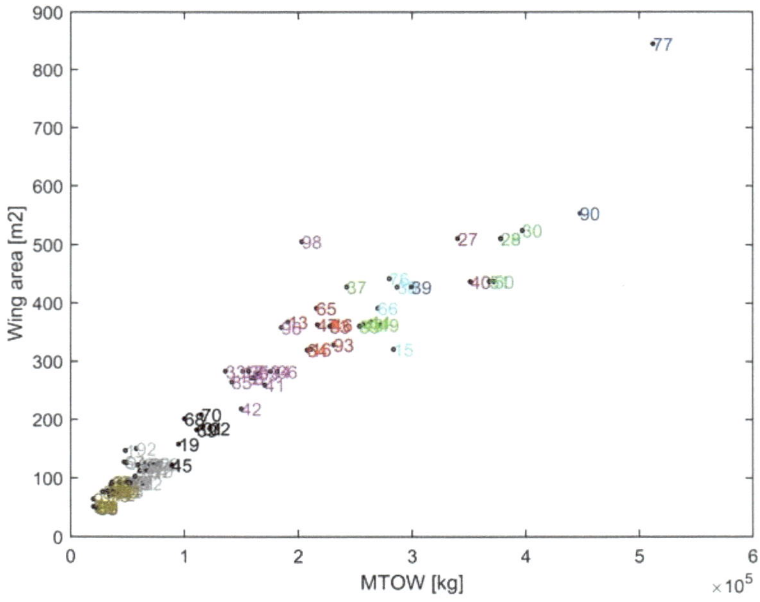

Fig. (3.8). Maximum takeoff weight and wing area for the 98 jet airliners used in the clustering analysis.

Table 3.4. Classification of airliners into 11 groups according to cluster analysis carried out in the present work.

McDonnell Douglas DC-10-10 Lockheed L-1011-100 A330-200 Ilyushin Il-86 Ilyushin Il-96-300 Boeing 787-8 Lockheed L-1011-500	**MD-11 / Boeing 777-200IGW Il-96M / Vickers VC-10 / Tupolev Tu-144 Concorde**	**Airbus A380 Boeing 747-8**
DC-10-30 Boeing 777-200 A340-200 A340-300 Boeing 787-9	**Boeing 777-300**	**Boeing 727-200Adv Boeing 757-200 Boeing 757-300 Airbus A321-200 Tu-154M Tu-204-200 Convair CV 990**
Boeing 747-200 Boeing 747-300 Boeing 747-400 Airbus A340-500 Airbus A340-600	**Boeing 747-100 Boeing 777-300ER**	**DC8-63 / DC8-73 Boeing 707-320C Boeing 767-200 Boeing 767-200ER Boeing 767-300 Boeing 767-300ER A300-600R A310-300 Il-62M MK Vickers VC-10 Concorde Tupolev Tu-144**
Caravelle VI DC 9-30 / DC 9-40 / DC 9-50 MD-81 / MD-82 / MD-83 / MD-87 MD-90-30 Boeing 717-200 737-200 737-300 737-400 737-500 737-600 737-700 737-800	**Douglas DC 9-10 RJ70 RJ85 RJ100 CRJ100ER CRJ100LR CRJ200ER CRJ200LR EMB-145ER Fokker F70 Fokker F100 EMBRAER E170 LR**	

(Table 3.4) contd.....

McDonnell Douglas DC-10-10 Lockheed L-1011-100 A330-200 Ilyushin Il-86 Ilyushin Il-96-300 Boeing 787-8 Lockheed L-1011-500	**MD-11 / Boeing 777-200IGW Il-96M / Vickers VC-10 / Tupolev Tu-144 Concorde**	**Airbus A380 Boeing 747-8**
A319-100 A320-200 RJ115 Tupolev Tu-134 Embraer E190LR Embraer 195LR Embraer E190E2 Airbus A318 Hawker-Siddeley Trident 1 Yakovlev Yak-42 Bombardier C-Series CS300 Bombardier C-Series CS100	**EMBRAER 175LR CRJ700 EMB-135LR EMB-140LR EMB-145XR EMB-145LR CRJ900ER Fokker F-28-1000 BAC-111/200 VFW-614**	

Table 3.5. Boeing 777 orders and deliveries on February 28, 2017 (Source: Wikipedia).

Version	Orders	Deliveries
777-200	88	88
777-200ER	422	422
777-200LR	59	59
777-300	60	60
777-300ER	807	709
777-F	161	129
777-X	306	–
Total	**1 903**	**1 467**

Using the same databank that was employed in the entropy statistics analysis the Euclidian distance between the airplanes was calculated and a dendrogram of the airplanes was then generated (Fig. **3.9**). Analyzing the plot of Fig. (**3.9** and Table **3.5**) it can be inferred that the linkage of the airplanes was precise, the supersonic airliners Tupolev Tu-144 and Concorde grouped in a pair as well as the Boeing 747 versions and variants. The calculated cophenetic correlation coefficient for this dendrogram is 0.90.

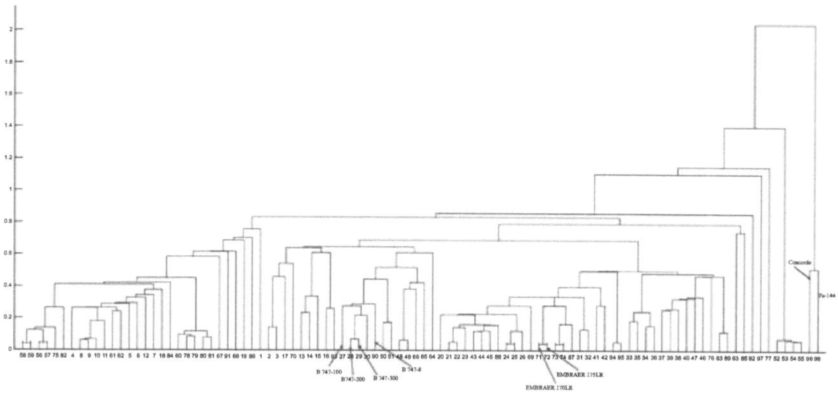

Fig. (3.9). Dendrogram of the airplanes used in the entropy statistics analysis.

Fighter Aircraft

The number aircraft in the database used in the simulations was considerably larger than that employed for the airliner classification: 281 instead of that of 98. However, just 18 parameters were employed for the fighter airplane representation.

The database was populated with aircraft of different nature. Rocket aircraft like the Messerschmitt Me 163 Komet and the Yokosuda Okha of World War II were included. Some bombers adapted for the night-fighter roles were included as well. This is the case of the Junkers Ju 88G, for instance. The Junkers Ju 88 (Fig. **3.10**) was an extremely versatile airplane and it was employed as a bomber, torpedo bomber, dive bomber, night fighter, in the reconnaissance role, and heavy fighter [21]. It saw service even as a flying bomb in the known *Mistel* combination [22]. Despite the approach of taking a broad number of concepts, no seaplanes were considered in the simulations.

The variables used to describe the fighter aircraft of the database are given below:

1. Year of introduction;
2. Engine type: =1 reciprocating; =2 turboprop; =3 rocket; =4 jet.
3. Number of engines;
4. Engine power [hp] or thrust [N];
5. Wing span [m];
6. Total length [m];
7. Total height [m];
8. Wing area (S) [m^2];

9. Lower wing-sweepback angle [degrees];
10. Higher wing-sweepback angle [degrees];
11. Empty weight [kg];
12. Maximum takeoff Weight (MTOW) [kg];
13. Maximum level speed (VMO)[km/h];
14. Service ceiling [m];
15. Range [km];
16. Full armament payload coefficient [kg];
17. Thrust to weight ratio (T/W);
18. Wing loading (W/S) [kg/m2].

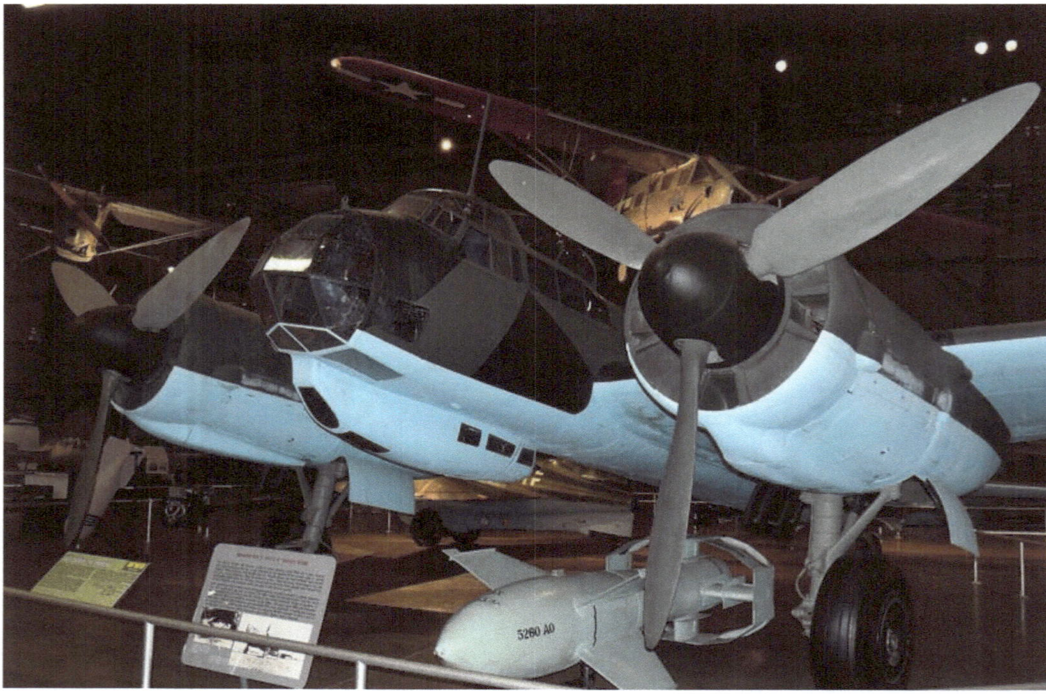

Fig. (3.10). Junkers Ju 88D at the National Museum of the United States Air Force (Photo: courtesy U.S. Air Force, public domain)

To properly consider airplanes with variable-sweep wings, the variables *9* and *10* represent the value of the wing sweep at the takeoff/landing and cruise conditions, respectively. Airplanes with no variable-sweep wings are represented with the same values for variables 9 and 10.

The thrust (*T*) for airplanes fitted with propeller are obtained using the following simple formula. Usually VMO is given at a determined altitude. To account the effects of power variation of power with altitude the following empirical formula was used [23]:

$$T = P_{sea\ level}\left(A_p \frac{\rho}{\rho_{sea\ level}} - (A_p - 1)\right)\frac{\eta_v}{VMO} \quad \textbf{(3.4)}$$

Where P is engine power, ρ is the air density and ηv is the viscous profile efficiency. A_p is a constant, of which a typical value of 1.132 is adopted. The propeller efficiency is highly dependent on the propeller type, basically fixed-pitch or constant speed ones. From **Eq. 3.4** it can observed that at altitude, the total shaft power is linear with density.

Some Featured Fighters and Attack Aircraft

Fokker E.I - This monoplane was essentially an armed version of the Fokker M.5K single-seat reconnaissance aircraft [24], which was in turn based on the French Morane-Saulnier Type H of 1913, nicknamed *The Bullet* [24]. Likewise, Morane-Saulnier, Fokker E.I featured a mid-braced wing with a box section fuselage and full movable horizontal and vertical stabilizers. Wing warping ensured control of the rolling motion, which was standard in airplanes at that time [24]. External cables attached to the wing rear spar handled the wing warping. The fuselage structure was fabric-covered with welded chromium-molybdenum steel tubing, thus accounting for the biggest difference between the Fokker and the Morane, which in contrast had an entirely wooden framework [24].

Westland Wyvern - Wyvern was a multi-role strike airplane featuring contra-rotating propellers (Fig. **3.11**). Its engine was placed behind the cockpit, driving a propeller in the nose, with a long shaft passing under the cockpit floor, like Bell P-39 Aircobra from World War II. All Wyverns were withdrawn from service by 1958. During its operational career, the type registered 68 accidents, of which 39 were hull losses. Those accidents are responsible for 13 fatalities [25].

Vought F7U Cutlass - The Vought F7U Cutlass was a United States Navy carrier-based jet fighter and fighter-bomber of the early Cold War era (Fig. **3.12**). Introduced in 1951, this elegant aircraft presented a highly unusual configuration, with no conventional horizontal stabilizer and a long nose landing gear; the latter tailored to provide higher angles of attack for shorter runs at takeoff [26]. A German engineer from World War II took part in the aircraft development, which utilized aerodynamic data and plans captured from the German Arado company at the end of World War II. The cockpit enabled good visibility for the pilot during aircraft carrier operations.

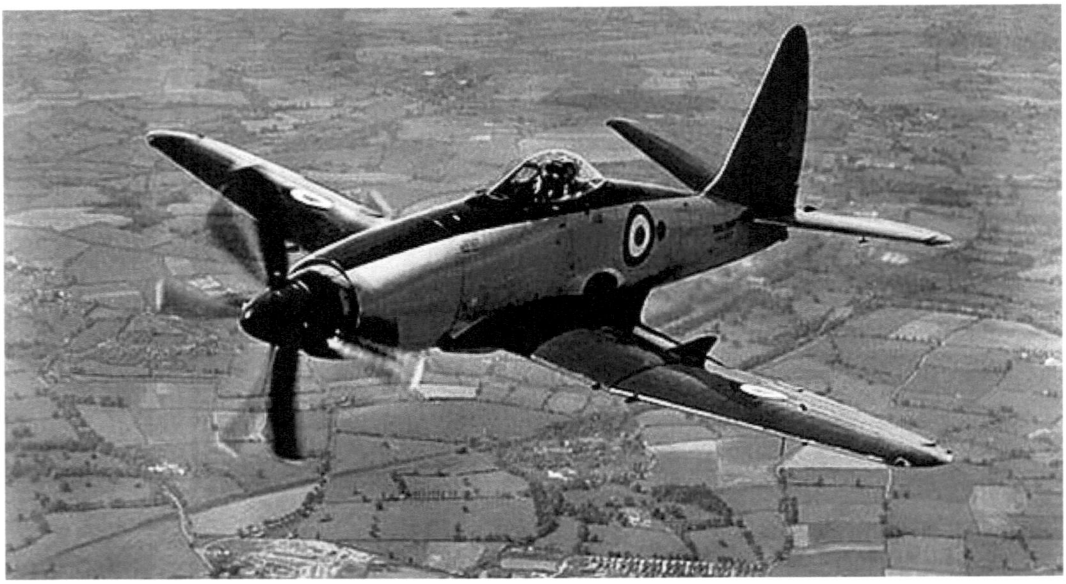

Fig. (3.11). Westland Wyvern (Public domain photo via Wikimedia Commons).

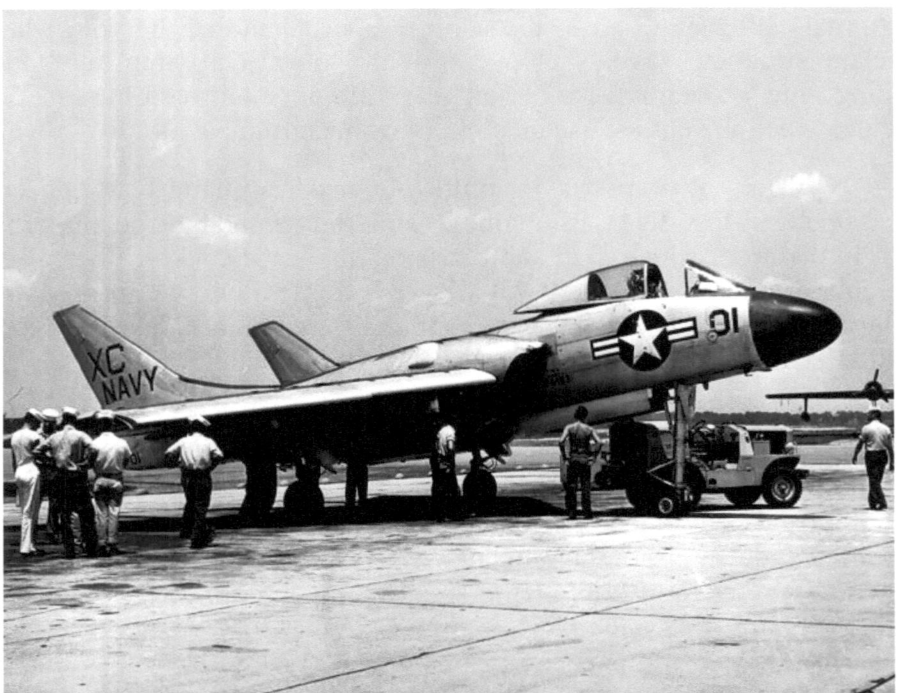

Fig. (3.12). Vought F7U Cutlass (Photo: U.S. Navy, public domain).

The Cutlass was fitted with a pressurized cockpit and ejection seats. The lack of conventional horizontal stabilizer led to necessity to the incorporation of an automatic fuel transfer system, to keep the center of gravity within acceptable margins. Besides its unusual configuration, the Cutlass fighter featured many innovations:

- First swept-wing naval aircraft.
- First production aircraft with afterburning.
- First fighter to carry radar-guided missiles.
- High-pressure hydraulic system (3000 psi).
- Tailless configuration.

Polikarpov I-16 - This light monoplane performed its maiden flight on December 31, 1933. The Polikarpov I-16 was the first in the world combining cantilever monoplane wings with retractable landing gear. By the time it started operations, I-16 was the fastest of its type [1]. The airplane had a good combat record against German aircraft during the Spanish Civil War (1936 to 1939), and against the Japanese Air Force in Manchuria in 1937 [27]. Although it was also highly maneuverable, possessing excellent climbing speed and roll rate, the Polykarpov fighter airplane was soon outperformed by newer German and Japanese designs that incorporated some of its features [1]. Due to its importance in terms the innovation, the Polykarpov I-16 fighter is of primary interest for analysis with the present methodology.

Douglas A-1 Skyraider - The piston-engine Skyraider was designed during World War II to meet United States Navy requirements for a carrier-based, single-seat, long-range, high performance dive/torpedo bomber, to follow-on from earlier types such as the Curtiss SB2C Helldiver and Grumman TBF Avenger [28]. The Douglas Skyraider attack aircraft began operations in 1946 and became a piston-powered, propeller-driven anachronism in the jet age [1].

Interpretation of the Results Obtained with the Fighter and Attack Aircraft Database

This analysis contains considerable more aircraft than that carried out for jet airliners. This and the results of the simulation help to evaluate the robustness of the codification and methodology used for airplane classification. The number of parameters to represent the fighter aircraft characteristics was slightly lower, 18, than those employed for the jet airliners. The timeframe chosen for the calculation of the convergence and diffusion indexes was 5 years. Fig. (**3.13**) contains two graphs that show the evolution of thrust-to-weight ratio (*T/W*) and wing loading (*W/S*) over the years for the aircraft in the database.

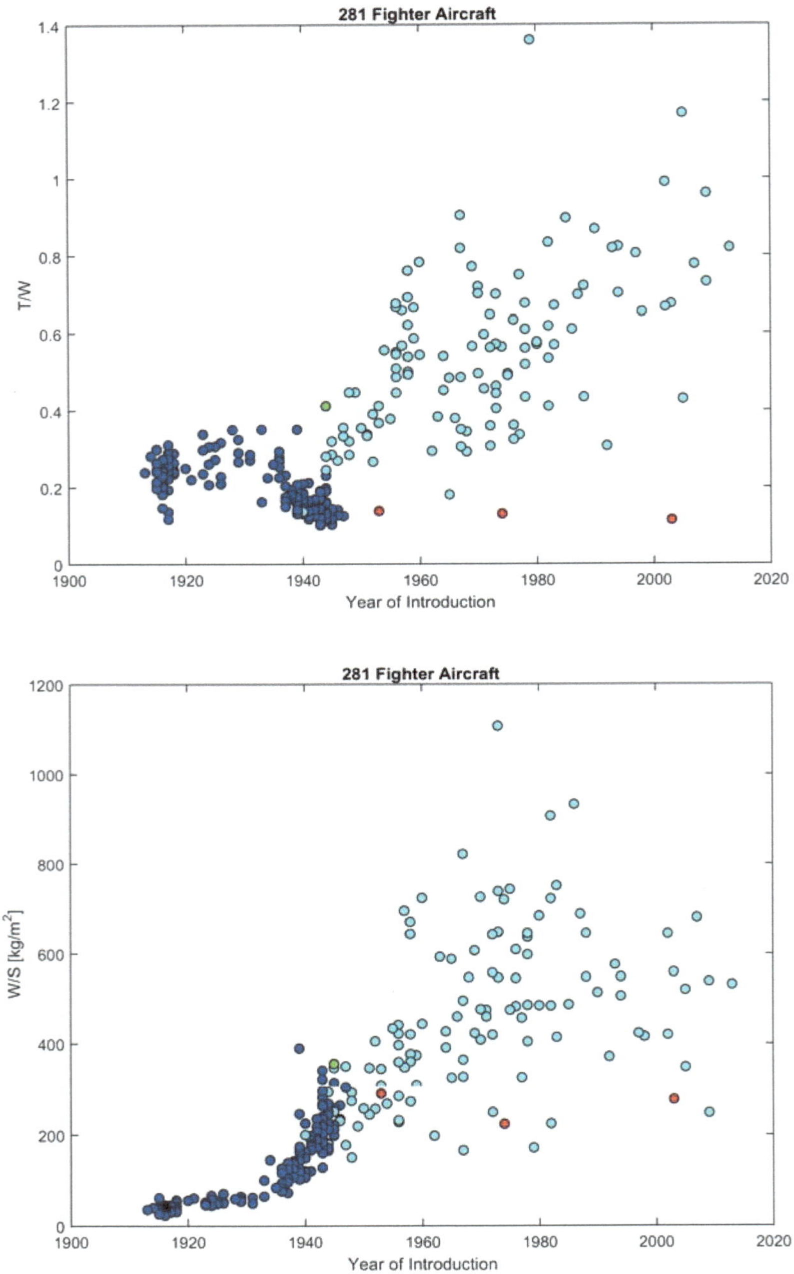

Fig. (3.13). Trust-to-weight ratio and wing loading of the fighters considered in the entropy statistics study (piston-powered airplanes are marked by dark blue circles; the jet aircraft by light blue ones).

After a certain stabilization in the interwar period, the average *T/W* begins to drop short before the start of World War II. A reasonable explanation to this trend is the fact that airplanes were becoming heavier, the wood and fabric construction being progressively replaced by metal structures. This can be easily verified in the graph of wing loading evolution. It clearly shows a sharp rise the *W/S* some years before the emergence of World War II. Besides the increase of aircraft weight, wings became smaller due to aerodynamic improvements, more powerful engines, and more efficient high-lift devices, contributing for an increase of *W/S* values.

The fighter aircraft analysis also revealed some significant differences regarding the previous study about the commercial aviation. The first difference can be seen in the diffusion graph, shown in Fig. (**3.14**). The difference of the effects that WWI (1914-1918) and WWII (1939-1945) exerted on fighter designs can be easily observed. The World War I triggered a huge batch of new concepts passing on their innovations, as can be observed by their low diffusion coefficients. This strength in new innovative concepts continued through World War II, more precisely until 1944. During the second half of WWII, the innovative concepts quickly spread its characteristics to other aircraft, these now possessing high-diffusion-index values, and this trend continued after the war. This is verified by the higher *I*-values in graph of Fig. (**3.14**). After a stabilization in the average value of the indexes in the period 1950-1975, the average diffusion-index value started to drop again from 1975 on.

The Polikarpov I-16 presents a low diffusion index, very like as that of its neighbors, indicating that it spread its characteristics to the following aircraft. The Vought F7U Cutlass represents a break of the diffusion-index rise after World War II. Its innovative features influenced fighters that came after it. Engines fitted with afterburners became an innate characteristic of fighter airplanes. Ground attack aircraft like the Argentinian Pucará, A-10A Thunderbolt II, and Cessna T-37 – this derived of the T-37A successful trainer - have high values of the diffusion index. The same can be applied to the naval strike Wyvern turboprop aircraft and the piston-powered Douglas Skyraider attack aircraft.

Indeed, the very stringent requirements that emerged during both wars tremendously accelerated aircraft development. After World War I, aircraft continue to evolve with little resemblance to the wartime airplanes. Contrary to this, some World War II aircraft presented a substantial rise in *I*-values, translating into a high degree of diffusion of previous concepts to them, a distinct pattern than that observed for WWI airplane evolution.

Tables **3.6** and **3.7** contains the airplanes presenting the highest and lowest diffusion indexes. All the airplanes of Table **3.6** are attack aircraft and that listed in T**able 3.7** were introduced before World War II.

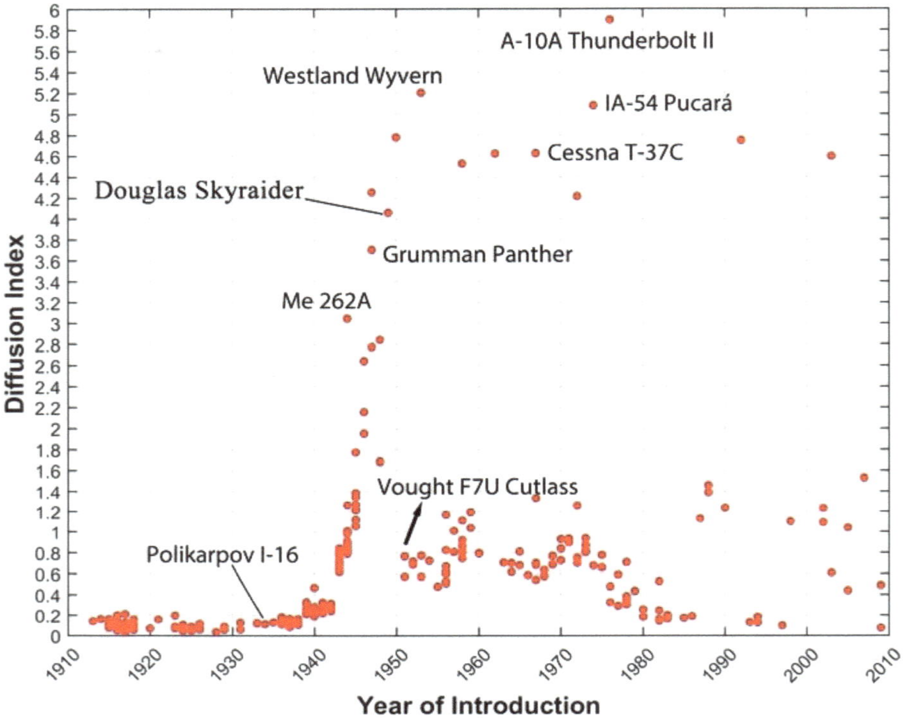

Fig. (3.14). Diffusion I-values for Fighter Aircraft.

Table 3.6. Highest diffusion values of fighter aircraft.

Airplane	Diffusion Index	Year of introduction
Tupolev I-4	0.037	1928
Albatros D.V	0.038	1917
Albatros D.III	0.040	1917
Pfalz D.III	0.041	1917
Royal Aircraft Factory S.E.5	0.045	1917
Grigorovitch I-2	0.046	1924
Nieuport 28	0.048	1917

Table 3.7. Highest diffusion values of fighter aircraft.

Airplane	Diffusion Index	Year of introduction
A-10A Thunderbolt II	5.91	1976
Westland Wyvern	5.21	1953
IA-54 Pucará	5.1	1974
Meteor NF Mark 11	4.78	1950
L-59 Super Albatros	4.75	1992
Cessna T-37C	4.63	1967
Aermacchi MB-326	4.62	1962

The convergence plot, as seen in Fig. (**3.15**), shows the same overall tendency seen in the diffusion graph (Fig. **3.14**), with low values of the index during the interwar period. However, the quantity of high-convergence indexes during and after World War II is not so massive as those seen in the diffusion graph. A peak during the 1950s can also be verified. The average value of the convergence index started to drop after 1960 and after 1980 it can be observed a dispersion of the *I*-values. Table **3.8** contains airplanes presenting the highest convergence *I*-values.

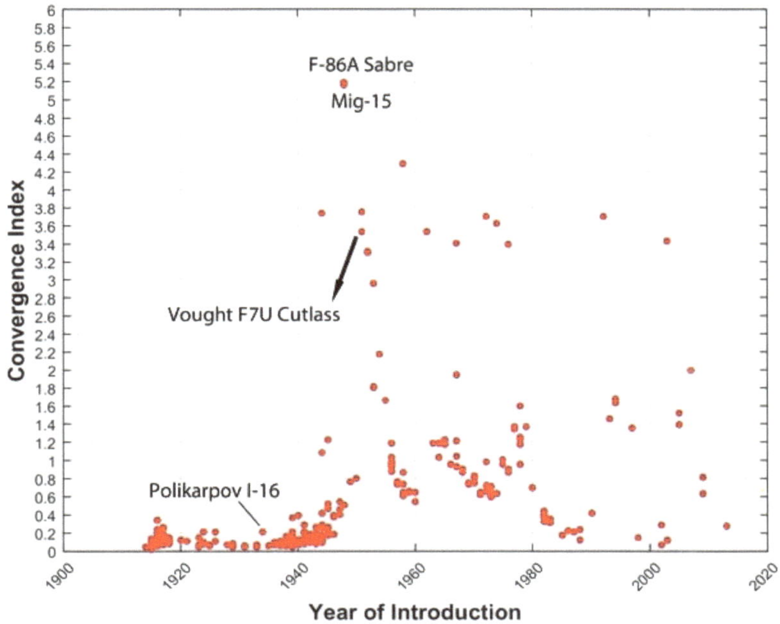

Fig. (3.15). Convergence I-values for Fighter Aircraft.

Table 3.8. Fighter aircraft presenting highest convergence values.

Airplane	Convergence Index	Year of Introduction
F-86A Sabre	5.185	1948
Mig-15	5.165	1948
F-104 Starfighter	4.292	1960
Saab J-29F Tunnan	3.749	1958
Me 262A	3.738	1944
L-39 Albatros	3.702	1972
L-59 Super Albatros	3.700	1992

Worthy of mention tis the fact that the convergence *I*-values during WWII are lower than the diffusion ones. This is somewhat expected considering that wars boost technological advances or improve previous designs considerably. The invention of the jet engine during World War II had longer impact on the aircraft development, enabling new concepts or other with improved performance as far the jet engine continued to improve.

The convergence and diffusion graphs reveal that aircraft manufacturers of the belligerent countries of the great wars developed a broad range of dominant designs for distinct reasons.

This was evident during WWI, as the powered heavier-than-air flight was only just beginning and therefore the differences among the airplanes was not so pronounced, most airplanes turning into classic ones. Beginning in 1950, the averaged *I*-value of the diffusion coefficient lowered because of constant technological evolution and the emergence of some dominant designs. During the 1990s, there was a drop of the *I*-values, revealing the presence of a dominant design.

Many aircraft are characterized by a low degree of diffusion (high *I*-value) into subsequent designs. This is the case for the A-1H Skyraider, one of the last piston-powered fighter/attack aircraft, whose development was initiated in WWII. Because it was the last one of its kind, it did not diffuse its technology onto later designs. Developed to satisfy a US Navy requirement of 1944 for a single-seat carrier-based dive bomber and torpedo carrier, the Douglas AD Skyraider materialized too late for operational service in World War II [28]. Ordered into production alongside the Martin AM Mauler, which had been developed to meet the same specification, it was to continue in production until 1957. The Skyraider reflected the navy's wartime experience gained in the Pacific theatre, where it had proved that the most important requirement for such aircraft was the ability to carry and deliver a heavy load of assorted weapons [28]. The Skyraider was also employed in the anticipated early warning (AEW) role (Fig. **3.16**). Facing Kamikaze threats in 1944, the United States Navy started the development of an airborne radar system to expand the radar horizon under which the Fleet was to operate during the series of campaigns through the Philippines and northwards to Japan. For this reason, the AN/APS-20 radar as fitted to the TBM-3W and PB-1W became the mainstay of AEW aircraft developments following WWII. While not designed specifically as an AEW aircraft, the Grumman AF-2W Guardian, when fitted with the AN/APS-20, had a secondary capability endowed by this system. Experience with the Guardian led to the development of an AEW variant of Douglas Skyraider. Once again the radar chosen was the AN/APS-20, with a large belly radome being fitted and a crew of three (one pilot and two operators) being carried. The Skyraider AEW was built in three versions, the AD-3W, AD-4W, and AD-5W. AEW aircraft is another example of divergence.

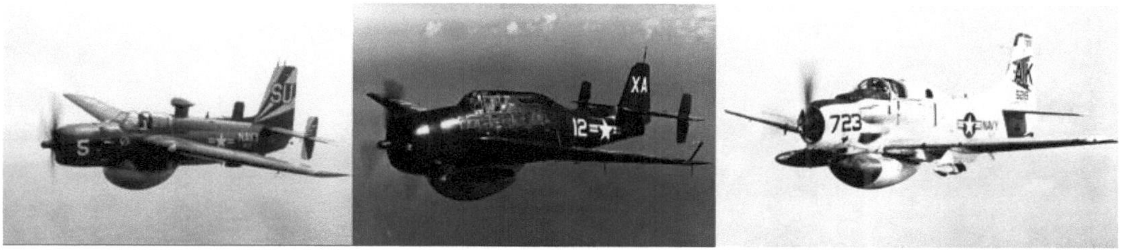

Fig. (3.16). The first early-warning and Control (AEW&C) aircraft of WWII. From left to right: AF-2W Guardian, Grumman TBM-3W Avenger and Douglas EA-1E Skyraider.

Most of the late propeller fighter designs have low diffusion, namely Republic P-47N, F4-U5 Hellcat, and North American P-51D. This also makes sense since they had not much in common with the jets that were being developed shortly thereafter. Another corner of the high-diffusion *I*-values is populated by some first-generation jets, such as Meteor Mk.8 and Yakovlev Yak-15. Fighters with low-diffusion *I*-values and high-convergence ones are the North American F-86A and Mig-15. This can be explained by the fact that a lot of their technology was passed on to later designs and they have little in common with their predecessors. The MiG-15 is considered, along with other opinions about the F-86 Sabre, as the best fighter aircraft of the Korean War [29]. It could expect such aircraft as Lockheed P-80 and the Messerschmitt Me 262 jet fighters to be in this category, but this is not the case because as pioneers most of their design ideas were not carried out, and the second generation is probably the one that contains better characteristics.

Fig. (**3.17**) displays the combined diffusion/convergence plot. Using the same classification technique of Table **3.2** we can categorize some aircraft. For example, the MiG-15 and Sabre F-86 are undoubtedly breakthrough designs of the second-generation of the military jet age. The Vought Cutlass was also labeled as a breakthrough, probably due to its engines fitted with afterburning. Low convergence and high diffusion of these planes place them in the breakthrough quadrant of Table **3.2**. Some Gloster Meteor variants are categorized as niche airplanes. The Me 262 was categorized as a "fuzzy" configuration, but it came close to the fuzzy/breakthrough boundary, which is a grey zone. Besides the consequences of the poor reliability of its engines, this jet fighter carried some characteristics of previous piston-powered airplanes and probably some of their drawbacks. Usually, this is the price to pay for some breakthrough concepts. Although classified as a breakthrough design, this is also the case of the Vought Cutlass, which recorded several accidents during its operational career.

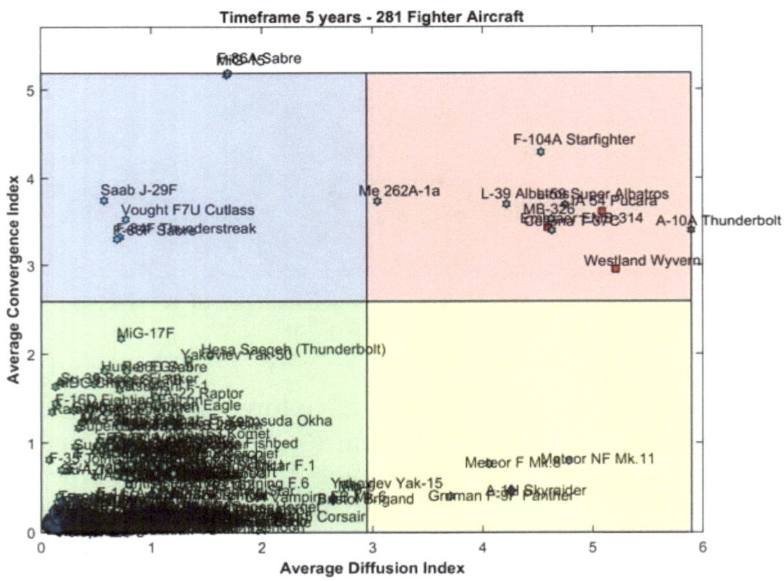

Fig. (3.17). Fighter aircraft classification by the entropy statistics analysis.

It is also worth mentioning the airplanes in the "fuzzy" quadrant: most are attack aircraft derived from trainer airplanes. Cessna T-37C is a variant of the successful T-37A side-by-side jet trainer; Embraer Super Tucano has considerably more weight than the EMB-312 Tucano (not in production anymore), of which it was based. However, wing planform and airfoils were inherited from the successful Embraer turboprop trainer, which presents impressive record sales. L-39, L-59, and MB-326 attack airplanes have almost the same configuration of the trainer airplanes that served as platform for them. However, the MB-326 presents a successful sales record being purchased by more than 10 countries and it was produced under license in Australia, Brazil (Fig. **3.18**) and South Africa [30]. In many countries, the MB-326 was used mainly in the advanced trainer role [31, 32].

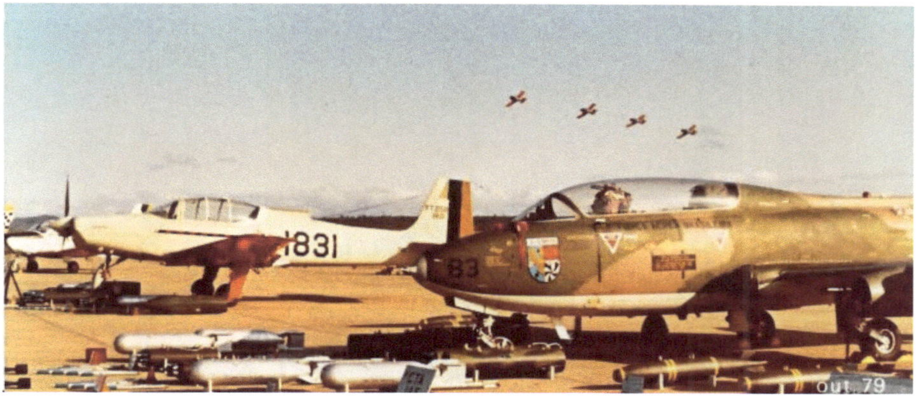

Fig. (3.18). From front to back: EMB-326GB Xavante, Neiva T-25 Universal, and Aerotec T-23 Uirapuru (Photo: ©1979 Bento Mattos).

Some dominant designs, are the Rafale C for the modern fighter jet, the F8-U Crusader for the Cold War fighters, the Bristol Bulldog for the pre-WWII era, and the Albatross D.III from WWI. During WWII, most aircraft stands out as a dominant design, becoming classical aircraft.

Entropy peaks can be found during the great wars as expected (Fig. **3.19**) with some minor ones in the interwar period. World War II is characterized or divided by two entropy peaks, indicating the introduction of many new aircraft types from the middle of that war. This entropy "footprint" indicates that the beginning of the war saw the introduction of new aircraft concepts probably integrating or consolidating the technology that emerged from the previous decade but that the war itself triggered a new wave of innovative concepts. This is what the second peak is indicating.

After calculating the Euclidian distance between the aircraft, a Dendrogram plot was generated with MATLAB® (Fig. **3.20**). The calculated cophenetic correlation coefficient for this Dendrogram is 0.96, indicating a very good correlation between the elements of the data sample. The maximum distance calculated is 10.25. Below one-third of this distance the groups can be differentiated by colors. On the left side of the plot of Fig. (**3.20**), most of World War I fighters are grouped. It can be noted a solo design by the black line between the yellow and green groups. This aircraft is the F-104 supersonic fighter. This agrees with the classification of Fig. (**3.17**) that labeled it as "fuzzy" concept.

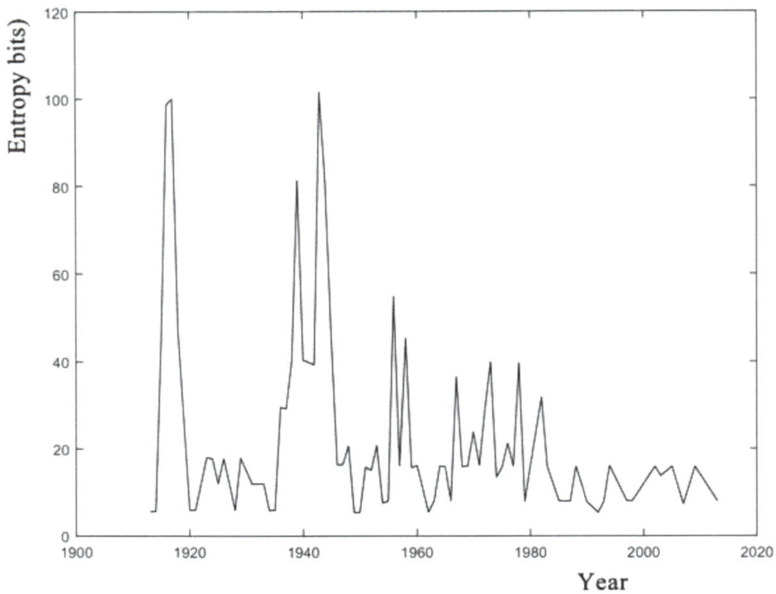

Fig. (3.19). Entropy of fighter aircraft over the years.

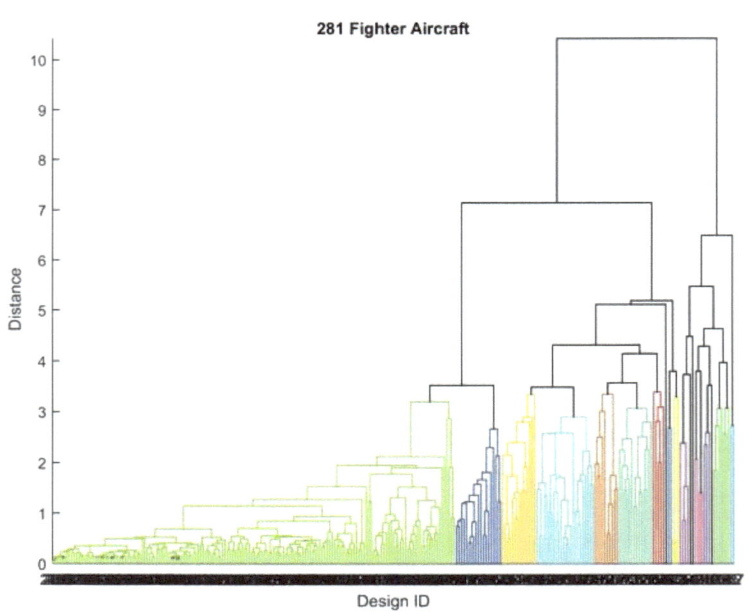

Fig. (3.20). Dendrogram obtained for the fighter aircraft from 1910 to 2013.

A close-up of two regions of the Dendrogram plot were selected for further analysis (Figs. **3.21** and **3.22**). The first region group adequately the L-29 and L-59 with the MB-326, ground-attack airplanes derived from trainer ones. Fig. (**3.22**) shows that similar aircraft were also correctly grouped.

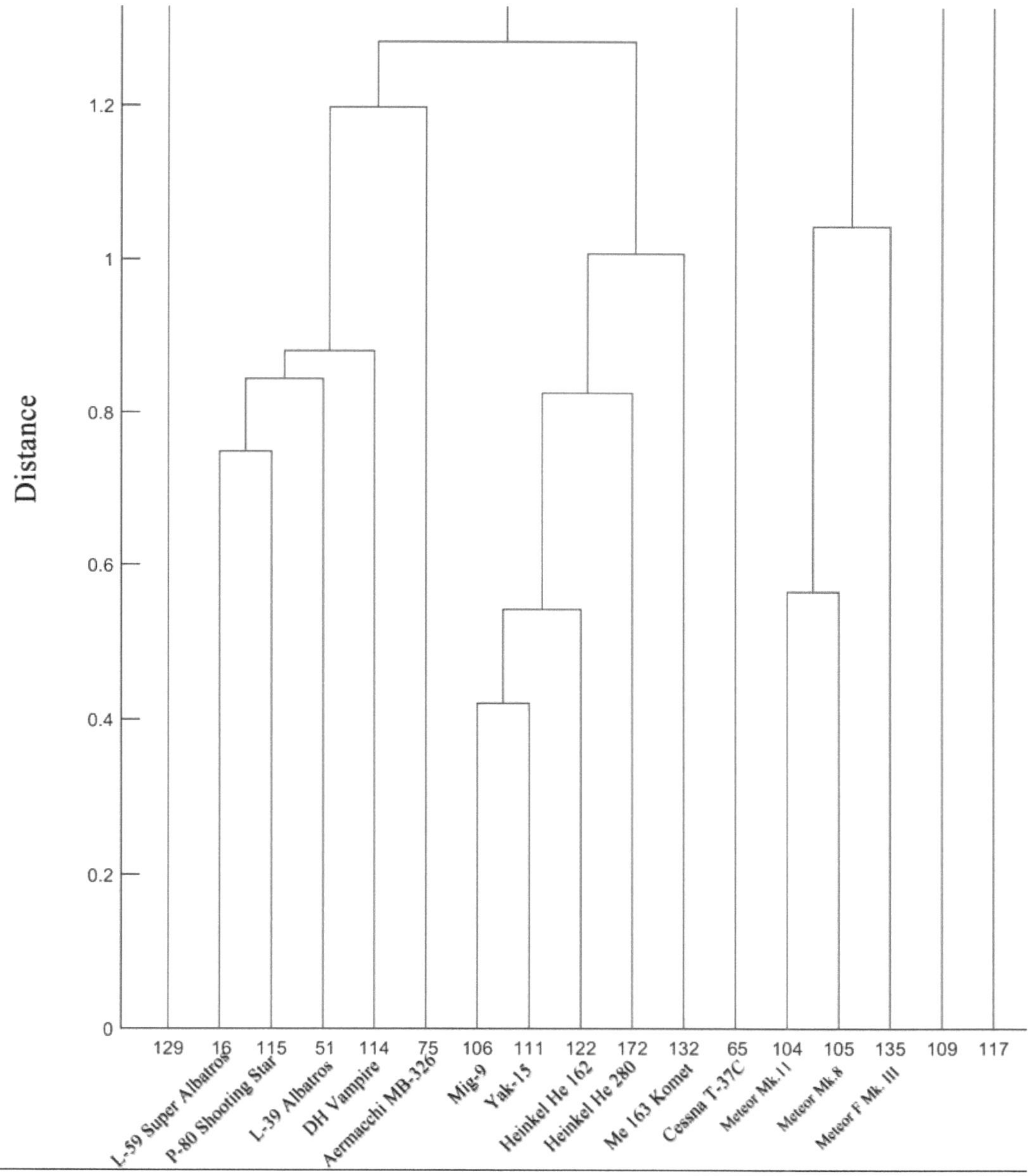

Fig. (3.21). a close-up of part of the Dendrogram plot.

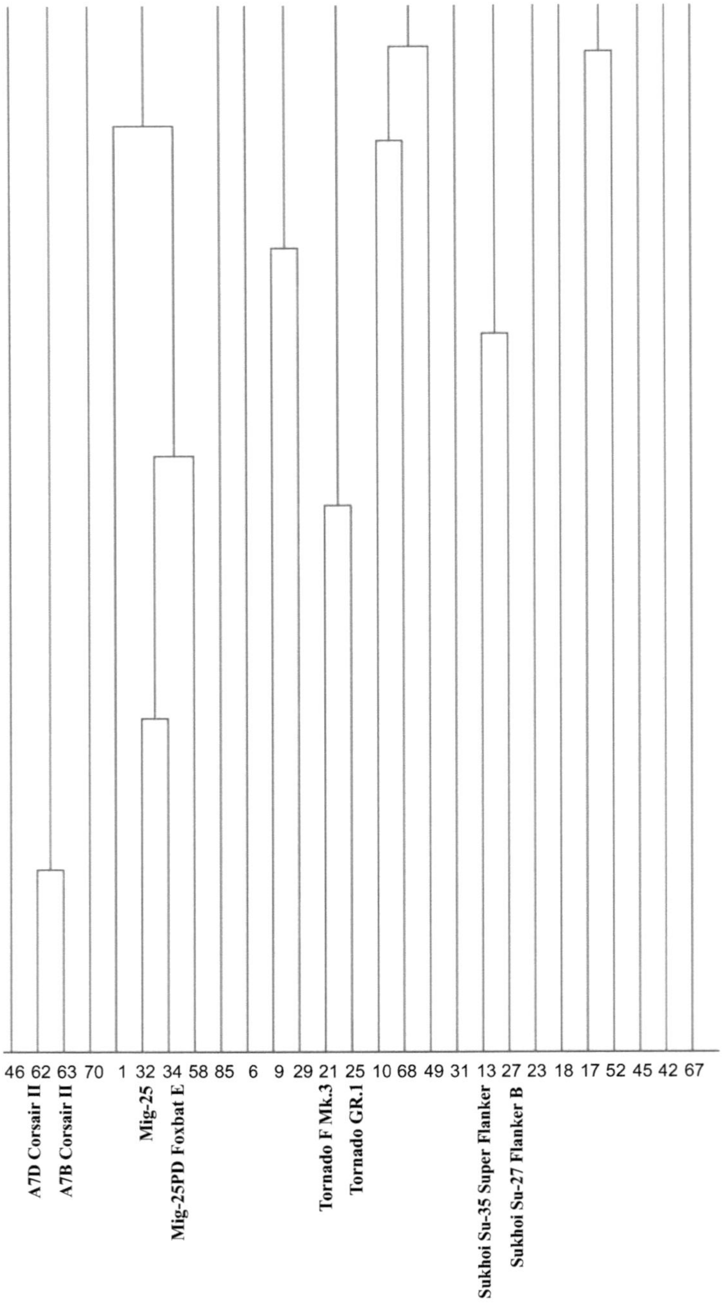

Fig. (3.22). a close-up of part of the Dendrogram plot.

CONCLUDING REMARKS

The combination of a seemingly unconnected mathematical theory and an empirical study of technological development a very useful qualitative analysis tool could be created. This computational tool can be used to assist technology assessment or as part of a corporate decision-making process.

As an academic tool, it is very interesting to use with a variety of seemingly unrelated products to study the effects of major events and breakthroughs on the timeline of technological evolution and the impact of political events like the 1978 Deregulation Act on airplane designs. If the same effect, such as a rise in diffusion or convergence I-values, can be observed for various products in the same timeframe, they might have some connection, such as events like a major war, or a major discovery. The possibilities are endless provided the product characteristics are well chosen and organized, and enough data points are gathered. This is particularly important as was seen in the fighter study.

If carefully analyzed, its results can substantially improve the firm's decision-making process. The classification method described in this paper allows a company to study how close it can get to its defined goal. With just the convergence results, that are more accurate for modern designs, one can sort out some unknowns from the process. It is simpler to think of a decision tree with two branches splitting into smaller branches each. If a strategy is known, say a breakthrough is the desired outcome of a future design, then a firm must aim for a low convergence level. On the other hand, if the company cannot afford any risk a high degree of converging technology is desired.

Trainer airplanes adapted to attack missions from 1960 on fitted in the "fuzzy" quadrant of the convergence/diffusion plot. This result deserves further analysis if this could indicate that attack variants from trainer airplanes could not be a good approach. This is a very relevant issue because many air forces around the world set or are considering establish requirements for airplanes with a dual role of trainer/counter-insurgency for budgetary reasons.

Estimating the information content on future competitors, and therefore calculate a preliminary diffusion value is a hard but doable task. Subsequently a complete classification can be obtained.

REFERENCES

[1] A. Bosquê, B.S. Mattos, and R.M. Girardi, "Entropy Statistics Applied to Airplane Evolution", *11th Brazilian Congress of Thermal Sciences and Engineering,* 2006 Curitiba, Brazil

[2] K. Frenken, and L. Leydesdorff, "Scaling Technologies in Civil Aviation (1931-1997)", *Res. Policy,* vol. 9, pp. 331-348, 1999.

[3] J. Schmookler, *Invention and Economic Growth.* Harvard University Press: Cambridge, MA, 1966. [http://dx.doi.org/10.4159/harvard.9780674432833]

[4] G. Dosi, "Technological Paradigms and Technological Trajectories", *Res. Policy,* vol. 11, pp. 147-162, 1982. [http://dx.doi.org/10.1016/0048-7333(82)90016-6]

[5] D. Mowery, and N. Rosemberg, "The influence of market demand upon innovation: A critical review of some recent empirical studies", *Res. Policy,* vol. 22, no. 2, pp. 107-108, 1993. [http://dx.doi.org/10.1016/0048-7333(93)90051-I]

[6] L. Ries, *The Origin of Brands: Discover the Natural Laws of Product Innovation and Business Survival.* HarperBusiness, 2004.

[7] J.M. Utterback, and J.W. Abernathy, "A Dynamic Model of Process and Product Innovation", *Int. J. Manag. Sci.,* vol. 3, no. 6, pp. 639-656, 1975.

[8] R.R. Nelson, and S.G. Winter, *An Evolucionary Theory of Economic Change.* Harvard University Press: Cambridge, MA, 1982.

[9] D. Sahal, "Technological Guideposts and Innovation Avenues", *Res. Policy,* vol. 14, pp. 61-82, 1985. [http://dx.doi.org/10.1016/0048-7333(85)90015-0]

[10] C.E. Shannon, "A Mathematical Theory of Communication", *Bell Syst. Tech. J.,* vol. 27, pp. 379-423, 1948. [http://dx.doi.org/10.1002/j.1538-7305.1948.tb01338.x]

[11] R. Clausius, The Mechanical Theory of Heat, W.R. Browne, Ed., Cambridge, Massaschusetts: Cambridge Press, 1879, p. 390.

[12] Wikipedia, The Free Encyclopedia, "Clausius Theorem," Wikipedia, 29 August 2017. [Online]. Available:, https://en.wikipedia.org/wiki/Clausius_theorem

[13] K. Frenken, and L. Leydesdorff, "Scaling Trajectories in Civil Aviation (1913-1997)", *Res. Policy,* vol. 29, pp. 331-348, 1999. [http://dx.doi.org/10.1016/S0048-7333(99)00037-2]

[14] A.P. Vale, *Teoria da Informação Aplicada na Análise da Evolução de Aeronaves Executivas.* Instituto Tecnológico de Aeronáutica: São José dos Campos, 2008.

[15] E. Mooi, and M. Sarstedt, *A Concise Guide to Market Research.* Springer Verlag: Berlin, Heidelberg, 2011. [http://dx.doi.org/10.1007/978-3-642-12541-6]

[16] S. Saraçli, N. Doğăn, and I. Doğăn, "Comparison of hierarchical cluster analysis methods by cophenetic correlation", *J. Inequal. Appl.,* 2013.

[17] Airfleets.net, *Production List: Canadair Regional Jet,* .

[18] Wikipedia, "Boeing 747," Wikipedia, 12 April 2-17. [Online]., Available: https://pt. wikipedia.org/wiki/Boeing_747

[19] Wikipedia, "Airbus A340," Wikipedia, 14 April 2017. [Online]., Available: https://en. wikipedia.org/wiki/Airbus_A340

[20] Wikipedia, The Free Encyclopedia, "Boeing 777," Wikipedia, 18 July 2017. [Online]. , Available: https://pt. wikipedia.org/wiki/Boeing_777

[21] Wikipedia, The Free Encyclopedia, "Junkers Ju 88," Wikipedia, 5 August 2017. [Online]. , Available: https://en. wikipedia.org/wiki/Junkers_Ju_88

[22] Wikipedia, The Free Encyclopedia, "Mistel," Wikipedia, 2017 July 2017. [Online], Available: https://en. wikipedia.org/wiki/Mistel

[23] F.H. Lutze, *AOE 3104 Vehicle Performance,* 2017. http://www. dept. aoe. vt.edu/ ~lutze/ AOE3104/

thrustmodels.pdf

[24] Wikipedia, The Free Encyclopedia, "Fokker E.I," Wikipedia, 9 June 2017. [Online], Available: https://en.wikipedia.org/wiki/Fokker_E.I

[25] Wikipedia, The Free Encyclopedia, "Westland Wyvern," Wikipedia, 3 July 2017. [Online], Available: https://en.wikipedia.org/wiki/Westland_Wyvern

[26] T.H. Thomason, *U.S. Naval Superiority: Development of Shipborne Jet Fighters 1943-1962.* Specialty Press, 2008.

[27] Wikipedia, The Free Encyclopedia, "Polykarpov I-16," Wikiepdia, 2017. [Online], Available: https://en.wikipedia.org/wiki/Polikarpov_I-16

[28] Wikipedia, The Free Encyclopedia, "Douglas A-1 Skyraider," Wikipedia, 25 August 2017. [Online], Available: https://en.wikipedia.org/wiki/Douglas_A-1_Skyraider

[29] E.R. McDowell, and R. Ward, North American F-86A-L Sabre.*USAF & Foreign Service.* vol. Vol. 17. Osprey Publications Ltd.: Canterbury, Kent, 1970.

[30] Wikipedia, The Free Encyclopedia, "Aermacchi MB-326," Wikipedia, September 2017. [Online], Available: https://en.wikipedia.org/wiki/Aermacchi_MB-326

[31] GlobalSecurity.org, *AT-26 Xavante,* 2013. https://www. globalsecurity. org/ military/ world/ brazil/ at26.htm

[32] A.C. Alamino, *EMB.326GB AT-26 Xavante,* 2017. http://www.rudnei.cunha.nom.br/ FAB/br/at-26.html

CHAPTER 4

Aircraft Design Phases

Abstract: Aircraft design is a complex and fascinating business and a field of research and many good books have been written about it. The very complex and dynamic nature of the subject means that no book can do justice to it. This chapter, therefore, will primarily act as an introduction to the whole field of aircraft design leading towards the main phases of an aircraft development program. It also provides information about the whole aircraft design process together with descriptions of the aircraft design phases. Certification is an important aspect of aircraft design process and therefore is covered in the present chapter with more details.

Keywords: Aircraft design phases, Conceptual design, Design requirements, Financial analysis.

DESIGNING AIRPLANES

Aircraft design is an extremely challenging task that requires compromising on solutions involving different disciplines. Aerodynamics, structures, aeroelasticity, landing gear and other systems, production and cost, propulsion system, and stability as well as control are only some of them. Moreover, there may be conflicting aspects within one and the same discipline. For instance, field and cruise performance demand conflicting airfoil shapes and wing planform. New challenges posed by new and tougher environmental requirements contribute to making this task even more complex. The Advisory Council for Aeronautics Research in Europe (ACARE), responsible for the definition of a strategic research agenda for all aeronautical research programs in Europe, established in 2001, a target for reduction of emitted airplane CO_2 by 50%, NO_x by 80% and external noise by 50% by the year 2020 [1].

Aircraft serial manufacturing is a huge investment for both the buyer and the manufacturer. It is thus imperative that the product meets customer needs and the development process cost be kept under control. Indeed, it is customary for commercial airframe manufacturers to secure purchase commitments from several airlines before deciding to commit to the production of an aircraft type. Basically, like any product, aircraft design originates from a set of requirements that drive the development process. These requirements may come from completely

Bento S. de Mattos, José A. T. G. Fregnani & Paulo Eduardo C. S. Magalhães

different areas such as operation, manufacturing, maintenance, certification, *etc.* As mentioned before, it is vital to listen to customers. A successful sale record will enable the manufacturer to improve its financial health and therefore to be able to develop new aircraft or improve existing products, while keeping or even increasing its market share. There are many cases of aircraft manufacturers that went out of business for offering an inappropriate product to the market. The military, on the other hand, will often create their own specifications in the form of a Request for Proposal (RFP). The RFP invites manufacturers to propose a design meeting the issued requirements. Each proposal is evaluated, and one is usually selected, turning the chosen manufacturer into the sole provider for the aircraft.

Aircraft manufacturers regularly conduct exploratory work on research, technology, and market analysis to evaluate if a new or improved product is worth being developed. Having determined the projected market for aircraft, the next stage is to examine the existing and under development competitors in that market. This will influence the product that will be developed.

Before a newly developed aircraft model enters operation, it must obtain a type certificate (TC) from the aviation regulatory agencies. A type certificate is issued to recognize the airworthiness of an aircraft manufacturing design. The certificate is issued by a regulating agency, and once it is issued, changes to the configuration will only be possible if a new, simplified certification process is followed, which can be an amendment to the type certificate, if carried out by the original manufacturer, or a Supplementary Type Certificate (STC), when it is performed by an operator or a third party. This Type Certificate reflects a determination stipulated by the regulating authority that the aircraft is manufactured according to an existing regulation basis, and that the design ensures compliance with airworthiness requirements.

Changes in configuration may take place in the last phases of the aircraft development program, impacting inevitably the certification process [2]. Performance and handling enhancements are usually the major causes of modifications, but often they are necessary to meet an unanticipated regulatory need, an excess drag or something as major as a system switch [2]. As exemplification, four commercial airplane programs that suffered delays or major redesign are analyzed below:

- During its development, the Eclipse 500 received new engines; Eclipse Aviation then switched from a small Williams International turbofan to the larger Pratt & Whitney Canada PW600 [2]. Excess drag accounted among other causes for this change that also led to a heavier airplane. Eclipse Aviation had therefore to

install tip tanks to attain performance goals [2].
- Dassault's Falcon 7X exceeded the performance goals after installation of a forward-fuselage fuel tank, modified winglets and redesigned empennage during the certification program [2]. Originally considered to offer a 5,700-nm range, the 7X was certified with a 5,950-nm maximum range with a payload of 8 passengers [2].
- In May 1999, EMBRAER expected the go-ahead for the ERJ-170 program in the second quarter of 1999 and forecasted that the initial deliveries of its ERJ-170 would take place in 2002 [3]. However, the type (later redesignated E-170) entered service with Polish Airlines only in May 2004 [4].
- The all-composite Boeing 787 Dreamliner suffered huge delays in its development program [5]. Software issues, load recalculation, airframe overweight, engine blowout during testing were major causes of delays [5]. Three years behind schedule, ANA received the first Dreamliner [5]. The aircraft also suffered from several in-service problems, including fires on board related to its lithium-ion batteries [6].

The aeronautical industry is linked to national industrial strategy, which in turn depends on country infrastructure, governmental policies (not just for ordering military aircraft), workforce capabilities, academic support in education and research, and natural resources. More than any other industry, the aerospace sector is linked to global trends. Commercial aviation is directly affected by recession, fuel price increases, spread of infectious diseases, and international politics. In addition to its importance for national security, the military aircraft sector is a key element in several of the world's largest economies.

Skilled labor force is essential, but it is not the only required condition for success of the aerospace industry, if there is no harmonization of activity with national policies. The basic three elements of the system must progress in a proper well-coordinated way: industry, government and research. Because large companies affect regional economic development and demand strong governmental support, they must share socio-economic responsibility for the region in which they are located.

Budget limitations, market requirements and global crisis set constraints on the design process and comprise the non-technical influences on aircraft design along with environmental factors. Competition leads companies to search for better efficiency in the aircraft configuration without compromising performance and incorporating new techniques and technology [7].

To keep risks as low as possible, a typical aircraft project contains the following distinctive features:

- Project is divided into phases.
- There are scheduled design reviews.
- Suppliers may become risk partners.
- Advanced engineering tools like computational fluid dynamics codes (CFD) and multi-disciplinary design and optimization (MDO) frameworks are employed.
- Extensive market studies are carried out.
- A launcher customer is sought and/or an expressive initial order must be consolidated.
- Manufacturing of some prototypes for ground and flight testing.
- Pioneering and creative concepts.
- Lessons learned from previous projects.
- Technology certification by technology demonstrators, laboratories, joint ventures, cooperative efforts with the academic community.

During the Cold War, a strong scientific and technological race between Western countries and the former Soviet Union took place. The landing of manned crew on the moon, the Internet, the Concorde supersonic airliner, all of these and much more are results from the Cold War. Indeed, in this scenario, even absurd like the very expensive nuclear-powered bomber program were considered. The advent of Intercontinental Ballistic Missiles (ICBMs) in the 1960s greatly diminished the tactical advantage of such aircraft, and related projects were cancelled. The Cold War came to an end with the dissolution of the Soviet Union. From 1992 on, military programs suffered deep cuts (Fig. **4.1**). However, according to the graph from Fig. (**4.1**), global and North American military expenditure surpassed 1988 levels in 2014. Anyway, civil programs that used to be beneficiaries of military technological developments also suffered from a decrease in innovations in the wake of budget cuts. Another consequence was that output and cost influenced a trend away from volume production and towards specialized manufacture of fewer types of airliners and military aircraft.

The aerospace industry acquired in the last two decades a set of unique characteristics in manufacturing and design [8]:

a. Performance demands for new systems require continual technological advancement, which in turn involves improved tools and methods of evaluation of uncertainty, risk, and economical feasibility. For the next decades, a bigger challenge is posed by environmental constraints such as noise and emissions.
b. Industry has increasingly sought academy to find solutions for improving its products. Government founded programs like the European Framework for Research Development seek a prominent level of collaboration and integration between industry and academy.

c. Because governments are the main customer, the military product line is subject to revisions on program levels occasioned by changing requirements and funding availability or the emergence of new threats.
d. Equipment that challenges the state of the art is necessarily costly, the more so because requirements generally dictate short production runs, negating the economies of large-scale production.
e. Technologically demanding programs require personnel emphasis on higher skill levels. Hence, labor input per unit of output is substantially larger than in other manufacturing industries [8].
f. The combination of technological uncertainty and long production time, about 7–10 years and frequently longer, between program start and completion, makes advanced estimation of costs particularly difficult. Inflation and varying exchange rates make cost estimation and its control within program budget an even bigger challenge.
g. There are now few customers and relatively few programs; competition for the business opportunities therefore is intense [8].
h. These characteristics contribute to exceptional demand for industry capital, yet profits as a percentage of sales are consistently well below the average for the remaining manufacturing industries [8].
i. Airplane lessors and companies that operate within fractional ownership business models are today big aircraft buyers. They have unique requirements for aircraft and many of them place big orders, demanding big discounts [8].

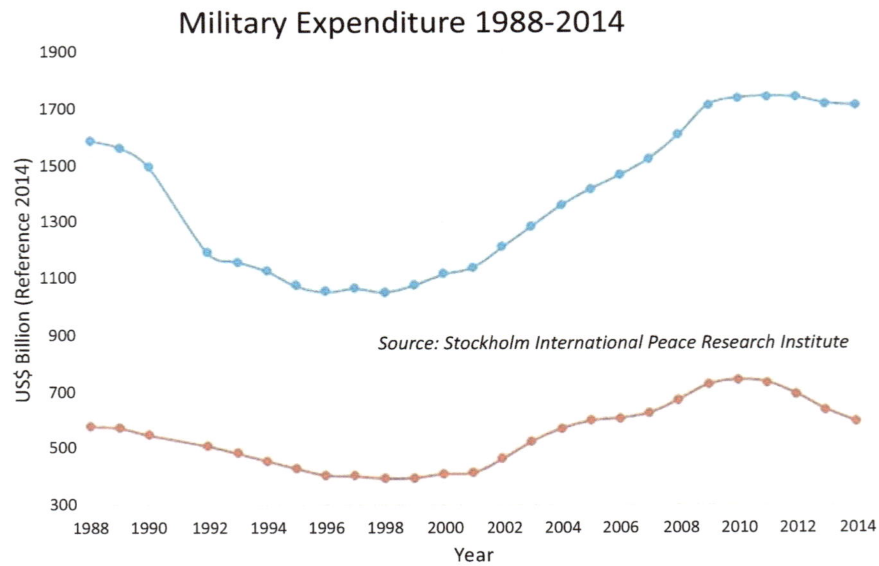

Fig. (4.1). Military expenditure in the 1998-2014 period (2014 dollar).

AIRCRAFT PROGRAM PHASES

Overview

Regarding the design phases, there are several approaches, which depend on each manufacturer organization. Fig. (**4.2**) shows the typical phases of an aircraft development program. Table **4.1** describes the activities and guidelines of the typical phases of an aircraft program. The following paragraphs of the present **Section** provide an overview of the phases.

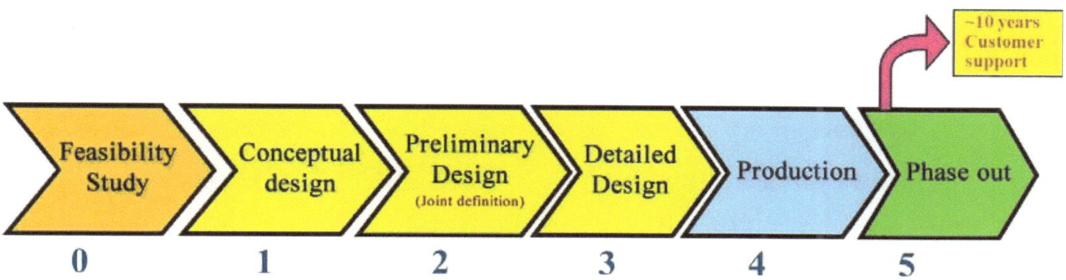

Fig. (4.2). Classical phase breakdown of aircraft development program.

Table 4.1. Phases of an aircraft project.

Phase	Activities	Guidelines
Feasibility study	Market analysis; business plan; technology assessment	Financing
Conceptual	Costs; performance; first wind-tunnel tests; CFD; MDO; layout of aircraft systems; partner and supplier selection	Aircraft configuration; sizing; engine selection
Preliminary design (Joint Definition Phase) *	System integration; mitigation of critical engineering problems;	Complete aircraft definition
Detailed design	Construction of prototypes; drawings (digital mockup); rigs; flight tests	Certification
Production	Production; preparation for entry into service; production plan; quality control	Manufacturing, production rate, Entry into service preparation
Operating life and phase out	Certification of maintenance shops; service bulletins; fatigue life; product improvement	Customer support/Recycling

(*Only some manufacturers use this approach).

There are several dedicated software and tools to assist program management. A Gantt chart (Fig. **4.3**) is a type of bar chart, adapted by both Karol Adamiecki in 1896 and independently by Henry Gantt in the 1910s, that illustrates a project schedule [9]. Gantt charts illustrate the start and closure dates of the terminal elements and summary elements of a project. Terminal elements and summary elements comprise the work breakdown structure of the project. Modern Gantt charts also show the dependency relationships between activities and contain important project dates and milestones.

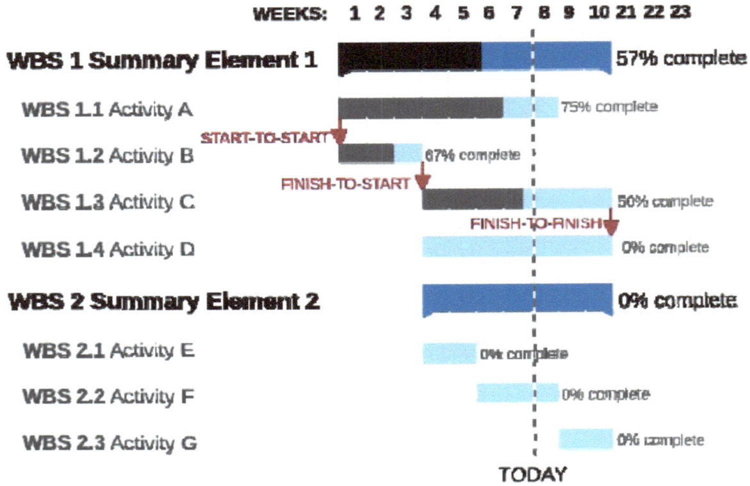

Fig. (4.3). Gantt chart showing three kinds of schedule dependencies (in red) and percent complete indications (Credit: Garry L. Booker, released to the public domain).

Another useful tool for project management is the critical path method (CPM), which is an algorithm for scheduling a set of project activities. It is a step-by-step project management technique for process planning that defines critical and non-critical tasks with the goal of prevent timeframe problems and process stagnation points.

The essential technique for using CPM is to construct a model of the project with the following content:

- A list of all activities required to complete the project. These activities are typically categorized within a work breakdown structure.
- The duration that each activity will take to complete.
- The dependencies between the activities.
- Logical end points such as milestones or deliverable items.
- Identification of the critical path.
- Critical path diagram to record project progress

The longest path of planned activities is calculated containing the logical end and start points of the project. In addition, the earliest and latest paths each activity can start and finish without making the project longer. This process determines which activities are "critical" (*i.e.*, on the longest path) and which have "total float" (*i.e.*, can be delayed without making the project longer). In project management, a critical path is the sequence of project network activities which add up to the longest overall duration, regardless if that longest duration has float or not. This determines the shortest time possible to complete the project. There can be 'total float' (unused time) within the critical path. For example, if a project is testing a solar panel and task 'B' requires 'sunrise', there could be a scheduling constraint on the testing activity so that it would not start until the scheduled time for sunrise. This might insert inactive time (total float) into the schedule for the activities on that path prior to the sunrise due to the necessary wait for this event. This path, with the constraint-generated total float would make the path longer, with total float being part of the shortest possible duration for the overall project. In other words, individual tasks on the critical path prior to the constraint might be able to be delayed without elongating the critical path; this is the 'total float' of that task. However, the time added to the project duration by the constraint is critical path drag, the amount by which the project's duration is extended by each critical path activity and constraint.

A project can have several, parallel, near critical paths; and some or all the tasks could have 'free float' and/or 'total float'. An additional parallel path through the network with the total durations shorter than the critical path is called a sub-critical or non-critical path. Activities on sub-critical paths have no drag, as they are not extending the project's duration.

Although the activity-on-arrow diagram, PERT Chart (Fig. **4.4**) is still used in a few places, it has generally been superseded by the activity-on-node diagram, where each activity is shown as a box or node and the arrows represent the logical relationships going from predecessor to successor as shown here in the "Activity-on-node diagram".

Feasibility Study

This is the phase where the airplane is first thought of. It starts with market analysis of what an interesting product for the current and forecasted market is, typically from 15 to 20 years in the future. Business opportunity may also come from an airline direct request, as was the case of the EMBRAER ERJ 140, a shortened version of the ERJ 145, developed to bypass scope clauses. There are virtually no scope limits to the number of 44-seat regional jets (RJ), while there is with the 50-seat ones. Bombardier Aerospace also has a 44-seat RJ model which is basically a CRJ-200 with 6 seats removed and certified as the CRJ-440. It was developed for Delta Airlines but Northwest ordered this version as well.

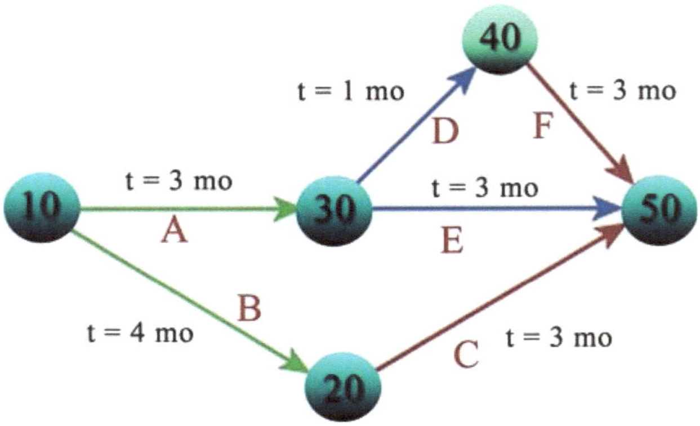

Fig. (4.4). PERT chart for a project with five milestones (10 through 50) and six activities (A through F). The project has two critical paths: activities B and C, or A, D, and F – giving a minimum project time of 7 months with fast tracking. Activity E is sub-critical, and has a float of 1 month (Credit: Jeremy Kemp, released to the public domain).

The aircraft development program usually consumes 5 years. Financial analysis (Fig. **4.5**) is carried out concerning product development, production and fleet support in this phase. The manufacturers will also seek means to finance their new or upgraded product. A business plan is the main deliverable of this phase. Once it is finished and the aircraft program could bring a target return of investment or the new product may be strategic for the company, the business plan is presented to the company board to obtain a decision whether to move forward with the program ("go ahead") or not.

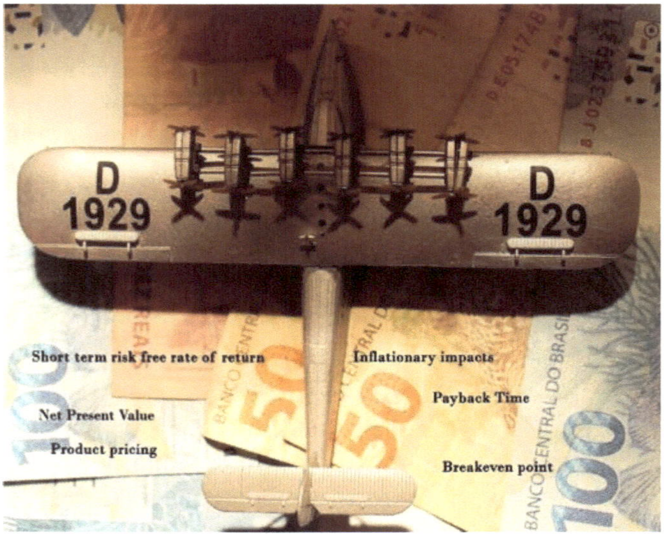

Fig. (4.5). Financial analysis will provide investment parameters (Photo: ©2015 Bento Mattos).

Market analysis should address:

- Trends and market dynamics.
- Existing fleet mapping.
- Market segmentation.
- Market potential.
- Market share.
- Elaboration of a database containing data and information about the competition (including other means of transportation).
- Competitive advantages.
- Potential customers.
- Market survey encompassing questionnaires and other sources to obtain key information.

The business plan usually comprises the following sections:

- Summary
- Description of the company
- Market analysis
- Business financial parameters
- Marketing strategy
- Product development plan
- Production scheme (required by certification authorities)
- Project management plan
- Master Phase Plan
- Risk assessment
- Financial analysis
- Capital amassment

Conceptual Studies

The conceptual design or, for many, the study of concepts, takes place after the feasibility study, which is the initial phase where the viability of an aircraft program is analyzed conclusively. In the conceptual phase, the aircraft configuration that best meets all the requirements is defined. Requirements are related to market, certification, manufacturing and others that may be established by the aircraft manufacturer.

Conceptual design activities are characterized by the definition and comparative evaluation of numerous alternative design concepts potentially satisfying an initial statement of design requirements. The conceptual design phase is iterative in nature. Modern aircraft design considers different configurations that comply with world scenarios raised by the company's strategic planning studies. The objective is the selection of concepts to explore their most relevant capabilities and meet the widest range of future challenges.

Design concepts are evaluated (Fig. **4.6**), compared to the requirements, revised, reevaluated, and so on until convergence to one or more satisfactory concepts is achieved. During this process, inconsistencies among the requirements are often exposed, so that the products of conceptual design frequently include a set of revised requirements. Table **4.2** contains the scope of this phase.

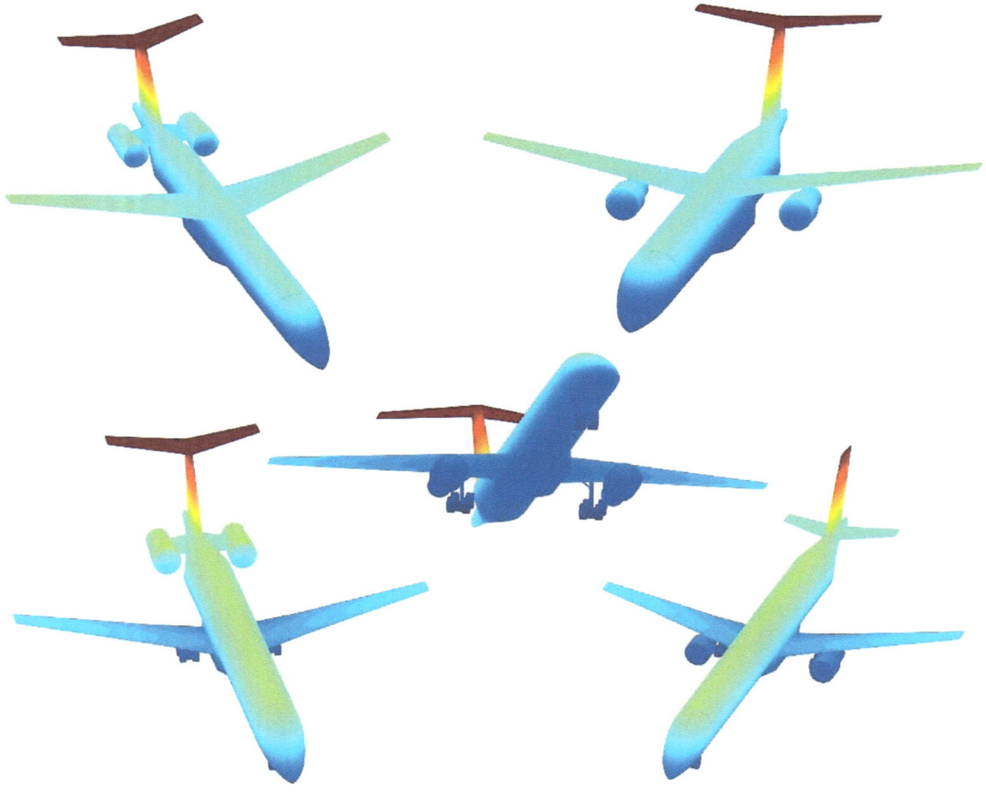

Fig. (4.6). During conceptual studies, several aircraft configurations are analyzed (Source: ITA/IEAP).

In the conceptual design phase, engine is selected, aircraft layout containing access panels is defined, the airplane is sized, and system architectures are established. Preliminary sizing of the airframe is also conducted in this phase.

Table 4.2. Conceptual design scope.

Item	Description
Requirement check	Requirements may suffer alterations and must be checked
Detailed budget	Budget from the previous phase is analyzed and detailed
Configuration study	Several configurations are proposed and one is selected according to the best compliance with requirements. Multi-disciplinary design and optimization and decision tools are used to choose the configuration that will be further studied
Sizing	Sizing and integration of aircraft parts
Structural layout	Aircraft structure layout with access panels is elaborated. There is a search for allocation of system components
Technical drawings, manuals and documents	Aircraft Technical Description: typical characteristics, including performance and systems description; used for marketing and customer prospection Aircraft Basic Data: detailed characteristics, used for data interchange among the different technologies involved in product design
Engine selection	The engine is chosen according to several criteria such as thrust, fuel consumption, size, bleed air capacity, easy and cheap maintenance, weight, *etc.*
Testing	Some wind-tunnel tests are performed

Aerodynamic analysis in the conceptual phase is usually carried out with numeric tools and wind-tunnel testing. The complexity of fluid flow is well demonstrated in many scientific papers and experiments. Most phenomena of fluid flow, such as shock waves and flow separation, are essentially nonlinear in nature and the variety of turbulence scales in the flow pattern is huge. Nowadays, computational fluid dynamics (CFD) is widely employed as a key tool for aircraft design (Fig. **4.7**). Reynolds Average Navier-Stokes (RANS) solutions are a common tool, as well as Euler and full potential formulations. Fig. (**4.8**) shows a hierarchy of several simplifications of the Navier-Stokes equations.

The length scale of the smallest persisting eddies in a turbulent flow can be estimated as of order of 1/Re3/4 in comparison with the macroscopic length scale. The solution of such scales for a complex aircraft configuration is still prohibitive. For this reason, simplified formulations are used in the aircraft industry. A computational grid with million cells are usually required for an external flow solution over a completed airplane configuration employing the RANS formulation.

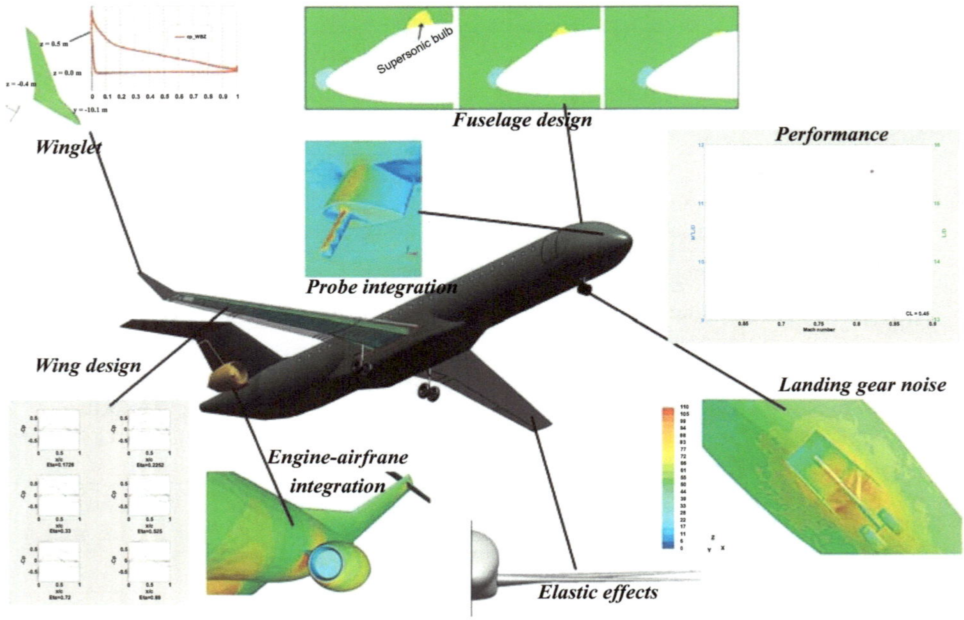

Fig. (4.7). Some CFD applications in aircraft design (Source: ITA/IEAP).

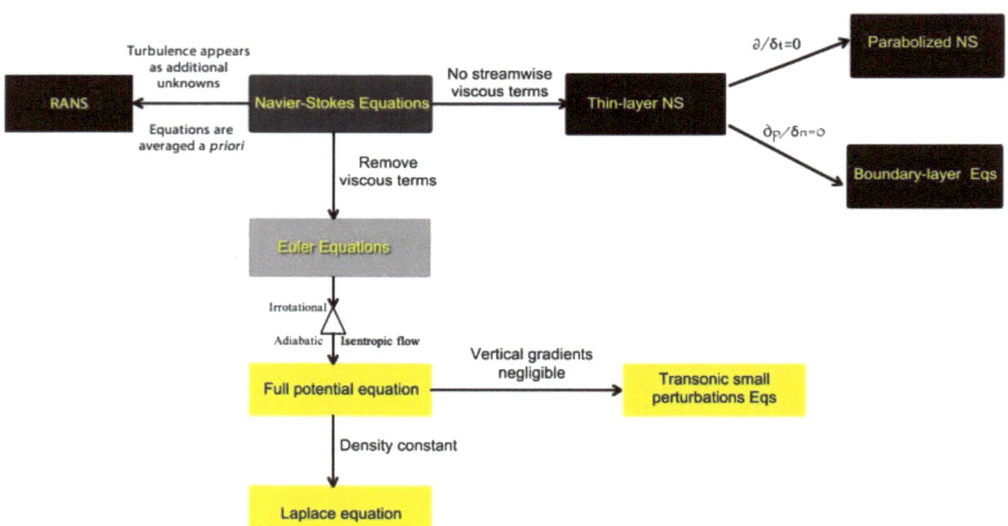

Fig. (4.8). Formulations for numerical flow analysis.

A viable alternative for MDO computations is the utilization of full potential codes with viscous corrections. Their cost benefit makes this formulation very attractive for higher fidelity aerodynamic computations in a MDO process, which requires extensive calls of the flow analysis codes for performance, load, and stability calculations. However, the extreme sensitive nature of transonic flow in regard the airplane geometry, in which variations in the order of boundary-layer thickness or lower lead to significant changes in pressure distribution, makes mandatory that integral boundary-layer routines to be coupled with the transonic potential and Euler codes. Besides delivering satisfactory profile drag values, the viscous coupled calculation shall also be able to handle shock-boundary layer interaction.

A comparison between a RANS code and a full-potential one [10] was carried-out for a twinjet airliner with rear-mounted engines (Fig. **4.9**). The RANS simulation employed the SST k-ω turbulence model and the hexahedral mesh that was created for the simulation was composed of approximately 2.1 million cells [11]. Making use of an implicit scheme for time marching, the convergence was reached after all residuals dropped to values below $1x10^{-4}$, which consumed 5675 iterations. Each iteration demanded in average 84 s on a desktop computer fitted with an Intel® Core™ i7-3820 processor. The full potential solution for the wing-fuselage combination took 25 secs to converge on the same machine. Fig. (**4.10**) shows a comparison between the results from the RANS and the full potential codes. There, Cp distributions for two wing stations of the airliner of Fig. (**4.9**) are shown. The agreement between the related Cp distributions is very good.

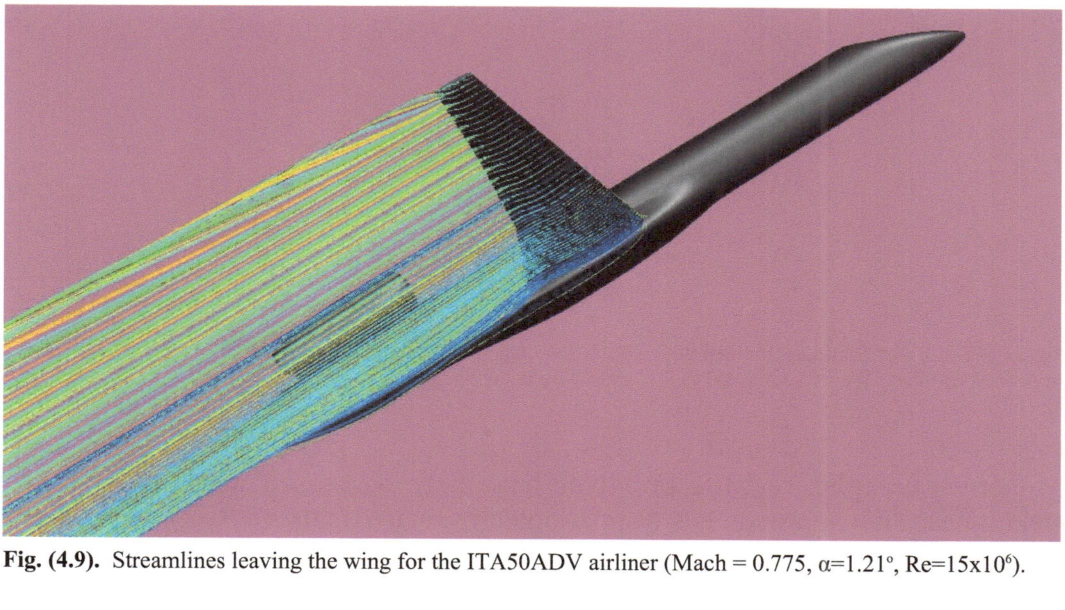

Fig. (4.9). Streamlines leaving the wing for the ITA50ADV airliner (Mach = 0.775, α=1.21°, Re=$15x10^6$).

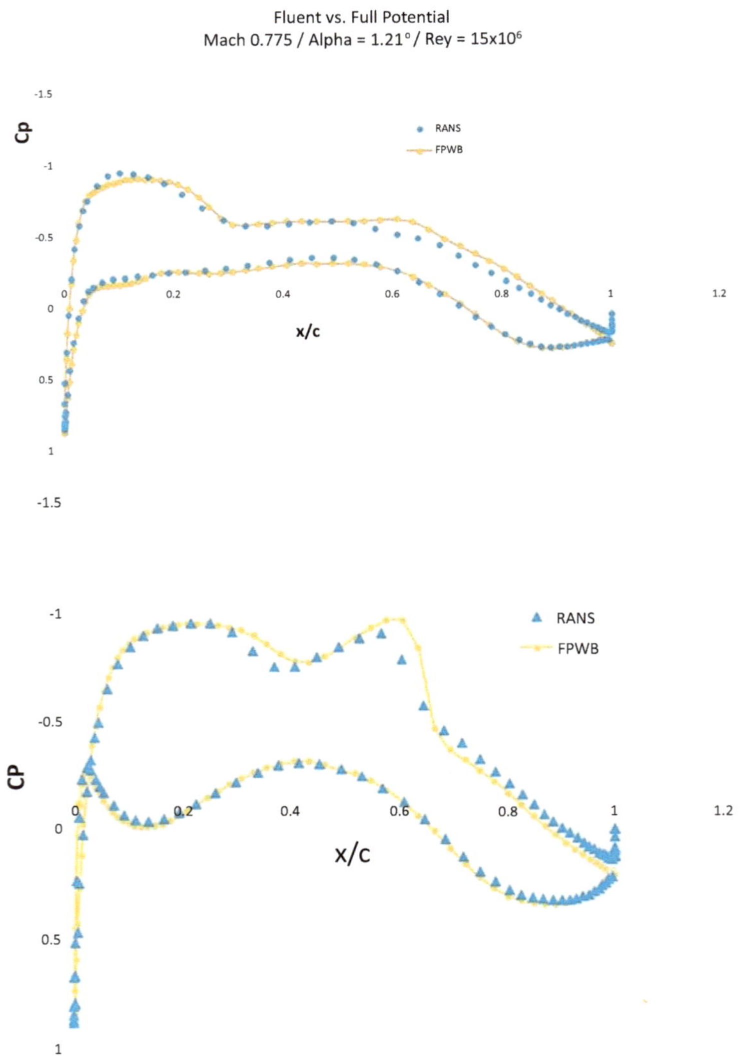

Fig. (4.10). Cp distributions obtained with a RANS code and a full potential one for the ITA50ADV airliner. At left, station a 22% of semispan; right, station located at 50% of semispan (Mach = 0.775, α=1.21°, Re=15x10[6]).

Numerous complex real-life problems have been addressed with optimization techniques. This approach has been adopted in many fields such as engineering, economics, and business, for problems that cannot be solved in a reasonable amount of time and at same time requiring a precise solution. Among other relevant aerospace applications, optimization techniques are employed to minimize engine emissions, noise footprint, development and production costs, or risk; and to maximize profit, performance, and aerodynamic efficiency. Indeed, aerospace problems are often highly nonlinear and encompass many disciplines and they are subjected to complex constraints. These constraints are either in the form of simple bounds such as flight quality, or in the form of nonlinear relationships such as maximum stress, maximum deflection, minimum noise levels, or geometrical configuration and topology.

Many optimization problems are solved by algorithms based on metaheuristics. Many fields including artificial intelligence, mathematical programming, and operational research utilize metaheuristics, which has been experiencing a huge development in the last 20 years [12]. Most metaheuristic algorithms are inspired by natural phenomena behaviors:

- Genetic Algorithm (GA) mimics the natural evolution process [13].
- Particle Swarm Optimization (PSO), proposed by Eberhart and Kennedy [14], is inspired by social behavior of flocks of birds searching for a landing spot.
- Every particle in the universe attracts every other particle, this rule based on the law of gravity and mass interactions is the one which Gravitational Search Algorithm (GSA) was developed [15].
- Developed by Karaboga, Artificial Bee Colony (ABC) models the foraging behavior of a bee colony [16].
- Ant colony (AC) is an optimization algorithm inspired by the foraging behavior of ant colonies [17].
- Cuckoo Search (CS) is another successful metaheuristic which mimics the cuckoo behavior reproduction strategy [18].
- ICA is the mathematical model and the computer simulation of human social evolution, while genetic algorithms are based on the biological evolution of species [19].
- Stocasthic Fractal Search (SFS) is based on the mathematical concept of fractal. Using the diffusion property seen regularly in random fractals, the particles in this algorithm explore the search space for an optimal solution [12].

Modern conceptual study employs multi-disciplinary design and optimization frameworks. They can handle diversity of configurations and the complex set of requirements that are embedded in aircraft design, including noise and emission constraints. Those frameworks embody several disciplines, including operational cost, and integrated them to comply with constrains and to search for optimal configurations under a multi-objective approach (Fig. **4.11**). Numerical optimization methods were initially applied to the design of optimally shaped airfoil sections. As computational capabilities increased, aerodynamicists tackled the design of optimally shaped wings. Recent advances in computer hardware and in parallel computing methods have placed engineers at the threshold of optimizing the shape of an entire aircraft configuration with a multi-disciplinary approach. The concept of system engineering and optimization has resulted in the inclusion of a host of engineering and non-engineering disciplines like manufacturing and program financial analysis under the umbrella of multidisciplinary design optimization.

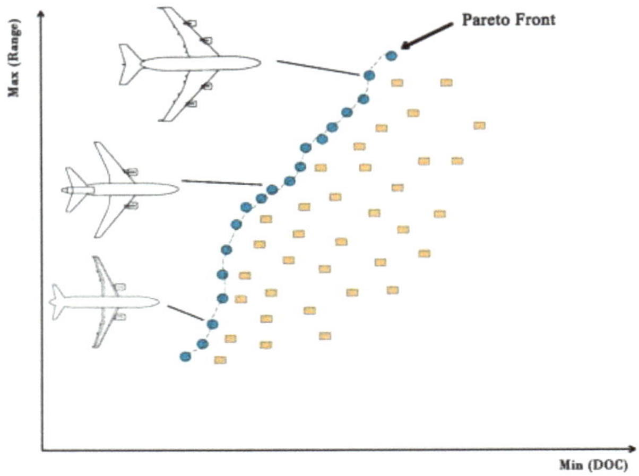

Fig. (4.11). Multi-disciplinary and multi-objective optimization is part of modern aircraft conceptual design as shown in this illustration.

After this phase, aircraft must look roughly according to Fig. **(4.12)**.

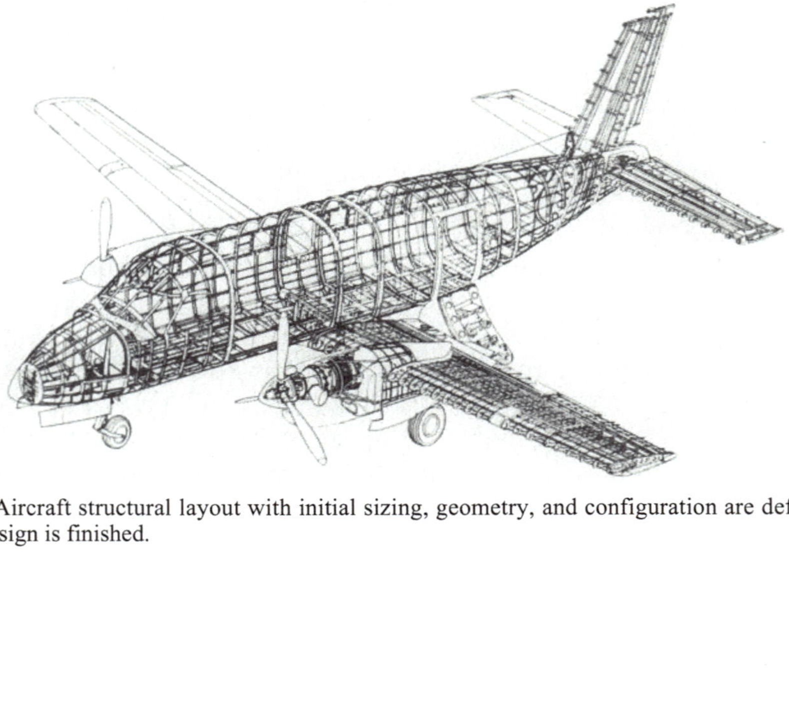

Fig. (4.12). Aircraft structural layout with initial sizing, geometry, and configuration are defined after the conceptual design is finished.

Preliminary Design

During preliminary design, one or more promising concepts from the conceptual design phase are subjected to more rigorous analysis and evaluation to define and validate the design that best meets the requirements. Extensive experimental efforts, including wind-tunnel testing and evaluation of any unique materials or structural concepts, are conducted during preliminary design so that key issues are addressed. All critical engineering problems are solved. The final product of preliminary design is a complete aircraft design description including all systems, and subsystems and their integration. The following items illustrate some of the deliverables of this phase (Figs. **4.13** - **4.18**):

- **Ground Servicing**

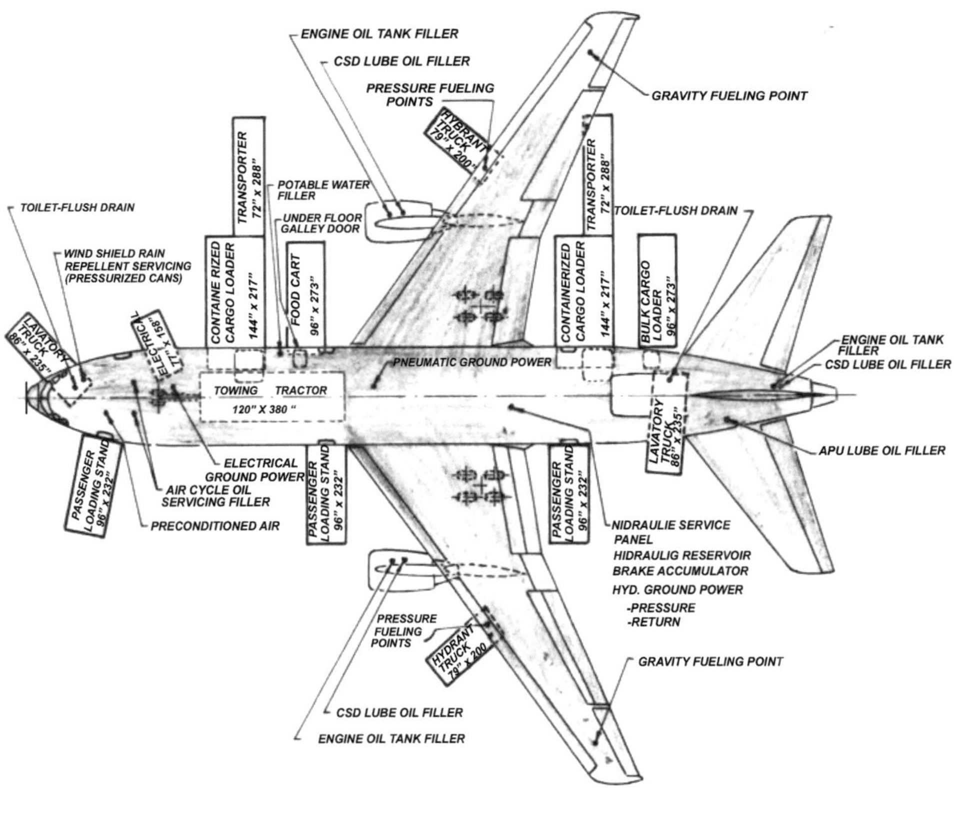

Fig. (4.13). Equipment for servicing a transport airplane on ground (Source: ITA/IEAP, Teodoro, 1971).

• Landing Gear Retraction and Accommodation

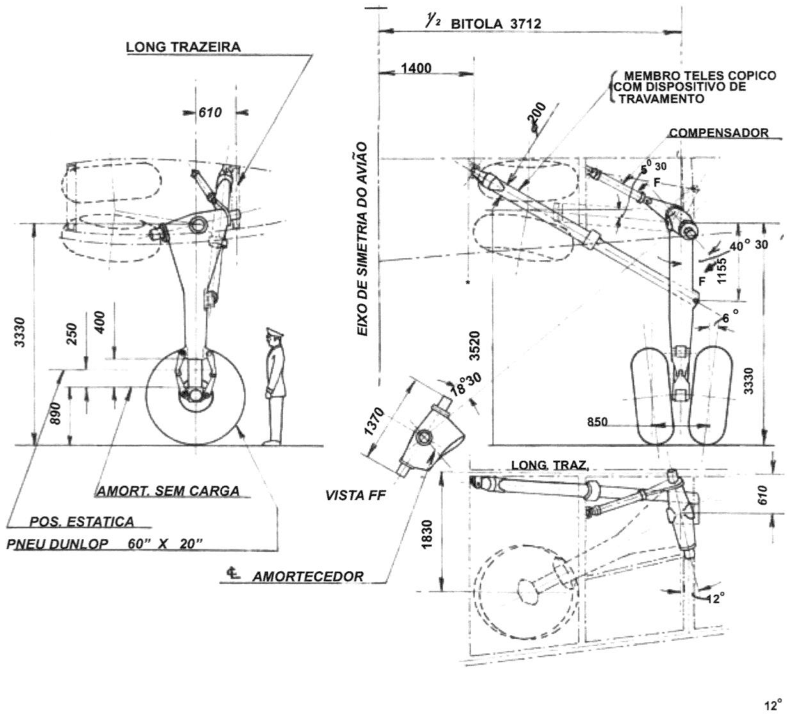

• Command Surfaces and High-lift System

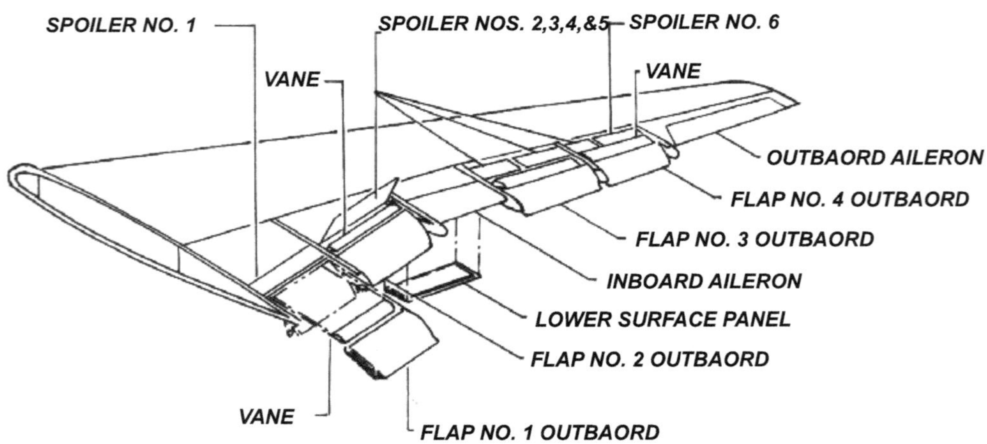

Fig. (4.15). Aileron, spoliler, flaps, and slats must be defined in the preliminary design phase (Source: ITA/IEAP, Teodoro, 1971).

- **Access to Aircraft Structure and its Systems**

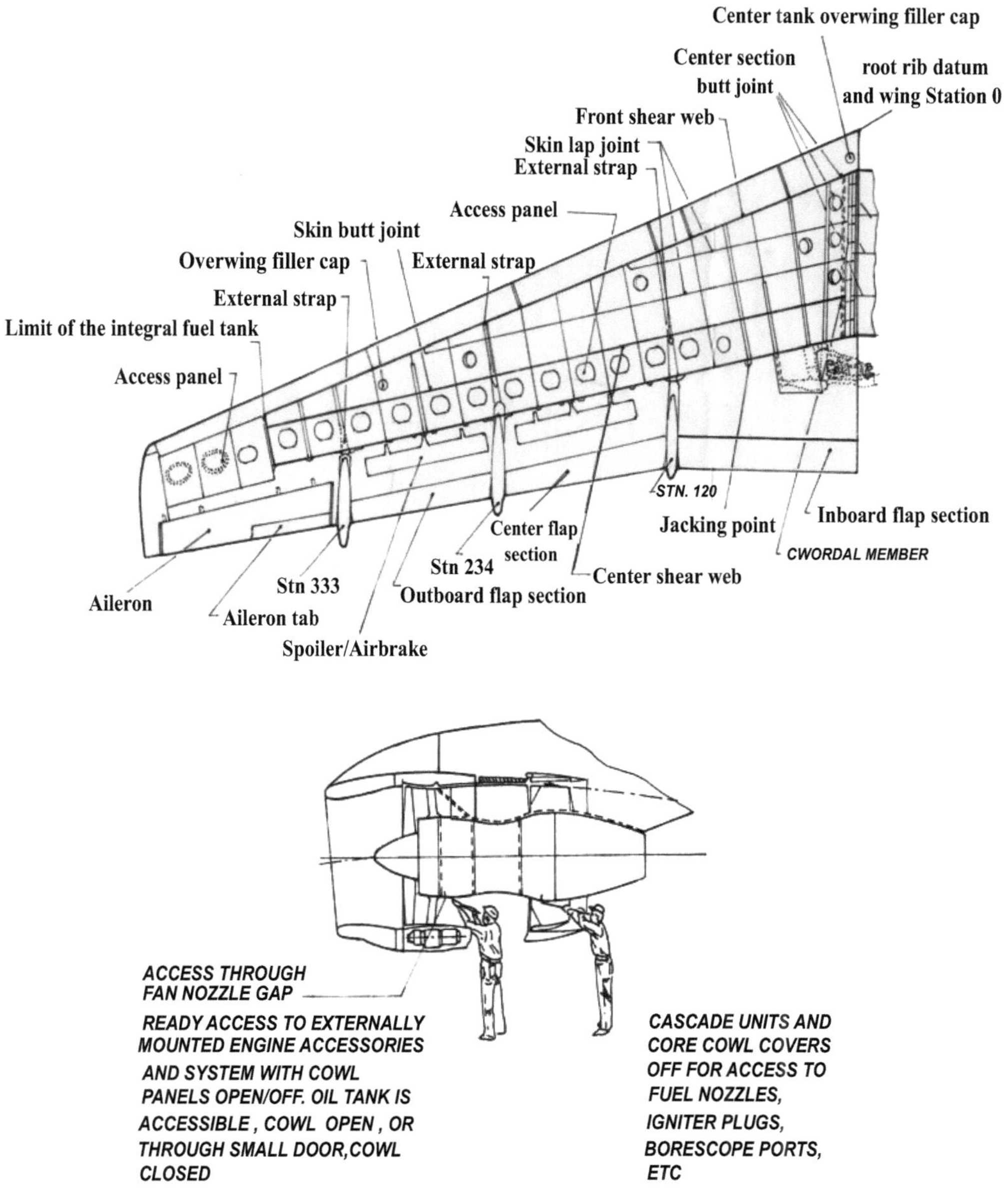

Fig. (4.16). Access to wing structure and engine (Source: ITA/IEAP, Teodoro, 1971).

• More Detailed Aircraft Structure

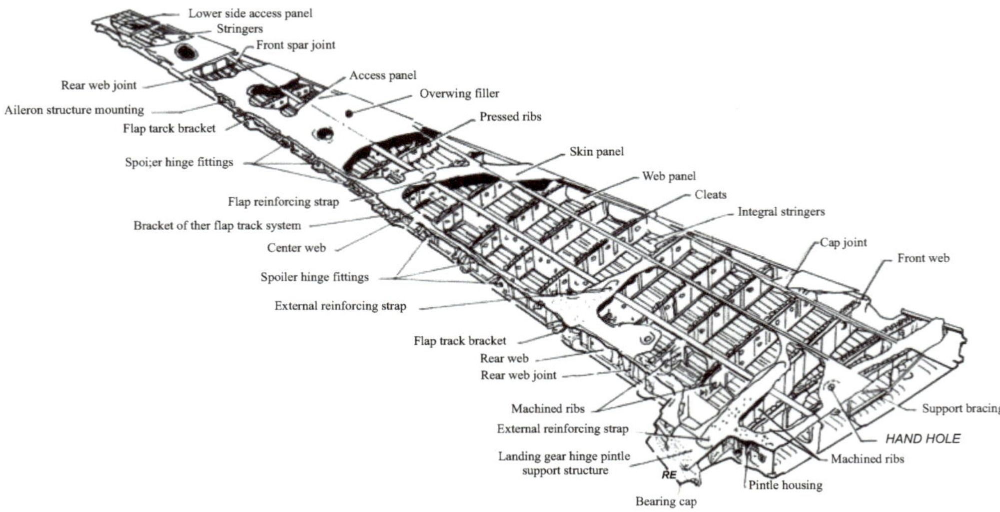

Fig. (4.17). Example of wing structure (Source: ITA/IEAP).

• System Integration

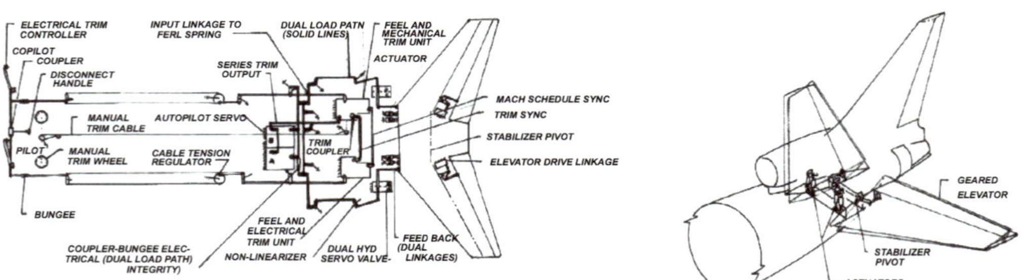

Horizontal stablizer and elevon actuation system

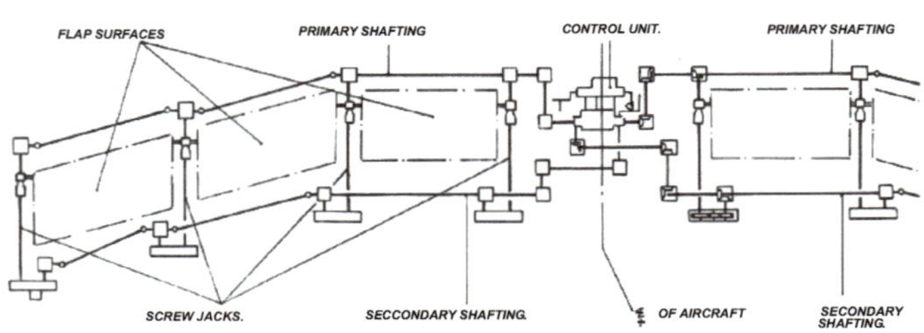

Flap actuation and retracting system

Fig. 4.18 contd.....

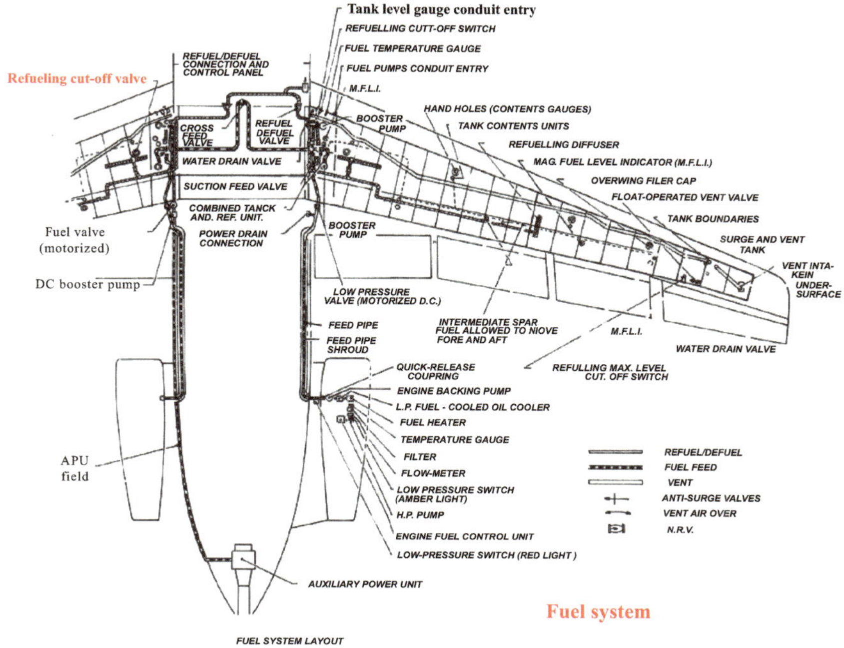

Fig. (4.18). Preliminary design is also concerned with system integration (Source: ITA/IEAP, Horley, 1971).

Detailed Design

During detailed design, the selected aircraft design is translated into the detailed engineering data required to support tooling and manufacturing activities. This process makes intensive use of tools such as CAD (Computer Aided Design). After freezing the airplane configuration, manufacturers move on to detail even further airplane parts and virtually assemble them using Computer Aided Design and Virtual Reality tools, so that a complete digital mock-up (DMU) of the airplane is obtained. The creation of a highly detailed single mock-up that is shared by all helps to speed up development, as everyone on the program – no matter where they are located – can work as a virtual team, sharing the very latest information during each phase of development and manufacturing. The DMU's functionality extends through to simulating and validating the industrial manufacturing processes at an early stage in development. It can also be used to show airlines what their aircraft's interior will look like, and even to train maintenance teams in advance. In addition, DMU is also useful to avoid spatial mismatch between elements of aircraft systems. (Fig. **4.19**)

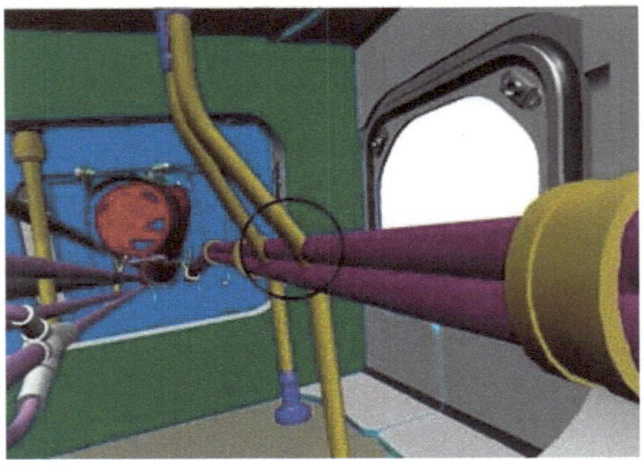

Fig. (4.19). Digital mock up is useful for identifying spatial mismatch between components of aircraft systems.

Other tools such as Virtual Reality may be used to assist engineers finalize the design (Fig. **4.20**). At this stage, parts start to be manufactured and the first prototypes are built. With the prototypes, the manufacturers start to test the airplane to validate assumptions and choices made during the previous phases. The aim of rig, ground, and flight-testing is to obtain a type certificate issued by certification authorities so that the airplane can be put into serial production, manufactured and delivered to owners and operators.

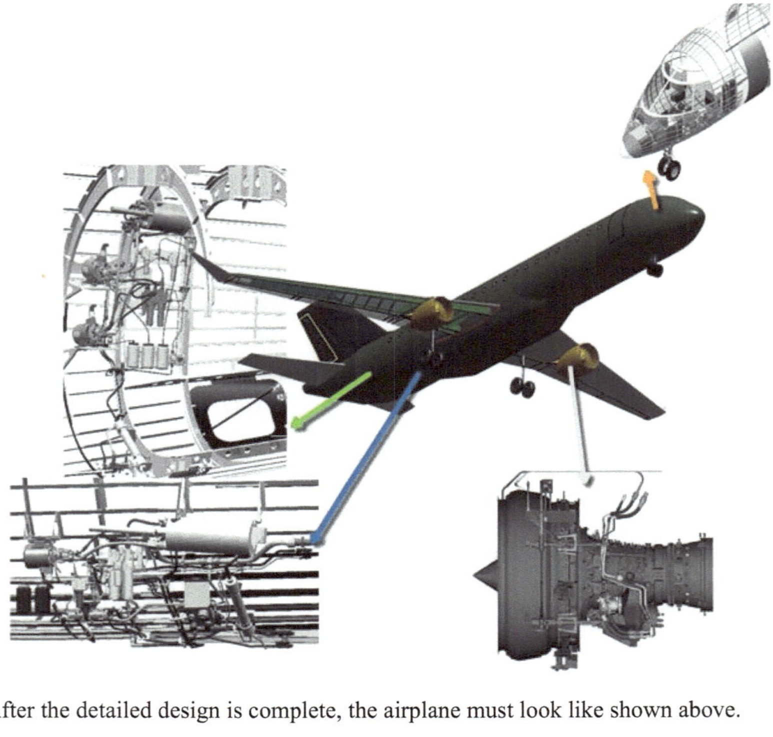

Fig. (4.20). After the detailed design is complete, the airplane must look like shown above.

Production

Materials

Weight is a critical issue for aerial vehicles. Aerospace manufacturers have developed new techniques for modifying the characteristics of materials that are employed in aerospace structures.

A composite material typically consists of relatively strong, stiff fibers in a tough resin matrix. The fibers are set into resin to form sheets which are laid on top of each other, bonded and then heated in a large oven, or "autoclave". The main materials used in aerospace composite structures are carbon- and glass-fiber reinforced plastic. They have several advantages over traditional aluminum alloys. As carbon composites are, in general, only 60% of the aluminum density and they provide a much better strength-to-weight ratio than metals: sometimes by as much as 20%. They can also be formed into more complex shapes than their metallic counterparts, reducing the number of fuselage parts and the need for fasteners and joints. Fig. (**4.21**) shows the percentage of composites used in modern aircraft [20]. Fig. (**4.22**) illustrates the distribution of materials that compose the structure of a proposed 150-seat airliner (a graduate student concept study).

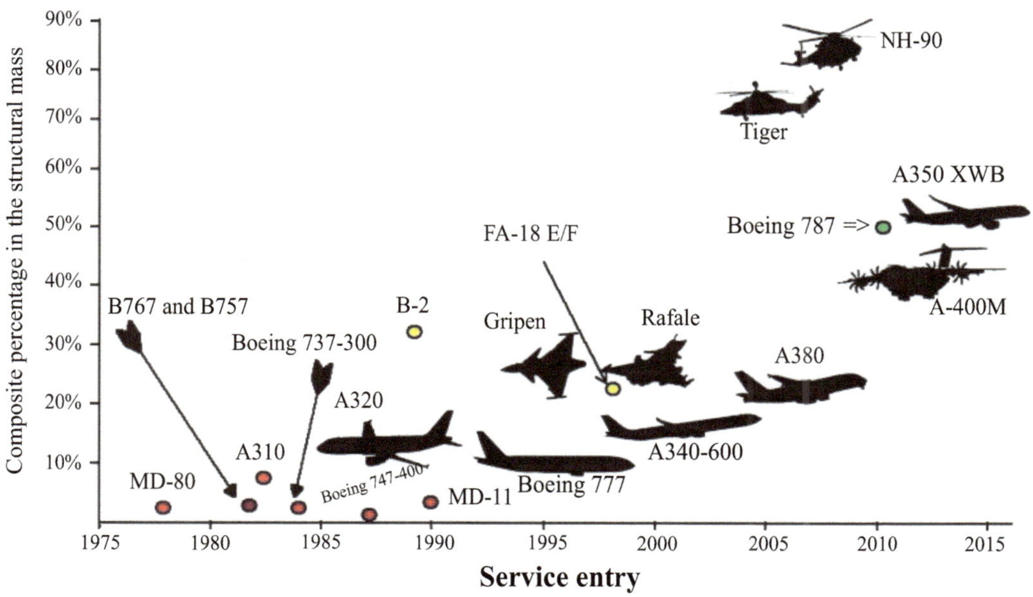

Fig. (4.21). Composite percentage employed in modern aircraft (Based on Planet Aerospace's data).

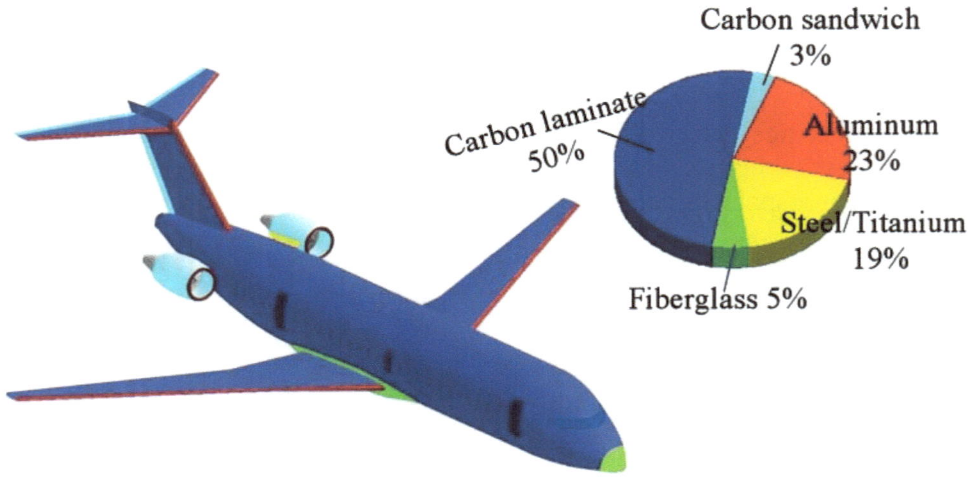

Fig. (4.22). materials considered for a 150-seat airliner concept.

The so-called honeycomb sandwich, which is far lighter than a metal plate of comparable thickness and has greater resistance to bending, consists of a honeycomb core, composed of rows of hollow hexagonal cells, bonded between extremely thin metal face sheets. Aluminum is the most extensively used metal in both core and face sheets, but the technique is applicable to a large variety of metallic and nonmetallic materials. Sandwich construction is now employed to some degree in almost every type of flight vehicle.

The strength/weight ratio is used as prime driver for material selections for both engines and aircraft [21]. This is still the first order of importance, alongside ease of assembly. However, although a lightweight structure is necessary, it is not sufficient anymore. Design criteria have become much more complex and multi-disciplinary and competitive aircraft now require innovative design methods as well as improved material and processing methods [21].

Materials play a key role not only in the fabrication methods used but also in the safety measures employed. For example, beryllium, whose combination of light weight, high strength, and high melting point makes it a valuable structural material, yields dust and chips during machining [22]. Because exposure to beryllium particles can cause adverse health effects, exceptional care is required to preclude their contamination of personnel or atmosphere [22]. Polymer-matrix composites also require special contamination protection because of the toxic character of the resins involved. Polymer-matrix composites are valued in the aerospace industry for their stiffness, lightness, and heat resistance. They are fabricated materials in which carbon, glass or Kevlar fibers (and sometimes metallic strands, filaments, or particles) are bonded together by polymer resins in either sheet or fiber-wound form. In the former, individual sheet elements are layered in metal, wood, or plastic molds and joined with adhesives. Applications for sheet composites include wing skins and fuselage bulkheads in aircraft and the underlying support for solar arrays in satellites. In fiber-wound forms, tubular or spherical shapes are fabricated by winding continuous fiber on a spinning mold (mandrel) with high-speed, computer-programmed precision, injecting liquid resin as the part is formed, and then curing the resin. This process is used for forming rocket motor casings; spherical containers for fuels, lubricants, and gases; and ducts for aircraft environmental systems.

Composites, making for lighter and more fuel-efficient aircraft, comprised roughly 50% of the airframe structure of Boeing's B787 Dreamliner (by weight), compared to about 5% in the original Boeing 747-100 from the late 1960s. Boeing itself lists its materials by weight as 50% composite, 20% aluminum, 15% titanium, 10% steel, and 5% other [23].

According to Boeing, experience with the Boeing 777 airliner demonstrated that composite structures require less scheduled maintenance than non-composite structures [23]. Although the 777 composite vertical tail is 25 percent larger than the 767 tail, which is made from aluminum, it requires 35 percent fewer scheduled maintenance labor hours [23]. This labor hour reduction is due to the result of a reduced risk of corrosion and fatigue of composites compared to metal [23].

Carbon and glass fiber composites - and, potentially more common - ceramic and metal matrix composites, are now being applied in an increasing number of airplane parts, including secondary structures, wing and fuselage and engine fan blades. In 2012, the global aerospace composites market was estimated at US$10.3 billion and demand for composite aircraft engine structures alone is forecast to grow by 7% annually through 2016 [24].

Batteries are used to power airplanes before the auxiliary power unit (APU) or engines are started. They also support ground operations such as refueling and powering brake systems when airplane is towed. However, the key role of batteries is to provide backup power for critical systems during flight in the extremely unlikely event of a power failure.

Lithium-ion batteries are used in many aircraft today. They present many advantages over traditional Ni-Cd batteries, such as:

- Higher power density, which is translated into smaller volume and weight (over 50% reduction compared to Ni-Cd batteries).

- Absence of lithium metal.
- Absence of toxic materials like cadmium, mercury and lead.
- No free liquids because of the use of a solid polymer electrolyte.
- No gas exerting pressure.
- No thermal runaway. Thermal runaway refers to a situation where an increase in temperature changes the conditions in a way that causes a further increase in temperature, often leading to a destructive result. It is a kind of uncontrolled positive feedback.
- No problem when submitted to incineration. No risk of explosion when batteries are exposed to short circuits, nail punctures, water immersion, overcharge, over discharge, and hydraulic pressures up to 1500 psi.
- Low-level heat generation.
- Operation at higher temperatures.
- Higher voltage. A single lithium ion cell generates a 3.7 V tension (average value), which is equal to either three nickel-cadmium or nickel-metal hydride cells serially connected.
- Long life cycle.
- No memory effects.
- Fast recharge.

The Boeing Company introduced several innovations into its Boeing 787 Dreamliner. Among 787 flight systems, a key change from traditional airliners is the electrical architecture. Bleed air and hydraulic power sources were replaced by electrically powered compressors and pumps, eliminating pneumatics and hydraulics from some subsystems, *e.g.*, engine starters or brakes [23]. However, in the first year of service, at least four 787 aircraft suffered from electrical system problems stemming from its lithium-ion batteries and the fleet was grounded. The Federal Aviation Administration (FAA) decided on April 19, 2013 to allow US Dreamliners to return to service after modifications were incorporated into their battery systems to better contain battery fires [25]. However, there are still concerns because the primary cause of the fires was not identified.

Nanotechnology is slowly being incorporated in aircraft - for example, carbon nano-tube-based materials or nanocoatings on electro-chromatic windows. EasyJet was among the first commercial airlines to use a “nano-coating” on its planes - a polymer coating used over a conventional film that repels dirt and dust to reduce drag, cutting fuel consumption [24].

Many materials used in the manufacturing process do not become part of the final airframe. Aircraft manufacturers may have tens of thousands of individual products approved for use in the manufacturing. A large quantity and variety of solvents are used, with environmentally damaging variants such as methyl ethyl ketone and Freon being replaced with more environmentally friendly solvents. Chromium- and nickel-containing steel alloys are used in tooling, and cobalt- and tungsten carbide-containing hard-metal bits are used in cutting tools. Lead, formerly used in metal-forming processes, is now rarely used, having been replaced with kirksite [20]. In total, the aerospace industry uses more than 5,000 chemicals and mixtures of chemical compounds, most from multiple suppliers, and with many compounds containing between five to ten ingredients [22].

Tooling

Aircraft manufacturing utilizes dedicated tooling in the assembly process to ensure the attainment of assembly tolerances and product quality. External surfaces are subjected to aerodynamic tolerances, in addition to assembly ones. The tighter the aerodynamic tolerance is, the costlier the manufacturing process is. Dedicated tooling clamps the aircraft parts to be assembled into the jig to enable assembly by riveting. However, increased competition in the aircraft industry has driven the need to improve assembly quality while reducing cost and, in turn, the need for innovative solutions to accomplish this. Today, robots are used to produce parts with increased accuracy. Due to the small product volumes in the aircraft industry, the jigs must be flexible to assemble more than one structure in each jig. Modern tooling also uses adjustable multi-point tooling technology. This innovative approach embraces the development of digitally adjustable multi-point tooling, the innovation of flexible fabrication tooling, applications of dieless forming tooling and jigless positioning tooling.

Assembly

Contrary to the automotive industry, where a vehicle is produced every minute, and approximately 1,000 cars are manufactured a day, an aircraft assembly line with high production rates produces one airplane per day. Assembly begins with the build-up of component parts into sub-assemblies. Major sub-assemblies include wings, stabilizers, fuselage sections, landing gear, doors and interior components. Wing assembly is particularly intensive, requiring many holes to be precisely drilled and counter-sunk in the skins, through which later rivets are driven. The finished wing is cleaned and sealed from the inside to ensure a leak-proof fuel compartment. Final assembly takes place in huge assembly halls (Fig. **4.23**), some of which are among the world's largest manufacturing buildings.

The assembly line comprises several sequential positions where the airframe remains for several days to more than a week while predetermined functions are performed. Numerous assembly operations take place simultaneously at each position, creating the potential for cross exposures to chemicals. Parts and sub-assemblies are moved on dollies, custom-built carriers and by overhead crane to the appropriate position. The airframe is moved between positions by overhead crane until the landing gears are installed. Subsequent movements are made by towing. During final assembly, the fuselage sections are riveted together around a supporting structure. Floor beams and stringers are installed and the interior coated with a corrosion-inhibiting compound. Fore and aft fuselage sections are joined to the wings and wing stub (a box-like structure that serves as a main fuel tank and the structural center of the aircraft). The fuselage interior is covered with blankets of fiberglass insulation, electrical wiring and air ducts are installed and interior surfaces are covered with decorative paneling. Storage bins, typically with integrated passenger lights and emergency oxygen supplies, are then installed. Pre-assembled seating, galleys and lavatories are moved by hand and secured to floor tracks, permitting the rapid reconfiguration of the passenger cabin to conform to air carrier needs. Powerplants and landing and nose gear are mounted, and avionic components are installed. The functioning of all components is thoroughly tested prior to towing the completed aircraft to a separate, well-ventilated paint hanger, where a protective primer coat is applied, followed by a decorative top-coat of urethane or epoxy paint. Prior to delivery of the aircraft, it is put through a rigorous series of ground and flight tests.

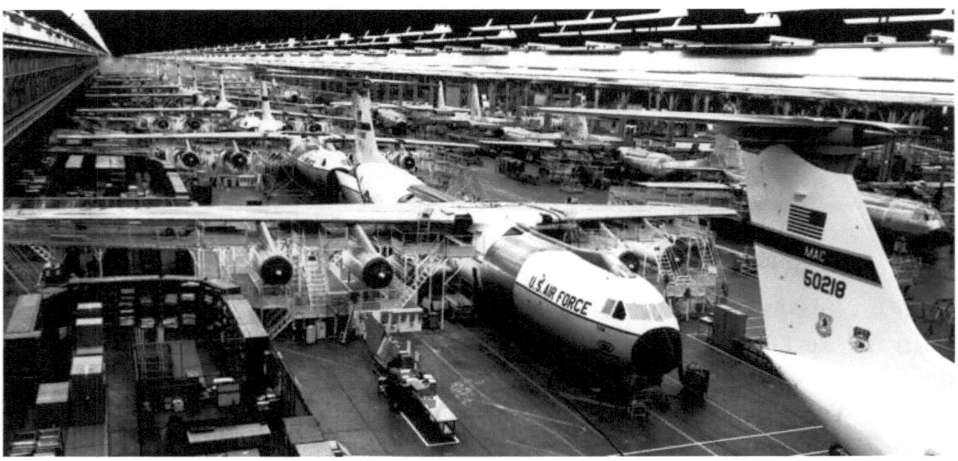

Fig. (4.23). Assembly Lockheed C-141 Starlifter aircraft plant in 1980 (Photo William G. Holder, public domain, via Wikimedia Commons).

A new, empty Boeing 777 weighs 166,441 kg and includes about 3 million parts [26]. Boeing employs a moving assembly line for the 777 twinjet, which is moved at 4.1 to 4.6 centimeters per minute during production [26]. According to Boeing, a moving line is a powerful tool available to identify and eliminate waste in a production system [26]. The manufacturer also states that it also drives efficiency throughout the system because it makes problems visible and creates a sense of urgency to fix the root causes of those problems. The moving line shortened the 777 final assembly process, the time it takes between the arrival of initial fuselage sections into systems installation to the day the completed jetliner rolls out the factory doors, from 26 days to 17 days [26].

Airbus' final assembly line in Toulouse for its A350 XWB airliner was conceived to present the lowest environmental footprint of any final assembly line ever built by Airbus [27]. The 72,000-m^2, L-shaped facility houses the initial stages of final assembly, involving the join-up of fuselage and wings. The assembly process for the A350 XWB allows teams to work in parallel, reducing the time from start of final assembly to aircraft delivery by 30 percent [27]. With a new lighting system, roof-mounted photovoltaic solar panels, translucent panels and glass arched roofs, the assembly facility can produce the equivalent of more than 50 per cent of its own energy [27]. Further increasing its status as the "greenest" final assembly line ever built by Airbus, many of the materials present on this site were recycled during the construction work.

Modern assembly lines use robots for automatic riveting and painting. Robots are also used to perform waterproofing and pressurization tests on fuselages, doors and windows – a meticulous process that is taxing on the human body. The robot tracks the entire perimeter of the part, centimeter by centimeter, recording and listening for noise that would indicate a leak or hole in the airframe.

Aircraft Delivery

For the operator and owner of a new aircraft, it is very important that the aircraft is inspected and checked during the assembly and acceptance phases. There are many steps a future owner should take prior to taking delivery of an airplane, from signing up for post-delivery product support programs to coordinating with certification authorities to ensure Reduced Vertical Separation Minima (RVSM) approval.

Delivery is a very important task in aircraft production process. Before taking delivery of an aircraft and signing the transfer of the title, the customer airline carries out a complete and detailed check. It is represented by a team of experts whose assignment is to check the conformity of the aircraft with the contractual specification. The delivery phase is usually spread over four or five days on average, dependent upon aircraft size and characteristics. A standard delivery procedure takes place as follows:

- 1st round: ground checks: external surfaces, bays and cabin visual inspection, static aircraft system and cockpit checks, engine tests.

- 2nd round: acceptance flight: checks during flight of all aircraft systems (including cabin systems) and aircraft behavior in the whole flight envelope. The aircraft evaluation flight is known as production flight.
- 3rd round: physical rework or provision of solutions for all technical and quality issues open in delivery.
- 4th round: completion of technical acceptance. Technical closure of the aircraft and all associated documents attesting the aircraft's compliance to the type certificate and conformity to the technical specification allowing the issuance of the Certificate of Airworthiness.
- 5th round: transfer of the aircraft's title deeds to the customer airline: the aircraft changes owner. Preparation of the aircraft for the ferry flight to its home base.

CERTIFICATION PROCESS

Overview

The aircraft manufacturer must present the project under consideration to the certification authority. An applicant's formal application for a Type Certificate includes an airplane description with a three-view drawing. After reaching a sufficient degree of maturity, the certification team set rules that are applicable to the certification of this specific aircraft type (Certification basis). The certification authority and the manufacturer define and agree on the means to demonstrate compliance of the aircraft type with each requirement of the Certification Basis.

The Certification Program Plan (CPP) is a key document. It contains the proposed certification basis, including noise and emission requirements. The plan also contemplates special conditions, exemptions, and equivalent level of safety findings. The use of delegations/designees is also planned.

The aircraft manufacturer must demonstrate compliance of its product with regulatory requirements: the structure, engines, control systems, electrical systems and the flight performance and handling qualities are analyzed according to the certification basis. This compliance demonstration is carried out by analyses during ground testing, such as tests on the structure to withstand bird strikes, fatigue tests and ground vibration tests (GVT). In addition, there is an extensive and expensive flight test campaign. Experts from the certification authority perform a detailed examination of this compliance demonstration, by means of document reviews in their offices and by attending some of these compliance demonstrations (test witnessing). This is the longest and probably the most demanding phase of the certification process. In the case of large aircraft, the period to complete the compliance demonstration is set at five years, which may be extended, if necessary.

The TC data sheet is part of the TC and it document conditions and limitations to meet certification requirements. If technically satisfied with the compliance demonstration by the manufacturer, the certification authority closes the investigation and issues the TC. The post certification activities include the Type Inspection Report (TIR), Certification Summary Report (CSR), and Post Certification Evaluation. Fig. (**4.24**) provides a summary of the certification phases.

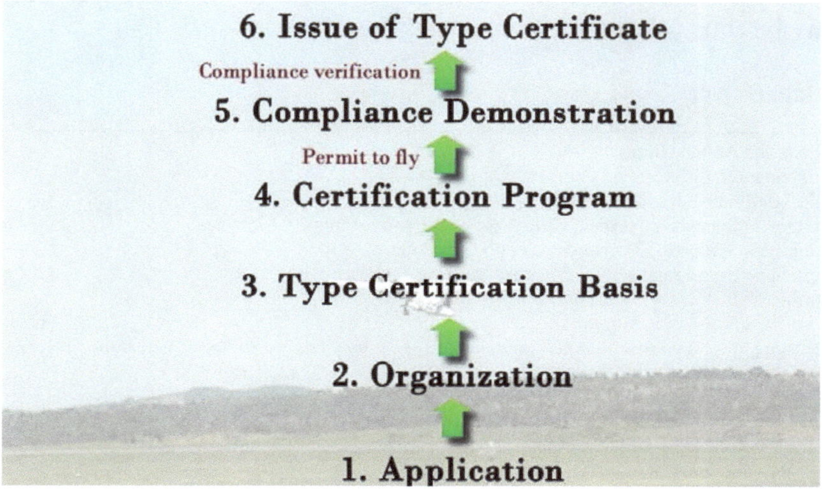

Fig. (4.24). Phases of certification process.

Certification Requirements

Each aviation authority defines its own set of requirements, which is organized into subsets covering the various aspects of aviation-related activities. One of the most comprehensive and well-organized set of requirements is that of the Federal Aviation Administration (USA), which is explained in the following paragraphs as an example.

Title 14 of the Code of Federal Regulations (14CFR) deals with aviation requirements [28]. Formerly known as Federal Aviation Regulations, or FARs, these rules prescribed by the Federal Aviation Administration (FAA) govern all aviation activities in the United States. A wide variety of activities are regulated, such as aircraft design and maintenance, typical airline flights, pilot training activities, hot-air ballooning, lighter-than-air aircraft, man-made structure heights, obstruction lighting and marking, and even model rocket launches, as well as model aircraft operation, and kite flying. These rules are designed to promote safe aviation, protecting pilots, flight attendants, passengers and the public from unnecessary risk. The FARs are organized into sections, called Parts, due to their organization within the CFR (Table **4.3**). Each part deals with a specific type of activity. For example, 14 CFR Part 141 contains rules for pilot training schools. The sections most relevant to aircraft pilots and AMTs (Aviation Maintenance Technicians) are listed in Table **4.3** [29]. Many parts of the FARs are designed to regulate certification of pilots, schools, or aircraft rather than the operation of airplanes [29]. Once an airplane design is certified by using some parts of these regulations, it is certified regardless of any future regulation changes. For that reason, newer planes are certified using newer versions of the FARs and in many aspects, may be thus considered safer designs.

Table 4.3. FAR Parts [29].

FAR Parts
Part 1 – Definitions and Abbreviations
Part 13 – Investigation and Enforcement Procedures
Part 21 – Certification Procedures for Products and Parts
Part 23 – Airworthiness Standards: Normal, Utility, Acrobatic and Commuter Airplanes
Part 25 – Airworthiness Standards: Transport Category Airplanes
Part 27 – Airworthiness Standards: Normal Category Rotorcraft
Part 29 – Airworthiness Standards: Transport Category Rotorcraft
Part 33 – Airworthiness Standards: Aircraft Engines
Part 34 – Fuel Venting and Exhaust Emission Requirements for Turbine Engine Powered Airplanes
Part 35 – Airworthiness Standards: Propellers
Part 39 – Airworthiness Directives
Part 43 – Maintenance, Preventive Maintenance, Rebuilding, and Alteration
Part 45 – Identification and Registration Marking
Part 47 – Aircraft Registration
Part 61 – Certification: Pilots, Flight Instructors, and Ground Instructors
Part 65 – Certification: Airmen Other Than Flight Crewmembers
Part 67 – Medical Standards and Certification
Part 71 – Designation of Class A, Class B, Class C, Class D, and Class E Airspace Areas; Airways; Routes; and Reporting Points
Part 73 – Special Use Airspace
Part 91 – General Operating and Flight Rules
Part 97 – Standard Instrument Approach Procedures
Part 101 – Moored Balloons, Kites, Unmanned Rockets and Unmanned Free Balloons
Part 103 – Ultralight Vehicles
Part 105 – Parachute Operations
Part 119 – Certification: Air Carriers and Commercial Operators
Part 121 – Operating Requirements: Domestic, Flag, and Supplemental Operations
Part 125 – Certification and Operations: Airplanes Having a Seating Capacity of 20 or More Passengers or a Payload Capacity of 6,000 lb or More
Part 129 – is a foreign carrier or operator of U.S. Aircraft
Part 133 – Rotorcraft External-Load Operations
Part 135 – Operating Requirements: Commuter and On Demand Operations and Rules Governing Persons on Board of Such Aircraft
Part 136 – Commercial Air Tours and National Parks Air Tour Management
Part 137 – Agricultural Aircraft Operations
Part 139 – Certification of Airports
Part 141 – Flight Schools
Part 142 – Training Centers
Part 145 – Repair Stations
Part 147 – Aviation Maintenance Technicians Schools
Part 183 – Representatives of The Administrator

FARs of direct interest for aircraft design are described in Part 21, 23, 25, 26, 27 and 29. They are described in the following paragraphs in more detail.

Part 21 – This Part describes the process to be followed to obtain a valid airworthiness type certificate.

Part 23 - Part 23 contains airworthiness standards for airplanes in the normal, utility, aerobatic, and commuter categories. It dictates the standards required for issuance and change of type certificates for airplanes in these categories. For instance, the maximum takeoff weight of an airplane in the normal, utility or acrobatic category cannot exceed 12,500 lb, while in the commuter category it may be up to 19,000 lb. This part has many regulations to ensure airworthiness in areas such as structural loads, airframe, controllability, performance, stability, and safety mechanisms, seat design, oxygen and air pressurization systems, fire prevention, escape hatches, flight management procedures, flight controls, communications, emergency landing procedures, and other limitations. In addition, it stipulates testing of all the aircraft systems. It also determines special aspects of aircraft performance such as stall speed (*e.g.*, for single engine airplanes – not more than 61 kts), rate of climb (not less than 300 ft/min), take-off speed, and weight of each pilot and passenger (170 lb for airplanes in the normal and commuter categories, and 190 lb for airplanes in the acrobatic and utility categories).

Cessna 177, EMBRAER Phenom 100, Cirrus SR20 and Piper PA-34 Seneca are well-known airplane types that were certificated according to FAR Part 23.

Most of the Federal Aviation Regulations, including Part 23, commenced on February 1, 1965. Prior to that date, airworthiness standards for airplanes in the normal, utility and acrobatic categories were promulgated in Part 3 of the US Civil Air Regulations. Many well-known types of light airplane are type certificated to CAR Part 3, even though they remained in production after 1965. For example, the Cessna 150 and Piper Cherokee are type certificated to CAR Part 3.

Part 25- This part contains airworthiness standards for airplanes in the transport category. Transport category airplanes are either:

- Jets with 10 or more seats or a maximum takeoff weight (MTOW) greater than 12,500 lb (5,670 kg); or
- Propeller-driven airplanes with greater than 19 seats or a MTOW greater than 19,000 lb (8,618 kg).

EMBRAER E-jets, Boeing 737 models, and Airbus A320 series, are well-known airplane types that were certificated to FAR Part 25.

Part 26 – This part covers the process and the requirements for continued airworthiness, which relate to changes and/or modifications to an already certificated aircraft.

Part 27 - This part contains airworthiness standards for rotorcraft in the normal category. Rotorcraft up to 7,000 lb Maximum Takeoff Weight (MTOW) and 9 or fewer passengers are type certified in this part. Examples of rotorcraft certified in this part are the Schweizer 300 and the Bell 429.

Part 29 – The applicability of these regulations is described below:

a. This part prescribes airworthiness standards for the issue of type certificates, and changes to those certificates, for transport category rotorcraft.
b. Transport category rotorcraft must be certificated in accordance with either the Category A or Category B requirements of this part. A multiengine rotorcraft may be type certificated as both Category A and Category B with appropriate and different operating limitations for each category.
c. Rotorcraft with a maximum weight greater than 20,000 lb and 10 or more passenger seats must be type certificated as Category A rotorcraft.
d. Rotorcraft with a maximum weight greater than 20,000 lb and nine or less passenger seats may be type certificated as Category B rotorcraft provided the Category A requirements of Subparts C, D, E, and F of this part are met.
e. Rotorcraft with a maximum weight of 20,000 lb or less but with 10 or more passenger seats may be type certificated as Category B rotorcraft provided the Category A requirements of §§29.67(a)(2), 29.87, 29.1517, and subparts C, D, E, and F of this part are met.
f. Rotorcraft with a maximum weight of 20,000 lb or less and nine or less passenger seats may be type certificated as Category B rotorcraft.
g. Each person who applies under Part 21 for a certificate or change described in paragraphs (a) through (f) of this section must show compliance with the applicable requirements of this part.

Environmental requirements: These are defined in Parts 34 (engine emissions) and 36 (noise). Aircraft designers must also pay close attention to the requirements contained in these Parts.

Operating Requirements: The airplane designer must also be familiar with operating requirements such as Parts 91, 121, and 135, as these requirements may impose constraints in aircraft design such as minimum cabin crew, fuel reserves, and landing distance factors among others. Part 91 contains the general requirements, which are applicable to all aircraft operations. Part 121 deals with commercial operations (essentially airline and charter operations) whereas Part 135 covers on-demand operations, such as that of air taxi companies.

Certification Tests

As part of the certification process, airplanes are flight tested to assess the outcome of all design choices. Such tests are usually divided into rig, ground and flight tests.

Rig testing is used to determine systems' characteristics and their integration. Each component, from the simplest (like a solenoid valve) to the most complex (such as a whole engine), must be tested within its defined operating range and specifications. It must be shown that the system is safe, reliable and works properly.

Ground testing consists of loads, materials and structures testing. Material properties, structure deformation under strain, fatigue testing, ground vibration tests (GVT), and landing gear drop tests are a few examples of ground testing.

Flight testing is performed to evaluate airplane aerodynamics, handling and performance. Tests, like braking, takeoff and landing, although performed on the ground, are also considered flight tests. As these tests deal primarily with the ultimate results of aircraft design, they will be discussed in more detail in the following paragraphs.

Aircraft manufacturer must build or contract the fabrication of test rigs to evaluate aircraft systems.

Bird strike can be critical for aircraft parts like the cockpit glazing and especially for engines and their first rotor, the engine fan. Regulations of certification authorities ensure a maximum of passenger safety, even when there is a major bird strike. According to current regulations, safe continuation of the flight must be guaranteed following a single bird strike. Specifically, Part 25 certification rules require that air transport aircraft can withstand impact at cruise speeds of a 4lb (1.8kg) bird on front part of the aircraft, including the windshields and wings, and an 8lb bird on the empennage. Despite all safety precautions, a multitude of bird strikes caused by a flock of bigger birds can in some seldom cases trigger a failure in one or even more engines. For any given impact, the most important determinant of damage potential is the speed of impact because the kinetic energy, which must be absorbed by the airframe or within the engine. The speed of the aircraft, rather than that of the bird, makes up nearly all the closing speed of impact so that, except for very small aircraft, aircraft speeds are directly proportional to the damage potential for collision with an object. Civil aircraft speeds are generally at their lowest where most birds are found - near the ground. Bird hazard disappears at somewhere above 2000 m.

Bird strike simulators or bird strike testing rigs can launch either real birds or gelatin substitutes at higher speeds, as, for instance, 650 km/h. For this reason, this testing apparatus is often called a "chicken gun." During tests, proximity sensors provide real-time velocity measurement of each shot. Data acquisition systems capture transient shock and load data, and high-speed video equipment monitors all impacts to provide important post-event analysis.

Iron Birds are used to minimize the development risk by testing fully integrated systems well in advance of the first test aircraft, but also to:

- Unload ground and flight testing.
- Perform Structural Fatigue.
- Conduct certification testing.

The primary focus of Iron Bird testing is to verify avionics, flight controls, landing gear, flight actuation components, and hydraulics, power systems, Heating, Ventilating and Air Conditioning (HVAC) Systems, *etc.*

Iron bird is a very important tool to confirm the characteristics of all system components, or to discover an incompatibility that may require modifications during early development stages. Additionally, the effects and subsequent treatment of failures introduced in the systems can be studied in full detail and recorded for analysis by using the Iron Bird as a testbed. Since all aircraft systems are controlled from the flight deck, the Iron Bird requires a cockpit for its control, which could be provided by flight simulators of fixed base, along with a mobile visual system.

Aircraft certification requires a costly an extensive flight test campaign. The airplane must exhibit acceptable flying qualities at the most critical loading within the ranges of speed and altitude for which certification is requested. The airline pilot is provided with a safe operational flight envelope (bounded by certificated limits) that must be thoroughly explored during flight-testing. The airplane is also test flown outside its operational envelope to account for inadvertent excursions beyond the certificated limits. Regarding handling qualities, the flight tests have the following goals:

- To demonstrate that the airplane can be safely controllable and maneuverable.
- To assure that no exceptional piloting skill, alertness and strength are required to fly the aircraft.
- To certify that the crew is capable of continued safe flight and landing following

any single failure or combination of failures not shown to be extremely improbable.

- The flying qualities requirements must be demonstrated throughout the flight envelope.

A typical handling qualities test campaign would address the following tests:

- Static, dynamic, and maneuvering stability.
- Longitudinal, directional and lateral control.
- Minimum control speeds.
- Trim and out-of-trim characteristics.
- Stall characteristics.
- Ground handling.
- Cross-wind.
- Buffeting and high-speed characteristics.

Several tests are carried out to determine the airplane flight performance. They are associated with flight phases:

- Takeoff tests
  - Takeoff speeds
  - Accelerate - Go
  - Accelerate - Stop
- Climb
  - Excess thrust and climb performance
  - Climb and cruise drag polars
- En Route (Engine performance, fuel consumption)
- Approach
  - Approach climb
  - Missed approaches
- Landing
  - Landing climb
  - Air, transition and braking distances

Performance testing involves assessment of the extremes of airplane operation. As such, these tests are often classified as substantial risk, both for the crew and the equipment. One of such tests is the accelerate-stop. In aviation terminology, a rejected takeoff (RTO) or aborted takeoff is the situation in which the pilot decides to abort the takeoff of an airplane. There can be many reasons for deciding to perform a rejected takeoff, but they are usually due to suspected or actual technical failures, like an engine failure. A rejected takeoff is normally performed only if the aircraft speed is below the takeoff decision speed (V_1), which is calculated before each flight begins. Below the decision speed, the airplane should be able to stop safely before the end of the runway. Above the decision speed, the airplane may overshoot the runway if the takeoff is aborted and therefore RTO should not be performed above this speed, unless the crew becomes aware that the airplane cannot fly. Single-engine aircraft rejects any takeoff after an engine failure, regardless of speed. Even if the airplane is already airborne and sufficient runway remains, an attempt to land straight ahead on the runway may be performed. This may also br applied to some light twin engine airplanes. Before the takeoff roll is started, the autobrake system of the aircraft, if available, is set to the RTO mode. The autobrake system will automatically apply maximum brakes if throttle is reduced to idle or reverse thrust during the takeoff roll. An RTO is usually seen as one of the hardest tests an airplane should undergo for its certification trials. RTO tests are performed under the worst possible conditions, with fully worn out brakes, the plane loaded to maximum takeoff weight and without use of thrust reversers. During an RTO test, most of the kinetic energy of the airplane is converted into heat by the brakes, which may cause the fusible plugs of the tires to melt, causing them to deflate. Small brake fires are acceptable if they do not spread to the airplane body within five minutes (the maximum likely time for arrival of the airport fire fighters).

The aircraft manufacturer should demonstrate that its product can be safely operated on wet runways. The water ingestion test validates how the aircraft would behave on a very rain-soaked runway, and verifies that neither the water under the aircraft nor the spray generated by the nose landing gear will enter the engines or APU. For the test, the "water trough" was created by applying to the runway's surface grooves and rubber strips inserted in the grooves to retain the water. The aircraft being evaluated must perform several runs as planned to test various cases, including the use of reverse thrust. According to Airbus, in the case of Airbus A350 evaluation (Fig. **4.25**), this pool measured 100 m long by 29 m wide [27].

VMU means mini5um unstick speed. It is the calibrated airspeed at and above which the airplane can safely lift off the ground and continue the takeoff. VMU speeds must be selected by the manufacturer throughout the range of thrust-t--weight ratios to be certified. Ground takeoff tests, where the airplane hits the ground are used to obtain these VMUs (Fig. **4.26**). These test series are one of the most demanding maneuvers of the entire test-program. The aerodynamic effect of the rudder is severely restricted due to the extremely low speed. There was the theoretical risk of seriously damaging the prototype, which could delay the entire certification program.

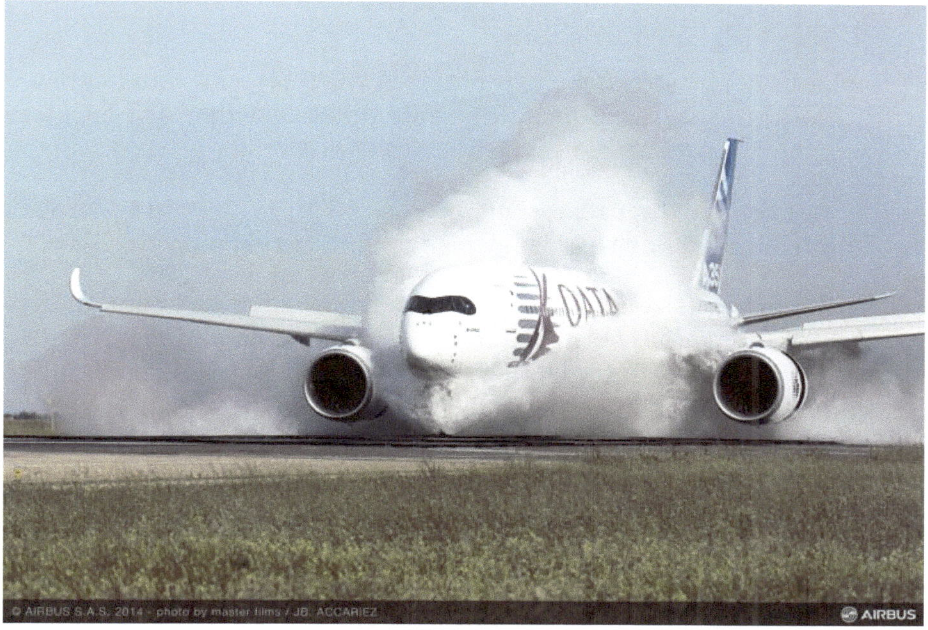

Fig. (4.25). Water ingestion test (Courtesy Airbus with permission).

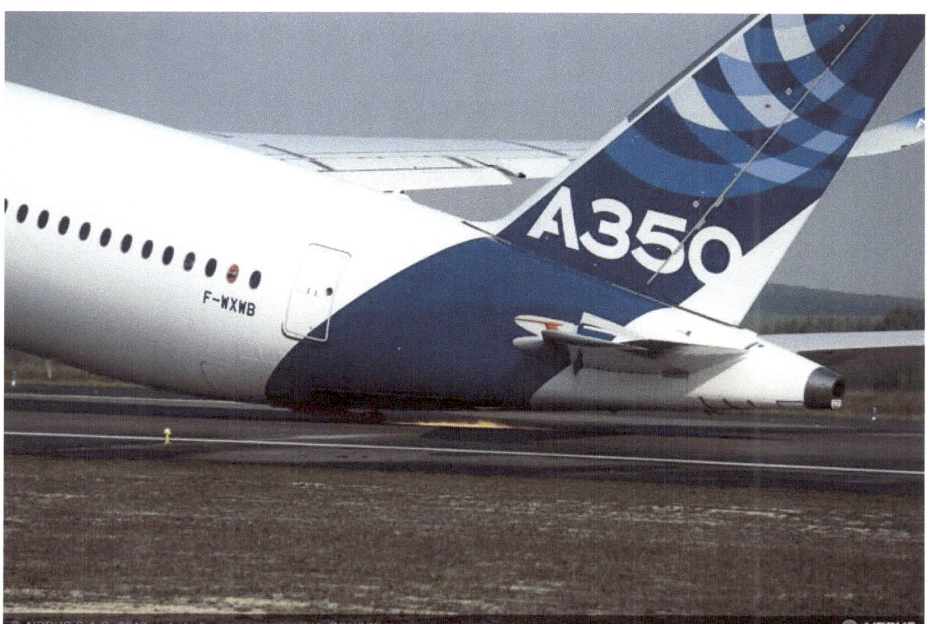

Fig. (4.26). Minimum unstick speed tests are required to obtain type certificate (Courtesy Airbus with permission).

CONCLUSION

The design phases of comercial aircraft program were described and commented. The certification process, its aplicability and flight test that are necessary to certify a commercial airplane comprised a large part of the present Chapter.

Considering that certification represents a great effort in designing airplanes, a brief description of regulations and some testing was carried out.

During the Cold War, a strong scientific and technological competition between Western countries and the former Soviet Union took place. The landing of manned crew on moon, the Internet, the Concorde supersonic airliner, all of this and much more are product from the Cold War. After the fall of the Berlin wall in 1989, the funding of military aircraft projects decreased substantially and most airlines lost their governmental protection in form of subsidies. This originated a deep impact on civil aircraft programs, that lost innovation content.

Multi-disciplinary optimization techniques have became a standard tool for engineering design. It was a long path for these methods to become well-used, and they, still, are not used everywhere. There are a host of reasons. First, the analysis, itself, of a complete aircraft configuration is rather complex, even without the optimization. Program size and complexity are such that only very well-documented and well-maintained computer programs can be used. These programs are often written by many people over many years and it is very difficult for an individual to know what the program can and cannot do. Many grandiose plans for completely integrated aircraft design systems have fallen by the wayside because they quickly become unmanageable. Although there is still a huge work to develop and turn fully functional efficient multi-disciplinary optimization they already belong to the evereday of large aerospace companies.

REFERENCES

[1] F. Quentin, "ACARE: The European Technology Platform for Aeronautics,", In: *Seminar of the Industrial Leaders of European technology Platforms*. Brussels, 2007

[2] M. Thurber, "The Aircraft Certification Process", Aviation International News, 2006. [Online]. Available: http://www.ainonline.com/ aviation-news/ aviation-international-news/ 2006-12-18/ aircraft- certification-process [Accessed December 2006].

[3] EMBRAER SA, *EMBRAER ERJ 170/190 Progress Report.* vol. Vol. 1. EMBRAER Newsletter: São José dos Campos, 1999.

[4] EMBRAER SA, *LOT Polish Airlines Welcomes its First EMBRAER 170 Jet* EMBRAER Press Release: São José dos Campos, 2004.

[5] C. Harress, "Boeing 787: A Complete Timeline of The Dreamliner's Legacy Of Failure, After Cracks Discovered In Wings", [Online]. Available: http://www.ibtimes.com/ boeing-787- complete-timeline-dreamliners- legacy-failure- after-cracks- discovered-wings- 1560491

[6] Wikipedia, "Boeing 787 Dreamliner", Wikipedia, the Free Encyclopedia, 2017. [Online]. Available: https://en.wikipedia.org/wiki/Boeing_787_Dreamliner. [Accessed 2017].

[7] L.R. Jenkinson, P. Simpkin, and D. Rhodes, *Civil Jet Aircraft Design.* Arnold Publishers, 1999. [http://dx.doi.org/10.2514/4.473500]

[8] J.G. Wensveen, *Air Transportation – A Management Perspective.* AshGate Publishing Ltd, 2007.

[9] P. Weaver, *"A Brief History of Scheduling," in my Primavera Conference.* Camberra: Australia, 2006.

[10] B.S. Mattos, *"Numerischer Entwurf von transsonischen Flügeln und Tragflügelprofilen unter Anwendung des AF2-Algorithmus zur Lösung de vollständigen Potentialgleichung,"*, Universität Stuttgart, PhD Thesis, Stuttgart, 1995.

[11] ANSYS Inc, *ANSYS 14 Fluent User Guide.* ANSYS Inc.: Canonsburg, PA, 2011.

[12] H. Salimi, *Stochastic Fractal Search: A powerful metaheuristic algorithm.* Knowl. Based Syst, 2014, pp. 1-18.

[13] M. Melamie, *An Introduction to Genetic Algorithms.* MIT Press: Cambridge, MA, 1998.

[14] R. Ebehardt, and J. Kennedy, "A New Optimizer Using Particle Swarm Theory", In: *Micro Machine and Human Science 95.* Nagoya, 1995.

[15] E. Rashedi, H. Nezamabadi-pour, and S. Saeid, "GSA: A Gravitational Search Algorithm", *Inf. Sci.,* vol. 179, no. 13, pp. 2232-2248, 2009. [http://dx.doi.org/10.1016/j.ins.2009.03.004]

[16] D. Karaboga, *An Idea Based on Honey Bee Swarm for Numerical Optimization.* Erciyes University, Engineering Faculty: Kayseri, 2005.

[17] M. Dorigo, *"Optimization, Learning and Natural Algorithms"*, Politecnico di Milano, PhD Thesis, Milan, 1992.

[18] S.-S. Yang, and D. Suash, "Engineering optimisation by cuckoo search", *International Journal of Mathematical Modelling and Numerical Optimisation,* 2010. [http://dx.doi.org/10.1504/IJMMNO.2010.035430]

[19] E. Atashpaz-Gargari, and C. Lucas, "Imperialist Competitive Algorithm: An algorithm for optimization inspired by imperialistic competition", *IEEE Congress on Evolutionary Computation,* 2007
[http://dx.doi.org/10.1109/CEC.2007.4425083]

[20] EADS, *Planet Aerospace.* EADS, 2007.

[21] J.C. Williams, and E.A. Starke, "Progress in Structural Materials for Aerospace Systems", *Acta Mater.,* vol. 51, pp. 5775-5799, 2003. [http://dx.doi.org/10.1016/j.actamat.2003.08.023]

[22] P. Roto, "Metal Processing and Metal Working Industry", In: *Encyclopedia of Occupational Health and Safety* 4th ed. International Labor Office, 1998.

[23] J. Hale, "Boeing 787 from Ground Up", In: *Boeing Aeromagazine, vol. 4th Quarter, 2006.* vol. 4th Quarter. , 2006.

[24] PwC Consulting, "Aviation Second Golden Age: Can the US Aircraft Industry Maintain Leadership?", 2013. [Online]. Available: https://www.pwc.com/ us/ en/ industrial-products/ publications/ assets/ pwc-commercial-aircraft-industry-future-report.pdf

[25] C. Drew, and J. Mouawad, "Boeing Fix for Battery is Approved by FAA", The New York Times, New York, 2016.

[26] E. Fetters-Walp, "Fine Line," Boeing Frontiers, no. 1st, 2010.

[27] "Airbus, A350 Test Programme and Certification", Airbus, 2016. [Online]. Available:

http://www.airbus.com/ company/ aircraft-manufacture/ how-is- an-aircraft- built/ test-programme-and- certification/ ?contentId=%5b_ TABLE%3Att_ content%3B_ FIELD%3Auid% 5d%2C& cHash= 22935adfac92fcbbd4ba4e1441d13383

[28] Federal Aviation Administration, "Title 14 of the Code of Federal Regulations (14 CFR)", 2016. [Online]. Available: https://www.faa.gov/ regulations_policies/ handbooks_manuals/ aircraft/ amt_handbook/ media/ faa-8083-30_ch12.pdf

[29] Federal Aviation Administration, "Historical CFR by Part", 2016. [Online]. Available: http://rgl.faa.gov/ Regulatory_ and_Guidance_ Library/ rgFAR.nsf/ MainFrame? OpenFrameSet

CHAPTER 5

Feasibility Study of an Airplane Development Program

Abstract: Aircraft design is a complex and fascinating business and field of research. Many good books have been written about it but most of them lack a comprehensive description about the feasibility phase of an aircraft development program. This chapter, therefore, will primarily act as an introduction to the elaboration of requirements for aircraft design leading towards the main steps of a viability analysis of an aircraft program. It will not attempt to duplicate the material found in the existing aircraft design books, but will give information about the financial analysis of a 50-seat airliner together with the descriptions of aircraft and component design. It also presents otherwise published and unpublished data and design methods that are suitable for feasibility studies, aircraft conceptual, preliminary and detail design activities. Examples of tasks carried out by under- and graduate students are presented. A viability of a new or re-engine program for a 75-seat airliner is explored using game theory.

Keywords: Aircraft design phases, Conceptual design, Design requirements, Financial analysis, Game theory, Market analysis.

OVERVIEW

As the feasibility study is the first of the aircraft development program, it is vital for its successful outcome. It provides most guidelines: strategy; financing; and the characterization of the product. This phase concludes if the aircraft program is viable. In addition, risks are evaluated to decide whether to proceed with the program or not. A business plan also results from this phase. It is the most important document that is produced, and it usually contains:

- Executive summary
- Description of the company
- Market analysis
- Competitive analysis
- Business financial parameters
- Marketing strategy
- Product development plan

Bento S. de Mattos, José A. T. G. Fregnani & Paulo Eduardo C. S. Magalhães

- Production scheme
- Project management plan
- Master Phase Plan
- Risk and obstacles assessment
- Financial analysis
- Capital amassment

No benefit will come from the development of a product with insufficient return on investment or technological unfeasibility. Spending any more time and resources attempting to develop such aircraft may lead the company to go out of business. Some revolutionary concepts initially attract interest but after a deeper analysis, they are impracticable or with no economic perspective. Feasibility study distinguishes between a creative and an impracticable design concept. Feasibility evaluation determines the degree to which each project satisfies the requirements and is economically viable. In the feasibility analysis, the answers to the following two questions are sought:

1. Are the goals achievable, are the objectives realistic, and can the design requirements be met?
2. Is the current design concept feasible? Is it strategically relevant and will it bring profit to the company if manufactured?

If the answer to the first question is negative, the following must happen: the design goal and objectives and hence the design requirements must be changed. Then, no matter what the source of the design requirements may have been - either customer survey or market analysis - they must be changed. When the answer to the second question is in negative, a new concept must be selected. Finding the answers to these questions is not always easy. To determine the answers other professionals beside design engineers - such as financial experts or manufacturing engineers - must often be involved in the feasibility study.

Some headlines in the press were selected to show the way aircraft manufacturers sometimes handle the study of new airplanes or airlines to analyze the incorporation of new airplanes into their fleets:

> *"Boeing Co. said it is not studying the resurrecting of its out-of-production 757 jetliner with new engines to plug a gap in its jetliner lineup between its largest single-aisle plane and its smallest wide-body models. According to Boeing that airplane had a very unique production system. It was relatively expensive to build."*
> Source: Reuters, 2015.

"India hopes to test fly its first indigenously-developed 90-seater regional transport aircraft (RTA) in the next five years. The 90-seater RTA will be developed as a team India initiative led by CSIR-National Aerospace Laboratory (NAL), which could also see some global participation."
Source: The Economic Times, 2011.

"Airbus believes there is a market for around 1,500 A380s over the next 20 years, about 10% of the total number of jet aircraft (excluding smaller regional jets) that it forecasts will be needed – whose need it forecasts. It reckons the market for several versions of its super-jumbo (possibly going up to 800 seats) will be worth $340 billion in total. Boeing claims there is a market for no more than 500 super-jumbos - hence its reluctance to launch a completely new product of its own."
Source: The Economist, 2012.

"We look at just about every type of airplane and the challenge we have right now is that we are too dependent on 50-seat RJs [regional jets]."
Chief Financial officer of United Airlines
Source: FlightGlobal, June 2015.

ESTABLISHING REQUIREMENTS

The Challenging Task of Establishing Proper Requirements

Conceptually, elaboration of requirements includes three types of activities:

- *Elicitation of requirements:* this concerns the task of communicating with users and customers for the preparation of terms of reference.
- *Requirement analysis:* determines whether the state of the requirements is unclear, incomplete, ambiguous, or contradictory and operates up to solving problems.
- *Records of requirements:* requirements can be documented in many ways, such as natural language documents, use cases, or specification process.

Requirements analysis can be a long and arduous process. New systems or products change the environment and relationships between people. Therefore, it is very important to identify all stakeholders, considering all their needs and aspirations, ensuring that they understood the implications of the new systems in question. Analysts can employ several techniques to elicit customer requirements. Historically, this involves activities such as organizing interviews or focus groups (workshops) and the creation of lists of requirements. More modern techniques include prototyping, scale models or building mock-ups, and using cases where the analyst will apply a combination of methods to establish the exact requirements of stakeholders; so that the system meets the business opportunity.

Some problems that can inhibit or hinder the attainment of goals:

- Customers do not know what they want.
- Users do not want to complete the writing of the set of requirements.
- Communication with the user is slow or broken.
- Users often do not participate in reviews or are unable to attend.
- Discussion partners are technically not qualified.
- Users do not understand the development process.
- Attachment to outdated dogmas and paradigms.

These issues could lead to situations where user requirements keep changing even when the development of the system or product has already begun. Next sections will analyze some airplane programs that suffered from the lack of establishment of proper requirements.

The problem statement describes the customer's needs, states the goals of the project, delineates the scope of the system, reports the concept of operations, describes the stakeholders, lists the deliverables and presents the key decisions that must be made.

The Failed Proposal of the Sonic Cruiser

Early in 2001, the Boeing Company announced the development of a wholly new high-speed aircraft, which was designated Sonic Cruiser. The most impressive features of this new concept were a range of up to 10,000 nm, a cruise Mach number of 0.98 and the claim of a significant reduction in flight time. Fig. (**5.1**) shows the geometry of Sonic Cruiser based on drawings released by Boeing. Martin Hepperle from the German research center DLR carried out a study to assess Sonic Cruiser performance [1]. One result from this study is that the reduction of flight time by increasing the cruise Mach number to number of Mach 0.98 is relatively small. A larger reduction of travel time seems to be possible only by using direct point-to-point services instead of hub and spoke connections. Another result is that the claimed range would be very hard to achieve flying close to the sound speed.

Table **5.1** compares Sonic Cruiser characteristics with two other Boeing airliners. The Concorde supersonic airliner offered a much higher cruise speed at the cost of a small passenger capacity, shorter range and higher fuel burn when compared to Sonic Cruiser; a typical airliner like the Boeing 767 operates very economically carrying a similar number of passengers like the Sonic Cruiser but at lower cruise Mach numbers. Sonic Cruiser's wingspan is slightly larger than that of a Boeing 767, but because of its high-speed cruise its fuselage is slenderer than that of Boeing 767. Boeing Co. ended the Sonic Cruiser project in December 2002 and shifted to the slower (Mach 0.85), but more fuel-efficient 7E7 (later named 787 Dreamliner) airliner.

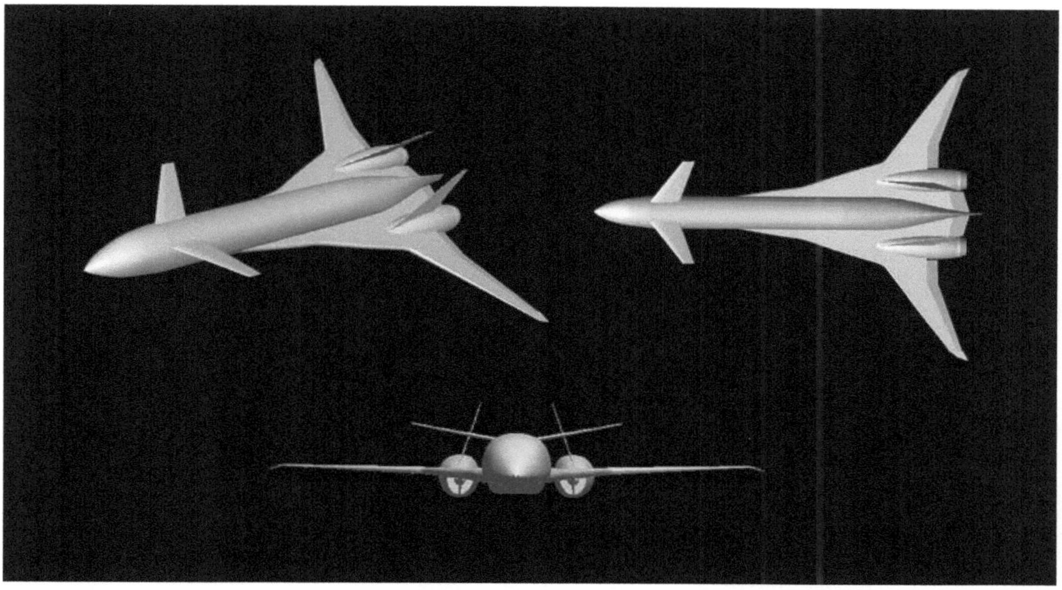

Fig. (5.1). Three-view of Boeing Sonic Cruiser.

Table 5.1. Characteristics of Sonic Cruiser compared to some existing airliners.

Parameter	Sonic Cruiser	B 767-200ER	B 777-200-IGW
Cruise Mach Number	0.96	0.80	0.82
Passengers	200	181	305
Wingspan (m)	50.0	47.6	60.9
Overall Length (m)	60.0	48.5	63.7
Fuselage Width (m)	5.1	5.0	6.2
Reference Area (m^2)	512	283	428
Range (nm)	6,500	6,600	7,150
Initial Cruise Altitude (ft)	40,000	35,000	34,100
Max. takeoff Mass (kg)	≈ 200,000	175,500	286,895
Max. Fuel Mass (kg)	≈ 90,000 kg	73,600	135,845

Chance-Vought Corsair: Grounded by Design

The Chance Vought F4U Corsair (Fig. **5.2**) was a fighter aircraft that saw service primarily in World War II and the Korean War. Demand for the airplane overwhelmed Vought's manufacturing capability, resulting in production by Goodyear and Brewster: Goodyear-built Corsairs were designated FG and Brewster-built aircraft F3A. From the first prototype delivery to the U.S. Navy in 1940 to final delivery in 1953 to the French, 12,571 F4U Corsairs were manufactured by Vought, in 16 separate models.

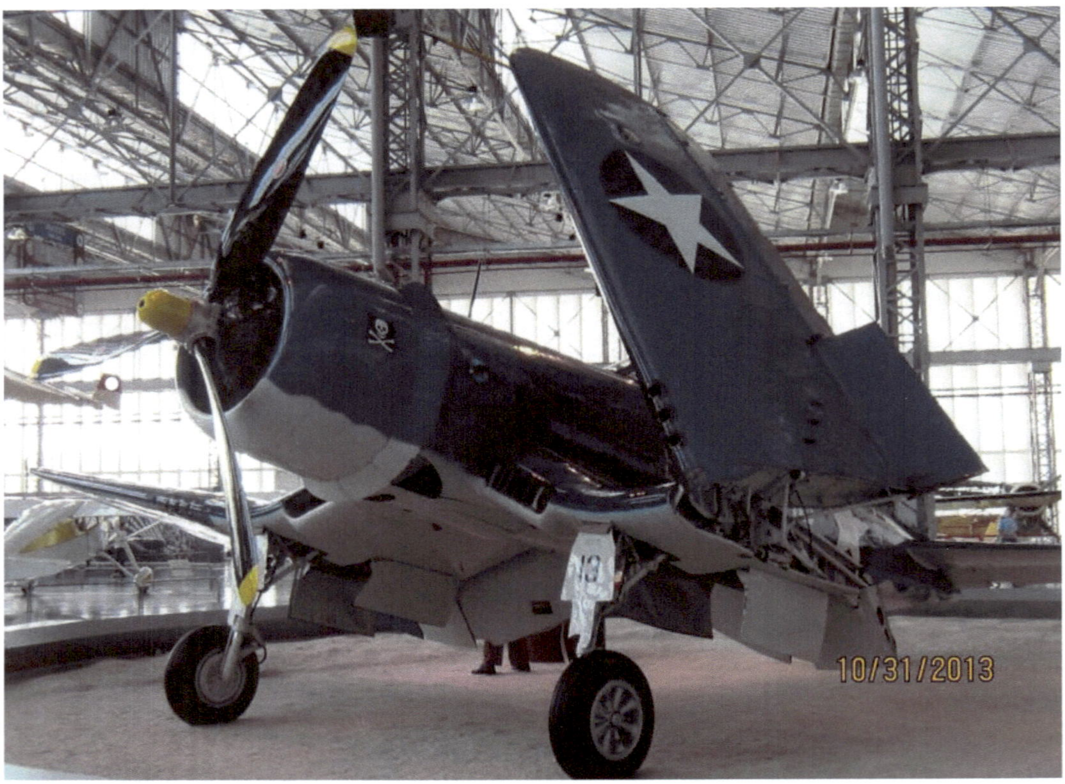

Fig. (5.2). Chance-Vought F4U Corsair (Photo: ©2013 Bento Mattos taken at TAM Museum, Brazil).

Corsair was fitted with a single Pratt & Whitney R-2800 Double Wasp radial engine. This 18-cylinder engine was the largest one available at the time. This required large propellers to obtain higher efficiency from this large amount of power. Later versions of this engine were capable to deliver 2000-hp of power.

Corsair's large fuselage panels were made of magnesium and were attached to the frames with the newly-developed technique of spot welding, thus mostly eliminating the use of rivets. An inverted gull wing, a similar layout to the one used by Germany's Junkers Ju 87 dive bomber, provided the F4U Corsair fighter with a considerably shortened length of the main gear legs. In addition, the wing-fuselage angle favored lower interference drag. Its long nose was the origin for poor visibility from the cockpit. This caused accidents at carrier operations. The combination of an aft cockpit and the Corsair's long nose made landings hazardous for newly-trained pilots. During landing approaches, it was found that oil from the hydraulic cowl flaps could spatter onto the windscreen, reducing visibility, and the undercarriage oil struts had bad rebound characteristics on landing, allowing the aircraft to bounce out of control down the carrier deck.

Originally designed as a carrier-capable fighter, it saw combat in Guadalcanal in 1943 as land-based fighter instead. Thus, the airplane was used in a combat environment completely different from what it had been designed for. Despite this, it was a very successful combat airplane. During World War II, Chance Vought produced 4,120 Corsairs of the initial F4U-1 version at the Stratford, Connecticut, plant.

Technology Assessment

Technology assessment during feasibility studies is mandatory. There are technologies or ideas that sound promising but may lead to big commercial failures of an aircraft program. An important problem concerning technology assessment is the so-called Collingridge dilemma: on the one hand, impacts of innovative technologies cannot be easily predicted until the technology is extensively developed and widely used; on the other hand, control or change of a technology is difficult as soon as it is widely used [2]. One example of this is the concept adopted for the business jet Hansa Jet (Fig. **5.3**), a German forward sweep wing airplane from the 1960s.

The HFB-320 Hansa Jet is an all-metal, twin-engine, 10-seat business jet built by German aircraft manufacturer Hamburger Flugzeugbau between 1964 and 1973. The most notable feature of the aircraft is its forward-swept wing, which is mid-mounted in the fuselage. This arrangement allows the wing spar to pass through the fuselage behind the passenger cabin providing more volume for it. Forward-sweep wing configurations are prone to aeroelastic problems. High-swept wings tend to be unstable at stall, since the tip stalls first cause (instead of causing) a pitch-up force, thus worsening the stall and making recovery difficult. This effect is more significant with forward sweep because the inner wing stall, first in a more severe way. The Visionaire Vantage single-engine jet airplane, designed by

Burt Rutan, also adopted this configuration and its program was restricted to a single prototype.

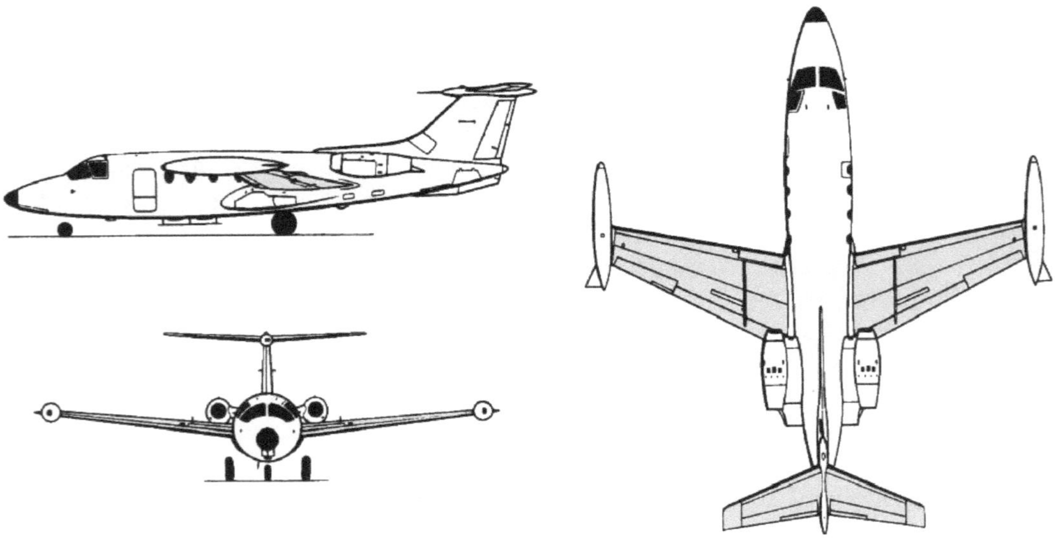

Fig. (5.3). Three-view of Hansa jet.

The Hansa Jet bizjet faced increased competition from new incoming executive jet models and a comparatively poor safety record led to disappointing orders, with production ceasing in 1973. The Aviation Safety Network lists a total of nine accidents (six fatal) for the type, an astounding 20 percent hull-loss rate, but only the crash of the prototype was directly attributable to the aircraft's design. Pilot error was blamed in most of the accidents.

The Grumman X-29 was an American experimental aircraft that tested a forward-swept wing, canard control surfaces, and other novel aircraft technologies. The X-29 was developed by Grumman, and the two types built were flown by NASA and the United States Air Force. The aerodynamic instability of the X-29's airframe required the use of computerized fly-by-wire control. Composite materials were used to control the aeroelastic divergent twisting experienced by forward-swept wings, and to reduce weight. The X-29 first flew in 1984.

There are some game-changing technologies, as well. The four-engine piston-powered Focke-Wulf 200 (Fig. **5.4**) is a good example of this. At the time that only dirigibles could fly non-stop between Europe and the Americas, the type performed a historical non-stop flight crossing the Atlantic on August 10-11, 1938. The German airliner took off from Berlin and landed at Floyd Bennett field in Brooklyn, New York. The Fw 200 was then the first land-based airliner to fly nonstop between Germany and the United States, making its flight a milestone in aviation [3]. The flight took 24 hours and 56 minutes; the return flight on 13 August 1938 took 19 hours and 47 minutes [3]. Despite the disaster with the Hindenburg in May 1937, the Fw 200 oceanic crossing signalized the definitive end of regular passenger transportation with airships. After World War II, line aviation with flying boats also ended, which made the land-based airplanes (becoming) the king of skies.

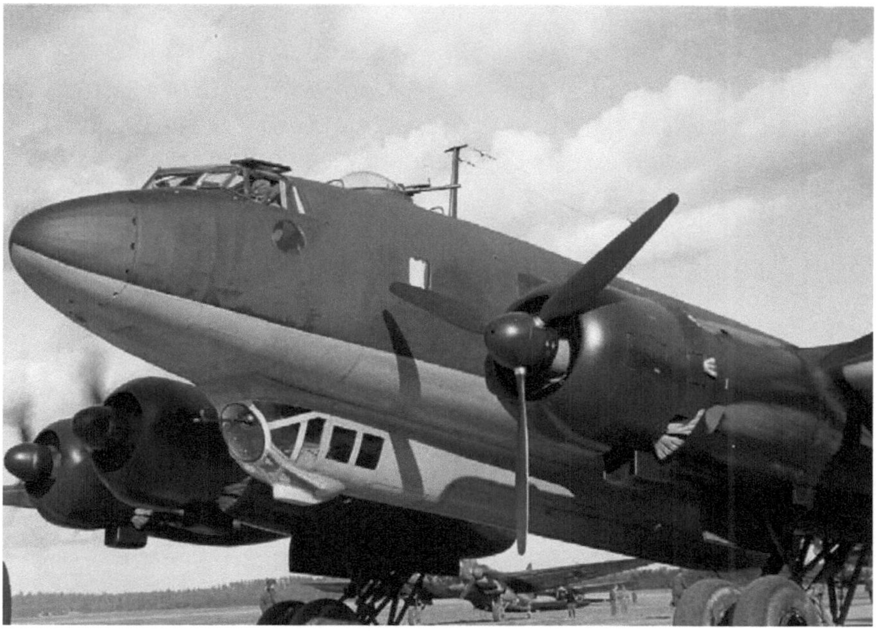

Fig. (5.4). Focke-Wulf 200C Condor (Photo: public domain, *via* Wikimedia Commons).

EMBRAER/FAMA CBA-123 AND SAAB 2000

Two cases about not understanding customer needs in a game changing environment

In the second half of the 1980s, EMBRAER was looking for a successor to the successful EMB-110 Bandeirante, of which 500 units were manufactured. Market surveys with potential operators indicated that the new generation of regional airplanes should provide greater comfort and fly faster than airplanes from previous generation. Thus, EMBRAER started conceptual studies considering a pressurized configuration with turboprop engines located at the aft fuselage, an unusual configuration. The model was designated EMB-123 by EMBRAER. The reason for the positioning of the engines at the rear of the aircraft was simple:

Because of the higher speed requirement, the engines needed to be more powerful (the EMB-123 was equipped with two 1,300-shp engines). Thus, if they were placed on the wing, the noise generated in the passenger cabin would cause much discomfort, compromising the requirement of comfort appointed by the operators. Moreover, in case of engine failure, the momentum caused by the remaining engine would require a large vertical stabilizer.

After the start of the program, the Brazilian President at the time, José Sarney, signed with Argentine President Raul Alfonsin a Brazil-Argentina cooperation agreement. From there, the Fabrica Militar de Aviones (FAMA) in Cordoba joined EMBRAER in the development of the airplane, which was then renamed CBA-123 (which stands for Brazil-Argentina Cooperation). The CBA-123 (Fig. **5.5**) also incorporated advanced systems like a carbon brake system and the rear fuselage was reshaped to improve the propeller's propulsive efficiency. The CBA-123 was to be sold at a very expensive list price of US$ 5.5 million, which put buyers off. The program was terminated in 1992 after the construction of three prototypes. One of them was restored and is in outdoor display within the area occupied by the Brazilian Aerospace Memorial (MAB), in São José dos Campos, São Paulo, Brazil.

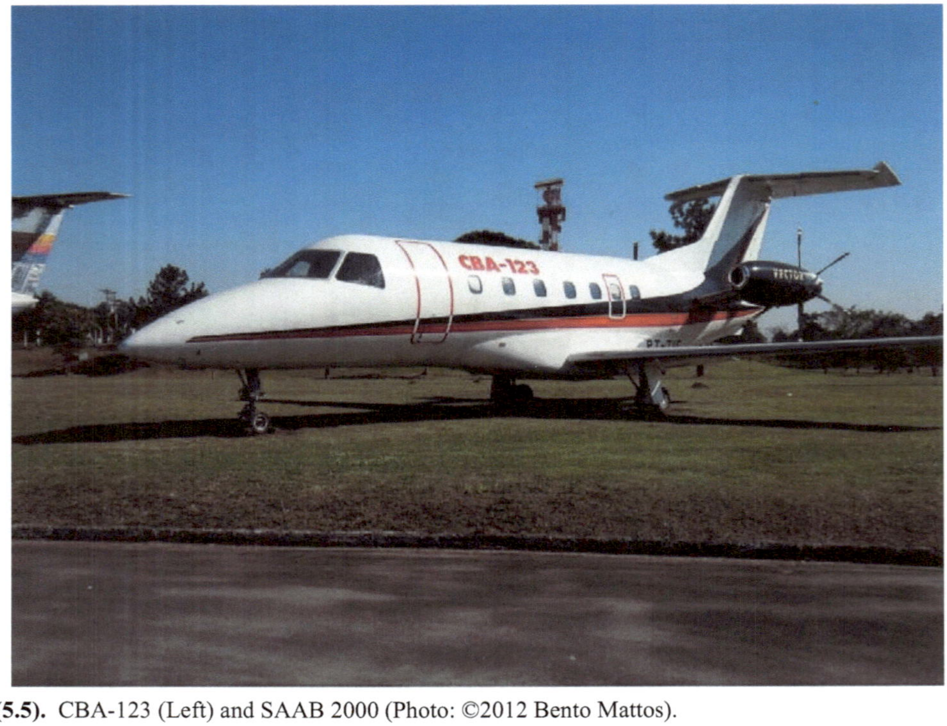

Fig. (5.5). CBA-123 (Left) and SAAB 2000 (Photo: ©2012 Bento Mattos).

CBA-123 design was continuously improved. Carbonfibre was used for the engine nacelle to reduce vibration propagation (Fig. **5.6**). EMBRAER undertook 1,900 h of wind-tunnel tests, necessary to achieve the envisaged high performance. The wing-to-fuselage fairing, originally based on that from the 30-seat Brasilia, was redesigned, and extended much further both ahead and behind the wing. Besides enabling the installation of two central fuel tanks with a total fuel capacity of 571 liters, a drag reduction of 20 drag counts was recorded in wind-tunnel tests.

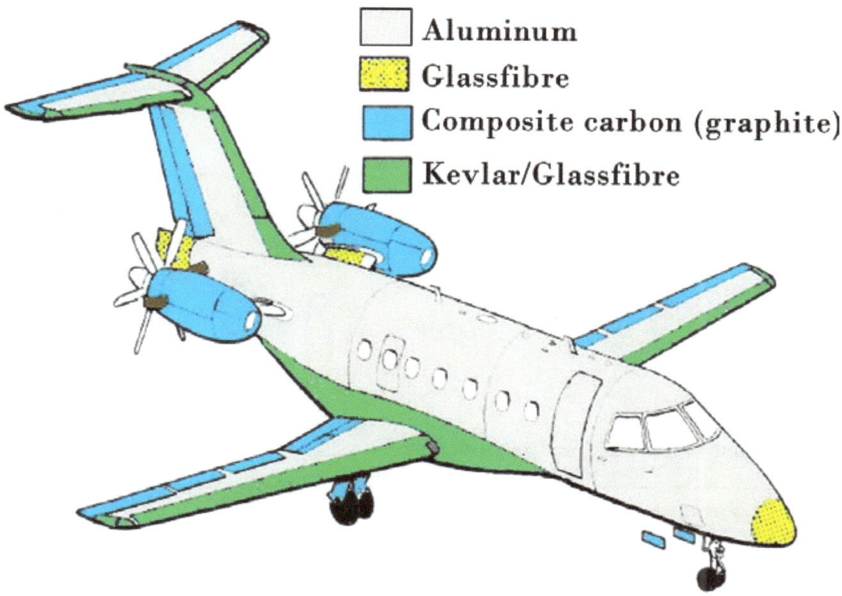

Fig. (5.6). CBA-123 structural materials (Source: FlightGlobal).

Spoilerons were eliminated by increasing wing and aileron spans. In a later redesign, engine pylons were slightly relocated in relation to the fuselage, and featured sweepback and dihedral angle. Engine nacelle also eliminated external exhaust ducts to reduce drag improved flow efficiency at the propellers. The vertical stabilizer was moved further aft to protect control cables against propeller blade failure, and to also protect the horizontal stabilizer (HT) from propeller thrown ice. The HT was modified, too: airfoils received a nose droop and a dog-tooth was added to its leading-edge. All this was carried out to improve HT maximum lift coefficient to avoid increasing its area to balance the airplane at takeoff and landings. CBA-123 strongest competitor in late 1980s was the Jetstream 31 (Fig. **5.7**). Table **5.2** compares CBA-123 characteristics with those from its main competitor.

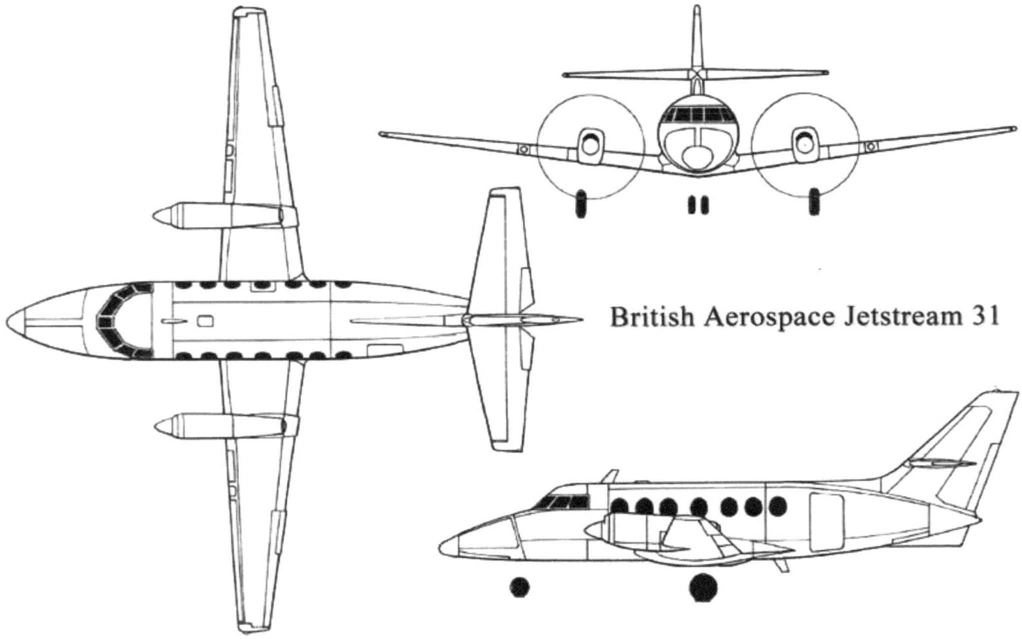

Fig. (5.7). Jetstream 31.

Table 5.2. Data relative to CBA-123 and Jetstream 31.

Parameter	CBA-123	Jetstream 31
Max. cruise speed	612 km/h	488 km/h
Range with maximum payload	925 km	1,260 km
Service ceiling	11,094 m (36,400 ft)	7.620 m (25,000 ft)
Wing area	27.2 m^2	25.2 m^2
Fuselage diameter	2.28 m	1.83 m
Maximum takeoff weight	7,711 kg	6,950 kg
Takeoff field length (MTOW, sea level, ISA)	1,300 m	1,030 m
Motorization	2 x Garret TPF351 with 1,300 shp each	2 x Garret TPE331 with 900 shp each

Like EMBRAER, the Swedish company SAAB conducted market studies and again, operators indicated they wanted aircraft with higher speed and greater passenger comfort. In 1988, SAAB began development of the SAAB 2000 turboprop airplane (Fig. **5.8**). SAAB 2000 is a pressurized airliner capable of carrying 50 passengers. It first flew in 1992 and became operational in 1994. The airplane can cruise at 665 km/h (370 knots). To meet the noise level requirement in the passenger cabin (comfort), SAAB introduced an active system to mitigate the background noise, with microphones and speakers distributed in the cabin. SAAB 2000 sales were disappointing. Crossair, a regional airline in which Swissair had 56% participation, placed the largest order for SAAB 2000. Due to the limited demand, SAAB ceased production of the SAAB 2000 in 1999. In 2000, 44 units of the SAAB 2000 were still in service. The failure of this airplane program led SAAB to leave the commercial aviation market.

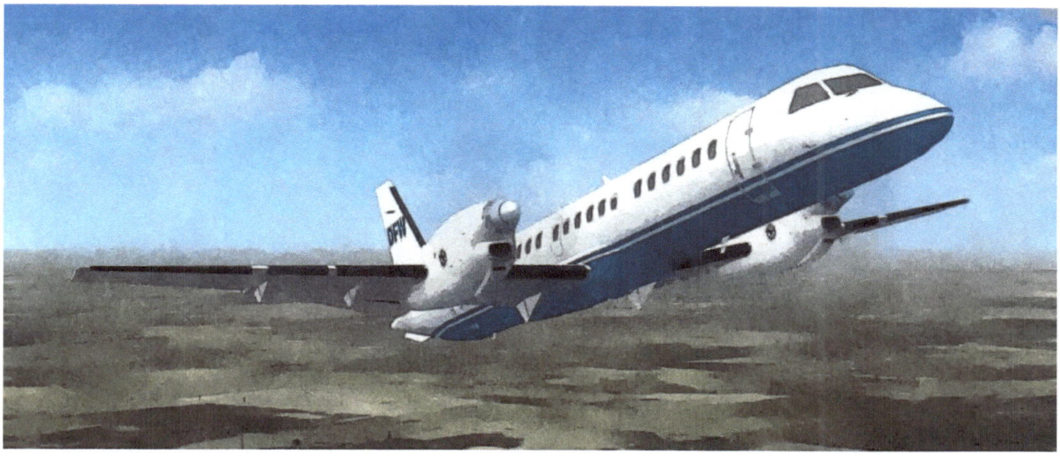

Fig. (5.8). SAAB 2000.

What were the reasons for the commercial failure of the CBA-123 and SAAB 2000? To help answer this question, some observations are made based on the information contained in reports that were published in various specialized magazines of aeronautics and aviation.

EMBRAER was promised that some government orders by Argentina and Brazil would be placed. However, that did not happen and the Brazilian company was forced to apply for private bank loans to continue with the CBA-123 development. This and the cost of developing the EMB-145 jet (Fig. **5.9**) led the company to a bankruptcy-like state, during which it had to rely on government assistance to survive, and which eventually resulted in its privatization late in 1994. In the late 1980s, Brazil was experiencing a severe financial crisis and this was the reason that EMBRAER lacked government support for the development of CBA-123.

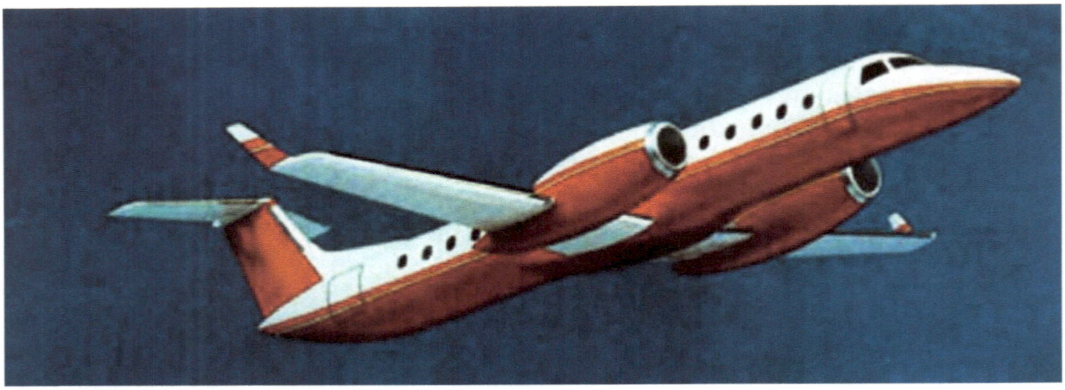

Fig. (5.9). EMBRAER first concept for its EMB-145.

Commonly, the 1980s are called the lost decade in terms of economic development. In Brazil and other Latin American countries, this period was marked by stagnation together with an aggressive decline in industrial production and global GDP. In most of these nations, the 1980s are a synonym for a crisis in the economy, inflation, low growth of gross domestic product (GDP), volatility of markets and increasing social inequality. Regarding the Brazilian economy during the 80s, reductions were observed in GDP, and the average growth that was 7% (1970) fell to 2% in the 1980s. The international interest rates that increased due to the U.S. inflation, caused the growth of Brazil's external debt with the U.S., and increased the public deficit. The domestic debt followed the same path, increasing gradually because of the expansionary fiscal policy of the Brazilian government. It is often said that the 1980s were the burial of the expansion experienced in the 1970s, which became known as the economic miracle. Thus, the economic and financial scenario at that time had a serious impact on the development of the CBA-123, which was considered too sophisticated and expensive for the market for which it was intended. EMBRAER had considered the redesign of the CBA-123 to make it less sophisticated and lowered the purchase price, but the lack of capital and investment needed for the EMB-145 program led to the abandonment of the CBA-123 program. The CBA-123 offered more comfort in the passenger cabin over existing aircraft, pressurized and non-pressurized, and better performance. However, the market was not willing to pay more for these benefits. The CBA-123 program's kiss of death came with the Gulf War in the early 1990s, which caused a huge downturn of the aviation market. The program, which was initiated in 1986, was canceled in 1992.

The confirmation that the market for CBA-123 was significant came with the good sales of the Beechcraft 1900 (Fig. **5.10**). This 19-seat pressurized airliner belongs to the CBA-123 category. According to Wikipedia, 695 units of

Beechcraft 1900 were manufactured. It originated from the Beechcraft Super King Air turboprop, which offers accommodation for 13 passengers. The 1900 made its first flight in 1992 and entered service in 1994. The pressurized competitors already in operation by the 1900 development were the Jetstream 31 and the Fairchild Swearingen Metroliner, the first with 386 and the latter with 600 units sold.

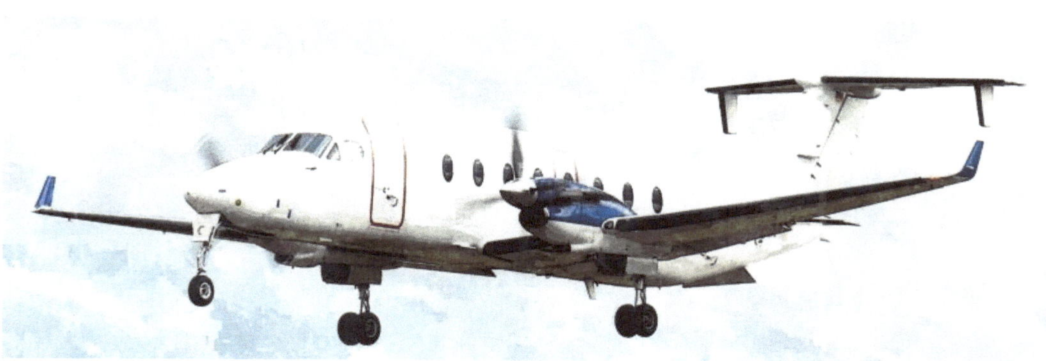

Fig. (5.10). Beechcraft 1900D.

Although EMBRAER was experiencing troubles with its CBA-123 twin-engine turboprop, the Swedish SAAB company had the same understanding about market needs, but incomplete. EMBRAER was not aware of the price limit that the market was willing to pay for a 19-seat high-performance airplane; and SAAB insisted on the development of a speedier 50-seat turboprop. However, the market was more prone to a jet airplane.

Some fatal accidents with turboprop airplanes in the United States in the early 1990s caused great fear of this type of aircraft among passengers. In addition, some jet engines for 50-seat airliners emerged on the market, among them the Allison AE 3007 and the General Electric CF-34, especially. These economic engines allowed the development of a new generation of jet aircraft, taking over the market share of turboprops. A pioneer in consideration of the introduction of the 50-seat jet in the 1990s was the American company COMAIR. COMAIR operated the turboprop EMB-120 Brasilia and for this reason started negotiations with EMBRAER for the purchase of 45-seat jet transport, which became the EMB-145 (renamed later to ERJ 145, with capacity increased to 50 seats). However, in the meantime EMBRAER faced a fiscal crisis as consequence of the CBA-123 development and from bad decisions regarding the EMB-145 configuration, which initially had engines on the wing (Fig. **5.9**). COMAIR and started to back Canadair (now Bombardier), which was developing the CRJ-100 airliner. COMAIR and Lufthansa pioneered the successful introduction of the 50-

seat regional jet, the CRJ-100, which entered service in 1992. EMBRAER continued with the development of the EMB-145, which came into operation in early 1997 with Continental Express (currently, Express Jet). In addition, the CRJ-100/200 (Fig. **5.11**) and ERJ 145 family aircraft reached the significant milestone of over 1000 units commercialized.

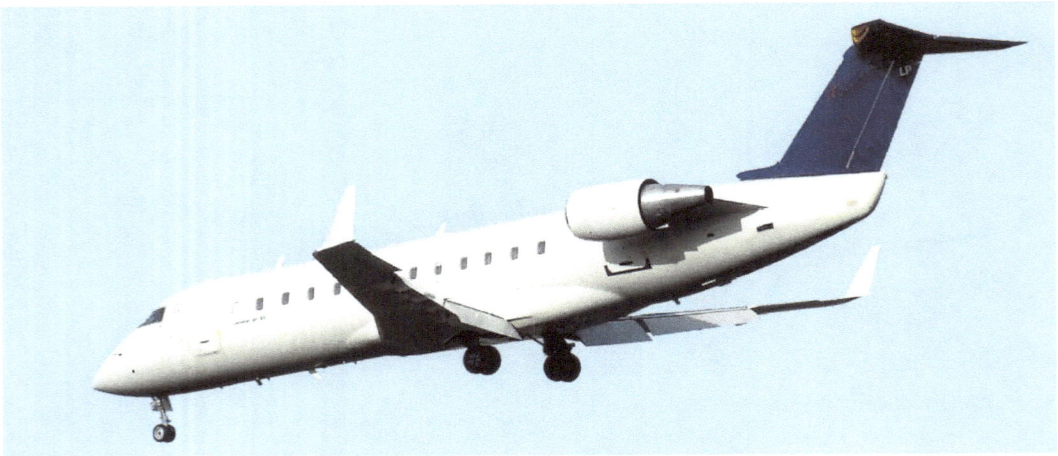

Fig. (5.11). Canadair CRJ-100.

The SAAB 2000 purchase cost was almost the same as that of a regional jet of the same capacity. However, thanks to higher speeds, the productivity of regional jets is higher, despite their higher fuel consumption. Indeed, they present a higher daily utilization rate thanks to their higher speed. Slowing sales of SAAB 2000 caused SAAB to leave the civil aviation market. This story illustrates the need to understand market requirements in a proper manner and to provide the right product at the right time.

VFW 614: AN INTERESTING CONCEPT AT THE WRONG TIME

The impressive success of the CRJ-100/200 and ERJ 145 family can be defined as the second jet age. The first jet age took place in the late 1950s through the emergence of the large-capacity jet market, dominated by Boeing 707 and Douglas DC-8. However, the CRJ and ERJ are not the pioneers of regional jets. At this point, it is important to mention the case of the regional jet VFW 614 (Fig. **5.12**), whose development began in 1961 and which entered service in 1975. The very long development time stands out, especially at a time during which aviation changed considerably. Thus, due to such a long development time, the initial requirements were no longer valid. It is important to remember that the world experienced the shock of a sudden oil price rise in 1973, which made the economic operation of the VFW 614 unfeasible. The twinjets of EMBRAER and Bombardier met success from early 1990s on because they were fitted with engines that enabled economical operation of 50-seat jet airplanes.

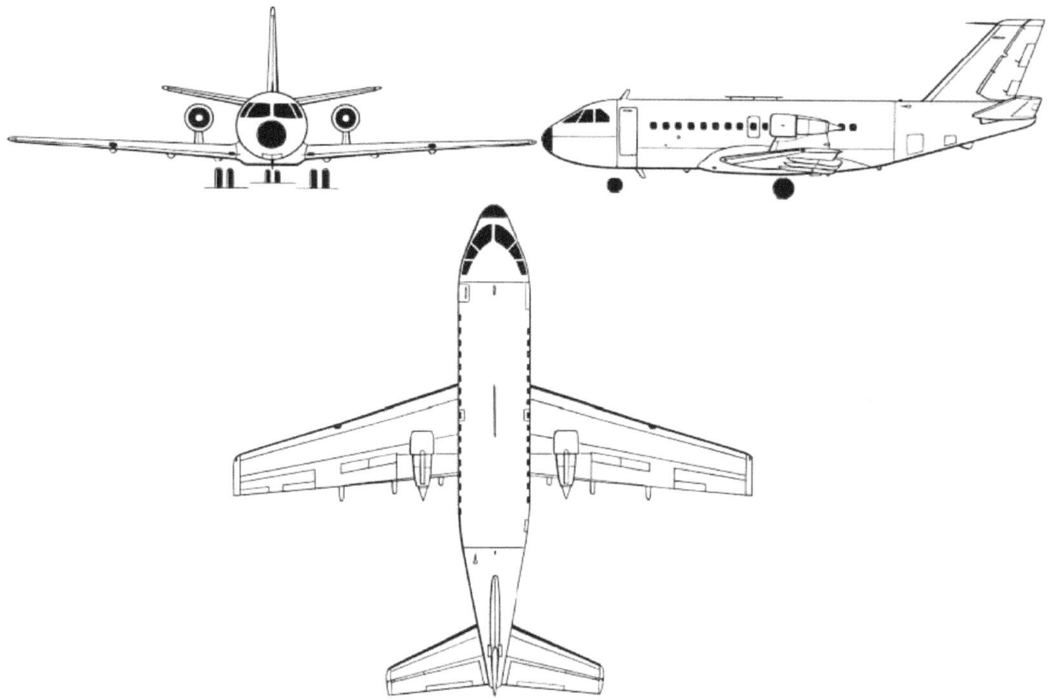

Fig. (5.12). VFW 614 development started in 1961.

The VFW 614 was originally proposed in 1961 by Entwicklungsring group Nord, comprising the Focke-Wulf Flugzeugbau Hamburger (HFB) and the Weser. Designated E.614, it was a transport airplane in the 36-40 seat range, powered by two low-bypass Lycoming PLF1B-2 turbofans. After a reorganization of the West German industry, the development of what was then known as VFW 614 continued.

Although Lycoming abandoned the development of PLF1, work with the VFW 614 continued due to the availability of the Rolls-Royce/SNECMA M45H turbofan, which was developed especially for the VFW 614. In 1968, the program received the green light, with 80% of financial contribution from the government of West Germany. Full-scale production was approved in 1970, a time when VFW merged with Fokker (a quite unfortunate arrangement that lasted only ten years). Also, risk partnership agreements had been concluded with SIAT in Germany, Fairey and SABCA in Belgium, and Shorts in the United Kingdom.

The final assembly of the aircraft was supposed to have taken place in Bremen. The first of three VFW 614 prototypes flew on July 14, 1971. The plane had an unconventional setting, with engines mounted on pylons M45H above the wings. This arrangement was used to avoid both the penalty of increased structural weight if the motors were positioned in rear fuselage and the debris ingestion problems if the engines were accommodated under the wings. This allowed a short and sturdy landing gear, especially suitable for operations on unprepared runways. The first of the three prototypes flew on July 14, 1971. The airplane had an unusual configuration with the M45H engines placed over the wings, supported by pylons. This configuration was chosen by VFW to avoid the weight penalty of fuselage rear-mounted engines and debris ingestion problems of underwing engine configurations. This allowed a short and robust landing gear assembly, especially suitable for operations on unprepared airfields.

The development of the airplane was slow and time-consuming, despite a strong advertising campaign. Their plight was worsened by the bankruptcy of Rolls-Royce in 1971, which threatened the supply of engines. In addition, the first prototype was lost on February 1st, 1972, due to the emergence of the elevator flutter, further damaging the order book. By February 1975, only ten aircraft had been sold. The first serial-manufactured VFW 614 flew in April 1975 and was delivered to Danish Cimber Air four months later. Only three airlines and the Luftwaffe (German Air Force) operated the 614s. The model was prone to engine problems and was too expensive to operate. The program was officially canceled in 1977 and the last aircraft available for sale flew in July 1978. Most aircraft were out of operation by 1981, with the manufacturer buying back the units that had been marketed.

EMBRAER ERJ 140: WHEN PILOTS DICTATE AIRCRAFT DESIGN

The ERJ 140 (Fig. **5.13**) also offers an interesting case for the study of requirements. American Eagle already operated the 50-seat jet ERJ 145 EMBRAER. The pilots of smaller capacity jets had considerably lower wages than those operating jets of medium and large capacity. As a result, the pilots' associations, which had considerably bargaining power at the time, imposed on airlines that regional jets operated a limited number of aircraft that could be acquired, which became known as scope clauses (arbitration clause).

There are virtually no scope limits to the number of 44-seat regional jets (RJ), while there is with the 50-seat ones. Bombardier Aerospace also has a 44-seat RJ model which is basically a CRJ-200 with 6 seats removed and certified as the CRJ-440 [4]. It was developed for Delta Airlines but Northwest ordered this version as well.

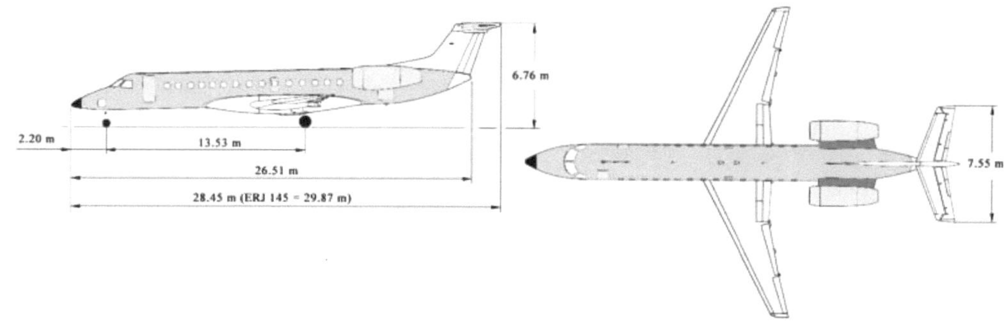

Fig. (5.13). ERJ 140 was a shortened variant of ERJ 145.

EMBRAER started to develop a shortened version of the ERJ 145, capable of carrying 44 passengers envisaging large orders from ERJ 145 operators like American Eagle. This way, the requirement to develop an airplane able to accommodate 44 passengers instead of 50 in a typical configuration arose. Of course, this was also the desire of some other U.S. airlines which were also subject to scope clauses with their respective riders.

Before the ERJ 140, EMBRAER developed the ERJ 135 for 37 passengers. Thus, one of the prototypes of the ERJ 145 (registration PT-ZJA) was shortened by 3.54 m for the certification campaign of the new model. The ERJ 135 was certified by the FAA in 1999. That same year, EMBRAER announced the development of the ERJ 140 to fulfill the request of some airlines as mentioned earlier. Again, the PZ-ZJA had been modified and was then extended to 2.12 m, leaving a total length of 28.45 m. The prototype of the ERJ 150 first flew on 27 June 2000. The ERJ 140 went into operation in 2001 with American Eagle. The cockpit, and therefore, the ERJ 140's instrumentation is the same as of its bigger brother, the 50-seat ERJ 145 airliner.

MARKET ANALYSIS

Introduction

Major aircraft manufacturers employ marketing departments that issue annual market outlooks for a 20-year timeframe. Aircraft manufacturers have to elaborate such reports because they commercialize shares on stock exchanges. Historical data are analyzed and extrapolated for the elaboration of market outlooks like, for example, world economic indicators. Fig. (**5.14**) shows the gross domestic product (GDP) and highlights the recent recessions. The estimation of the future market is essential for any company and therefore the monitoring of demand indicators is important for decision-making about the direction to be followed by the company.

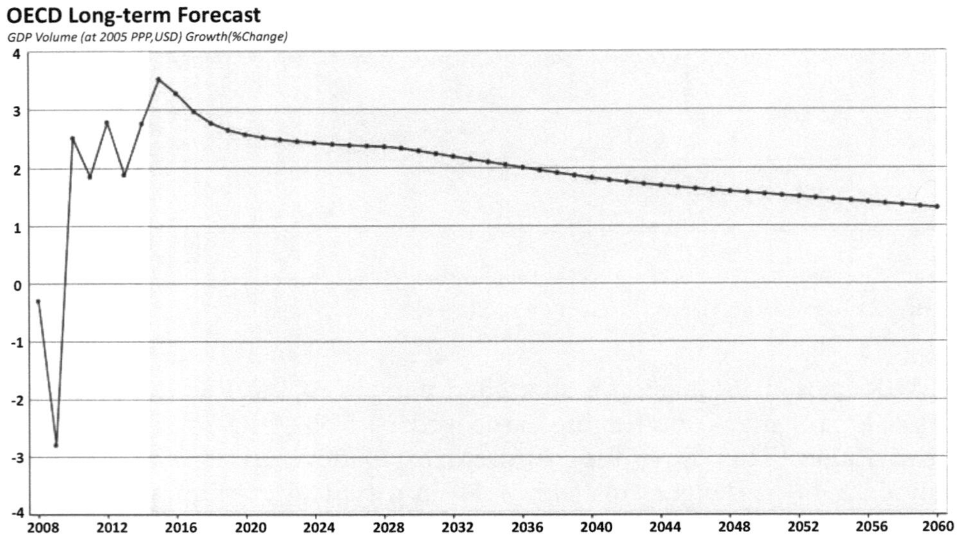

Fig. (5.14). Long-term world`s GDP projection (Source: OECD).

In the airline industry, a very well-done study of the future demand for aircraft is even more crucial due to many factors such as:

- There are many variables that can influence the global demand for air travel, from the growth of world urbanization to the average price of airline tickets, which in turn is related to the price of a barrel of oil, for example;
- the aircraft development time from design to manufacturing in series often takes years;
- the development of products whose market demand is lower than expected can cause the manufacturer serious financial trouble.

In the 1990s, EMBRAER developed in partnership with Argentina the CBA-123, an airplane with technological innovations in avionics, aerodynamics, comfort, and propulsion integration. Although demand for a 19-seat airplane existed, the airlines were not keen to pay for the sophistication offered by the CBA-123. Similarly, SAAB developed a high-performance turboprop that cost the same as jets presenting the same capacity.

The cases of CBA-123 and SAAB 2000 are good examples of poor understanding of market requirements. The failure of both programs caused the insolvency of EMBRAER and led SAAB to leave the civil aviation market.

The Brazilian company could survive thanks to massive governmental support; SAAB had recorded before a sales success with its SAAB 340 airliner.

There are generally four areas in which aircraft are deployed; they consist of:

1. **New markets** - Greater liberalization of aviation market is often a driver for aviation growth and the development of new markets through the opening of new air routes between growing numbers of origins and destinations. The impact of liberalization is particularly dramatic in the case of low-cost airlines, which are stimulating air travel by lowering fares and opening new markets [5].
2. **Replacement/Retirements** - Replacements are a key part of any forecast, as the time at which aircraft leave passenger service to retire or be converted to other uses has an impact on the level of demand for new aircraft deliveries. High fuel costs and the need to meet new environmental regulations are compelling airlines to accelerate replacement of older airplanes [5].
3. **Natural Growth** - Worldwide economic activity is the most powerful driver of natural growth in commercial air transport and the resulting demand for airplanes. World GDP is expected to grow at over 3% per year on average in the next ten years.
4. **Right-Sizing** - Using right sized equipment allows airlines to maximize operational efficiency and profitability by optimizing capacity to demand. Adequate airplanes provide operators with an optimally designed aircraft to target routes/frequencies [5].

SWOT MATRIX

SWOT analysis (alternatively SWOT Matrix) is a tool for auditing an organization and its environment (Table **5.3**). It is the first stage of planning and helps marketers to focus on key issues. This is a very effective way of identifying Strengths and Weaknesses (internal factors) and examining the Opportunities and Threats (external factors) faced by a company [6]. Basically, internal factors are fully influenced by a company itself while external ones cannot be controlled by it. After identifying these points, the next stage is to analyze the relation between them, in order to evaluate necessary strategies that must be implemented to do good business [6].

As an example, for the elaboration of a SWOT matrix, a 50-seat airliner development program is analyzed. The SWOT matrix shown in Table **5.4** was adapted from a 2006 report elaborated by a design team composed by graduate students. It was then considered that students' company already had been engaged in the manufacture of a 70-seat airliner and they had to decide on the introduction of a 50-seat twinjet on the market.

Table 5.3. SWOT Matrix.

	Helpful in Achieving Objectives	Harmful in Achieving Objectives
Internal Origins	Strengths	Weakness
External Origins	Opportunities	Threats

Table 5.4. SWOT Matrix for the 50-seat program.

	Helpful	Harmful
Internal Origins	1. Strong collaboration with academia in research programs 2. Risk partnerships with major suppliers in the 70-seater program 3. Focus on regional jets 4. Flexibility and agility to introduce product modifications 5. High-skilled manpower 6. Global presence 7. Customer base 8. Keep existing workforce (jobs) 9. Provide strength to brand name	1. No military product (technology transfer to civil products) 2. Small portfolio of products 3. Huge capital investment needed 4. Lack of experience in developing turboprop airplanes
External Origins	1. Provide new technology for the 30-50 seat capacity market segment and provide an environmental friendly airplane 2. Huge 50-seat fleet will need replacement 3. Emerging markets in India and China and other countries in the Pacific region 4. Stay ahead of competition 5. Development of existing market	1. Strong competition in the 70-110 seat capacity market segment 2. Increase of oil price 3. Competition is strongly subsidized 4. Menace of big terrorist attack with global consequences on travel 5. Governmental support of the competition 6. High interest rates in Brazil

Table 5.5. Strategy matrix.

	Opportunities	Threats
Strengths	O-S strategies: O1 ↔ S1/S2/S4/S5 O2 ↔ S3/S7/S9 O3 ↔ S6	T-S strategies: T1 ↔ S1/S4/S7 T2 ↔ S1/S2/S4
Weakness	O-W strategies: O4 ↔ W2 O5 ↔ W4	T-W strategies: T2 ↔ W4 T3 ↔ W3 T4 ↔ W2 T5 ↔ W1 T6 ↔ W3

In SWOT Matrix, there are four SWOT cells that are comparisons of opportunities, strengths, threats and weakness as seen before. Besides the SWOT analysis, the analysis of SWOT Matrix cells is subjective and could be made from many different points of view. These cells yield a variety of matches that helps generating the strategies. Table **5.5** shows the strategy matrix with some considered for the 50-seat program.

Regarding the O-S strategies, the company should pursue opportunities that are a good fit to its strengths. Below, the description of some considered in the strategy matrix of Table **5.5**:

- **O1↔ S1/S2/S4/S5:** The aircraft development program is an extremely complex and challenging task. The airplane has to meet customers' needs and satisfy environmental requirements and offer a considerably lower operating cost when compared with existing airliners. The incorporation of new technologies, new manufacturing processes, advanced design tools, software development and other issues must be addressed. New concepts for the 30-50 seat market segment will be required both to provide lower operational costs, more passenger comfort, and airplanes with lower noise footprint and emission levels. A new opportunity may be could reveal economically viable and heavy competitors might be slow to react and fulfil it. There are basically four issues:
    1. The gap between capacity and demand is growing;
    2. Some operators use aircraft with too much capacity;
    3. New operations are pushing the limits of regional jets;
    4. Commercial fleet in the segment is aging.

  Besides strengthening the collaboration with research centers, new alliances with suppliers must also be established, increasing the accessibility to innovative technologies and encouraging them to develop new ones. All company's strengths allied with the opportunity to develop a modern product will certainly optimize the airline's profits by means of right-sizing their fleet in the untapped 70 to 110 seat market, helping the airlines to achieve operational efficiency without compromising performance or passenger comfort.
- **O3 ↔ S6:** Considering that the Asia Pacific market represents about 20% of the world's Revenue Passenger kilometers (RPK) in the 30-120 seat category, a participation that will be growing during the next twenty years, the development of a new fuel-efficient 50-seat airliner certainly represents a great opportunity for new businesses. Thus, the company can increase its presence in this region, and in other parts of the world, also preventing newcomers to enter the aircraft manufacturing club with a relatively low-cost aircraft program. There is a need to establish new offices and maintenance shops in the region.

By adopting O-W Strategies, the company should attempt to overcome weaknesses by taking advantage of opportunities. Addressing one contained in Table **5.5**:

- **O4 ↔ W2:** With just a 70-seat airplane and a stretch able to accommodate 80 passengers in a single class configuration, the portfolio of products is limited and must be expanded. A new business jet could also be developed from the 50-seat airliner (or from a shortened version of it), increasing even more the participation in the civil aviation market. Consumer needs and wants continuously changes. Firms should respond to these changes through their products and services. Otherwise consumers will switch to competitor products that satisfy their needs and wants.

T-S Strategies: the company should identify ways for using its strengths in order to reduce its vulnerability to external threats. Again, the description of one of those shown in Table **5.5**:

- **T2 ↔ S1/S2/S4:** 50-seat jets are more expensive to operate on a per seat basis, even though they operate in a single class configuration while the larger ones have First and Premium Economy, making them less dense. To remain competitive in a high-oil price scenario, they must be extremely fuel-efficient. This requires investment in innovative technologies, which turn the aircraft development program costlier and riskier. This will require a strong cooperation and collaboration with research centers and risk partners. The opposite scenario, if a significant drop in oil prices takes place, airlines will process with a fleet reorganization keeping older fuel-thirsty airplanes. Suddenly, customers may notice that the airplanes they are boarding might be somewhat older. The value of older aircraft currently in service rises with lower fuel costs. Specifically, it becomes attractive to either extend the use of older aircraft or lease older airplanes that may otherwise be pegged for decommissioning. Although reduced fuel prices may slow the purchase of new aircraft, an extended period of higher margins could also unlock capital for investment. Airlines could then get a push to modernize their fleets.

T-W Strategies: the company establishes a defensive plan to minimize its weaknesses from making it highly susceptible to external threats.

- **T2 ↔ W4:** Turboprop may represent the optimal airplane if a huge surge in oil price occurs. However, turboprop acquisition costs must remain in line with those of larger jets on a per-seat basis, according to some consulting companies specialized in the aviation market.

A 50-seat New Airplane Program

Two market analyzes are presented in this section relative to a 50-seat regional jet program [7]. Two teams of aeronautical engineering undergraduate students who took the tests in 2013 carried out the studies. The original text was somewhat changed by the author of this Chapter for purposes of text clarity and precision. The requirements that were provided to the design teams are summarized in Table **5.6**.

Table 5.6. Requirements set for the market analysis of a 50-seat regional jet [7].

Parameter		Figure
Maximum operating Mach number		Somewhat in the range 0.70 - 0.85
Passenger capacity		50
Service ceiling		Choice by design team
Takeoff field length (MTOW, ISA, sea level)		≤ 1700 m
Range with maximum payload		≥ 1600 nm
Direct Operating Cost (DOC) (900nm stage length)		20% lower than that of ERJ 145XR
Cabin comfort	Windows pax cabin	Dimming electronic system
	Aisle width	≥ 0,50 m
	Internal noise at wing-fuselage junction station	-15 dB lower than that from ERJ 145LR
Emissions LTO NO_X		30% lower than that from ERJ 145XR
Noise signature at ICAO points		Stage 4 - 15 dB

Team 1 Report on 50-seat Regional Jet

The successful regional jet seats emerged in the early 1990s, complementing the market for turboprop and replacing them on many routes. The need for less expensive flights on regional routes was an opportunity for companies such as EMBRAER and Canadair (later acquired by Bombardier) to share the small jet market with their ERJ 145 family jets and CRJ-100/200, respectively. These small aircraft boosted the aviation market creating wealth in medium-sized cities, facilitating tourism and increasing business. The operating companies were intrinsically low-cost airlines, which obtained higher profits due to low operational cost of these aircraft, lower wages for pilots and high average occupancy rates. However, the use of these planes has decreased substantially after the 2008 crisis, caused by neoliberal policies and oil price hikes. Tables **5.7a** and **5.7b** show the main types of aircraft removed from service and stationed in places with low humidity to aid in their conservation [8, 9].

Table 5.7a. Out of operation airliners.

Aircraft Type	2010	2009	2008
MD-80	288	304	282
Boeing 737 (CFMI)	265	303	247
Boeing 737 (JT8D)	218	244	244
Boeing 747	193	201	157
DC-9	171	189	196
Tupolev Tu-154	164	189	153
Boeing 727	160	165	217
Bombardier CRJ	144	105	100
Antonov An-26	117	125	138
Yakolev Yak-40	103	128	104
Airbus A320	100	99	53
Airbus A340	99	101	100
Boeing 757	97	95	85
Antonov An-24	93	108	126

(Source: AviationWeek, http://aviationweek.com/awin/parting-ways)

Regional jets (RJs) were stored in the desert based on their cost of operation. Jets with 50 seats or less greatly suffered from the sharp rise of oil price in the 2000s (Fig. **5.15**). In 2014, oil barrel price exceeded US$ 120, so that smaller capacity aircraft became unfeasible to operate as evidenced by Table **5.7a** and **5.7b**. Another reason that the airlines have discarded 50-seat airliners and even smaller ones was the relaxation of various scope clauses by several airlines in the United States (Table **5.8**). Scope clauses are contractual agreements between airlines and pilot associations that impose restrictions on the quantity and size of aircraft that a regional airline can operate [10]. The large number of airlines that have filed for bankruptcy, has led to the relaxation of scope clauses, allowing 70-seat or larger aircraft to be operated [10].

Table 5.7b. Data for North-American regional jet fleet in 2014 (Source: Airfleets.net).

Airline	Aircraft	In operation	In storage
American Eagle	ERJ 135	0	36
American Eagle	ATR 42	0	3
American Eagle	ATR 72	0	16
American Eagle	SAAB 340	0	54

(Table 5.7b) contd.....

Airline	Aircraft	In operation	In storage
Comair	CRJ-100	0	77
Comair	EMB-120 Brasilia	0	7
ExpressJet	CRJ-200	92	9
ExpressJet	ERJ 135	8	22
ExpressJet	ERJ 145	240	2
Republic Airways	Dash 8-400	20	3
Republic Airways	EMBRAER 190	8	1

Fig. (**5.16**) plots energy efficiency, *i.e.*, the mass of fuel required to move a passenger a mile, for various transport jets. It can be seen that the maximum efficiency occurs with aircraft which have about 3000 nm range with typical payload, such as the Boeing 767-200. From there, the efficiency falls again with increased range up to about 5200 nm. Again, we see an improvement in efficiency until we reach the Boeing 777-200LR. Regional jets typically present a typical range of 2000 nm. The plot reveals that RJs have low energy efficiency when compared to aircraft of greater capacity. The Fokker 70 has the same wing of the larger Fokker 100. Thus, its structure is oversized to carry 79 passengers in a single class and, therefore, reveals a relatively poor energy efficiency index compared with the airplanes listed in the chart of Fig. (**5.16**).

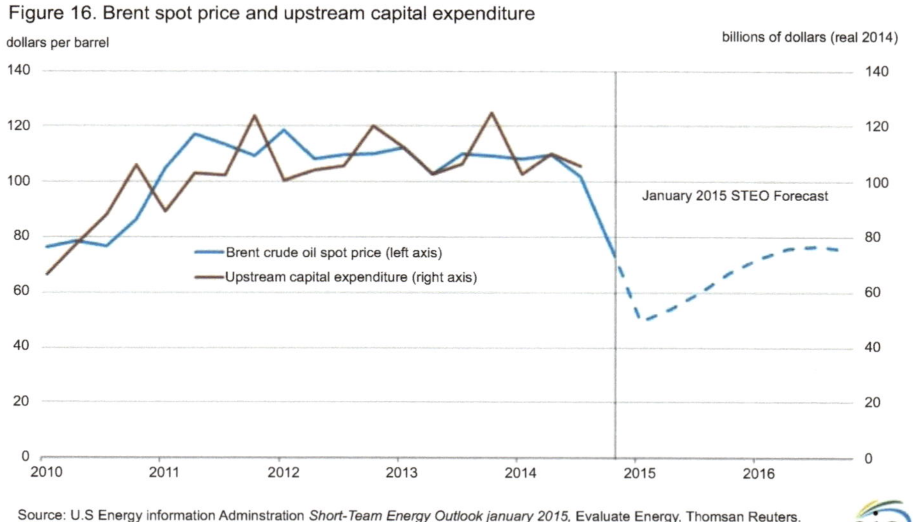

Fig. (5.15). Price evolution of Brent crude oil barrel.
(Source: U.S. Energy Information Administration)

Table 5.8. This 2012 analysis shows the effects of changing scope clauses, which were indicating that 75-seat jets would embrace 70% of the market below 90 seats [9, 10].

	2000	2001
United	100% jets between 30-60 seats	54% jets between 61-90 seats 46% jets between 30-60 seats
Continental	100% jets between 30-60 seats	100%
Us Airways	100% jets between 30-60 seats	61% jets between 61-90 seats 39% jets between 30-60 seats
Delta	100% jets between 30-60 seats	60% jets between 61-90 seats 40% jets between 30-60 seats
American	100% jets between 30-60 seats	29% jets between 61-90 seats 71% jets between 30-60 seats

(Source: EMBRAER)

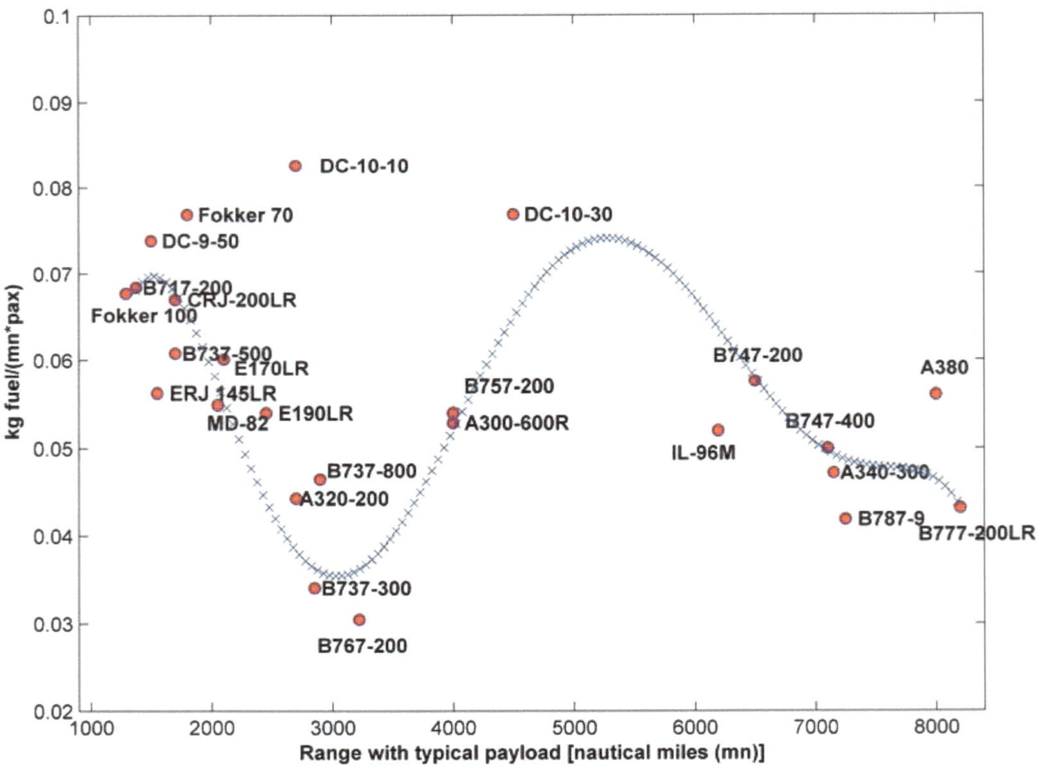

Fig. (5.16). Energy efficiency plot for some airliners.

The Federal Aviation Administration (FAA) yearly issues a forecast for the aerospace sector. According to FAA, U.S. domestic capacity decreased by 7.7 percent in the 2007-2012 period [11]; and mainline carriers reduced their domestic capacity by 9.2 percent with share decreases by network carriers more than offsetting the growth of low-cost carriers [11]. Regional airlines expanded capacity 2.4 percent since 2007. During the same period, mainline carrier Revenue Passenger Miles (RPMs) decreased 5.0 percent, while enplanements have fallen 7.3 percent [11]. In comparison, regional carrier RPMs and enplanements increased 5.3 percent and 1.8 percent, respectively [11]. As a result, mainline carrier domestic capacity share has fallen from 87.6 percent in 2007 to 85.7 percent in 2012, with the share of domestic RPMs flown by mainline carriers dropping from 88.3 percent to 86.8 percent during the same period.

At first glance, the market outlook for airplanes seating up to 50 passengers is not promising [10]. The analysis of this type of market requires attention to the US market, since it has the largest regional fleet, comprising 80% of the world. Of this regional market, 42.6% are composed of 50-seat jets. But one cannot fail to analyze the emerging market countries, where really good business opportunities can be found.

Oil barrel topped US$ 140 in 2008. Consequently, due to the huge increase in fuel prices, operating costs of jets with 50 seats or lower also increased considerably. In this panorama, Bombardier closed the assembly line of the CRJ-200; EMBRAER did not receive any more orders for the ERJ 145 aircraft family. Nevertheless, the Brazilian company still kept the models in its portfolio of marketable products in 2014.

To amortize the increase in operating direct cost, DOC, airlines have operated and made requests for jets in the range of 70-80 seats, especially for routes where there is sufficient demand to maintain higher load factors. Although the larger aircraft present the greatest absolute DOC, the cost is diluted among a higher number of seats [11]. For example, the DOC per seat E715LR is 14.3% lower than that for the ERJ 145LR [12] (Fig. **5.17**). Furthermore, revenue with the E175 was larger for the same occupancy rate. To ensure high profit margins, the goal of the companies is precisely to maintain this load factor for the largest passenger capacity aircraft. Despite the pessimistic current situation, forecasts carried out by JADC (Japan Aircraft Development Corporation) indicated in 2008 that by 2028 there would be a demand for 2,081 airplanes (1,108 new ones) in the range of 20-59 seats [13], shown in Fig. (**5.18**). Based on this document, Team No. 1's market research concludes, considering the size of the U.S. market in 2013, that 1000 of these aircraft would be 50-seat jets. Therefore, according to them, if their company could ensure a substantial share in this market, a great opportunity for profit, with a market estimated at 25.5 billion dollars, would emerge. Another important aspect to consider is the obsolescence of 50-seat airliners, which were designed in the early 1990s and have not received any significant technology upgrades until recent times. Thus, the current models will be even more outdated further in the future. In addition, no aircraft manufacturer has shown interest in investing in new concepts for the 50-seat aircraft.

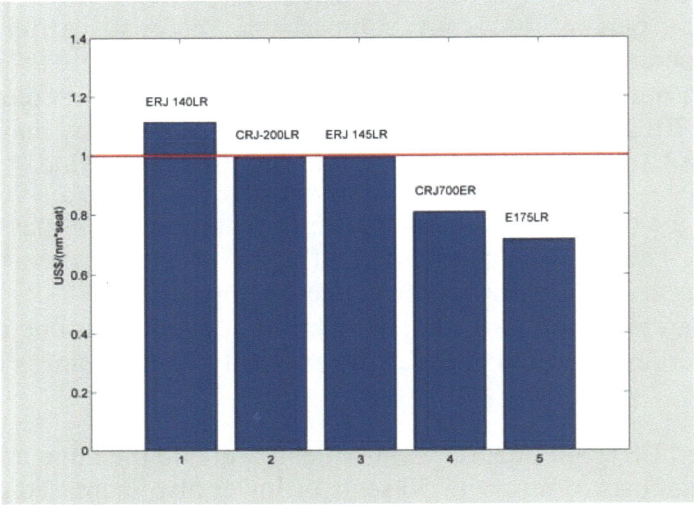

Fig. (5.17). Comparative DOC per seat for some regional jets (ERJ 145LR =1) [11].

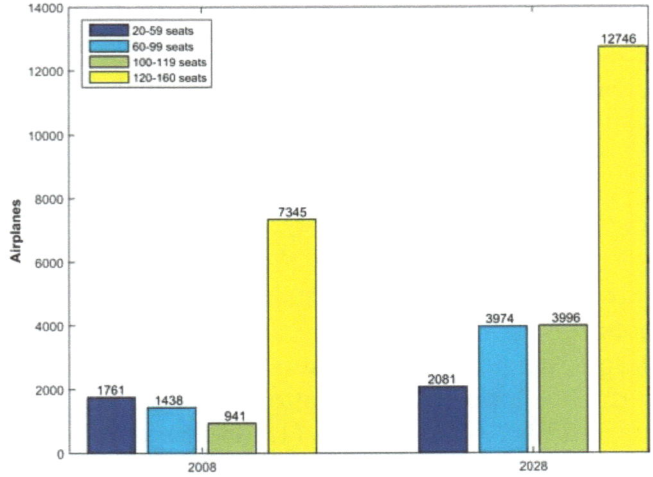

Fig. (5.18). Market forecast for transport airplanes carried out by Japan Aircraft Development Corporation in 2008 [12]. Numbers indicate the sum of new plus retained airplanes.

"Therefore, there would be a large market opportunity for a company that is able to develop a 50-seat jet with considerably lower DOC. It will have a great chance to be hegemonic in this sector."
Team no. 1

JADC published a report in 2013 in which the future demand for jets in the range of 20-59 seats was completely revised: the previous/original estimation of 1,108 new aircraft contained in the 2008 report, changed to only 146 (319 in total) in 2028 [14] (Fig. **5.19**). According to the JADC new scenario in their new report, the development of a 50-seat jet program would not be feasible. However, the Team 1 analysis was based on the 2008 JADC report. This report had concluded that the demand for 50-seat aircraft was promising because the regional market had enormous potential in emerging markets such as Africa, Latin America and Eastern Europe with the strengthening of their respective regional markets in the coming years. Then a global economic-financial crisis started in 2008. This crisis led fuel prices to skyrocket and the global economy almost came to a standstill, with dozens of millions of people losing their jobs. Thus, the operation of smaller airplane became unprofitable on many routes.

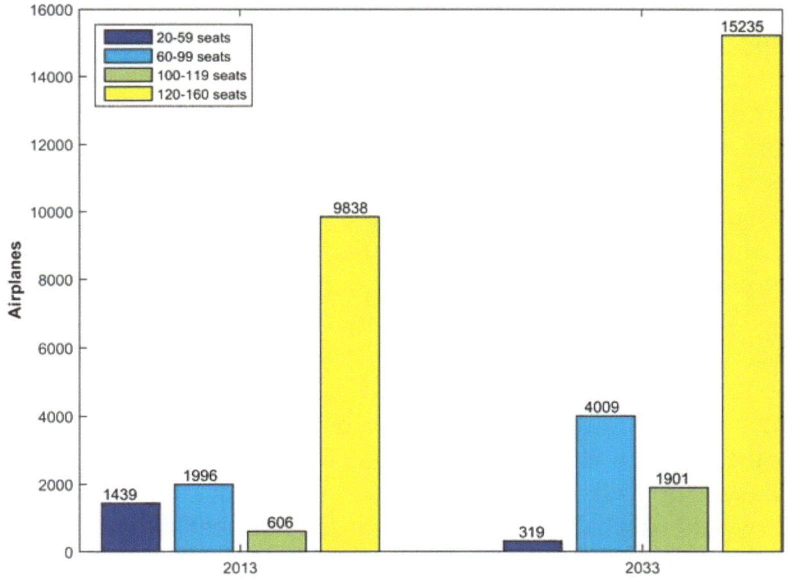

Fig. (5.19). Market forecast for airliners carried out by Japan Aircraft Development Corporation in 2013 [13]. Numbers indicate the sum of new plus retained airplanes.

The conclusions of the Team 1 were based on the 2008 JADC report, and they stated:

> *"Available data reveal that the general outlook for the aviation market is promising to consider the optimistic expectation of world economic growth until 2029. Considering the trend of economic growth, more airlines will be founded, that will be eager to make good profit. In this more competitive environment, airlines will probably have to invest in alternative routes to conquer customers. By having 50-seat airplanes, they can guarantee a higher load factor for specific routes. Given these arguments, it is noted that the1, 108 new aircraft that will be needed according to JDAC totally encourages an investment analysis for a new product. This number can even be considered pessimistic market estimation. In general, business for a 50-seat airliner can be promising, so the development program of a 50-seat jet is recommended."*

The Brazilian Federal Government announced an investment package valued R$ 7.3 billion for the expansion of regional aviation, with mesh increase of regional airports in all regions of the country. The project also included renovations and expansions of airport infrastructure in Brazil [15]. Likewise, airport data revealed that airport infrastructure expansions in China and India are also strongly occurring [16]. This is consistent with the expected growth of regional airport markets in emerging markets. Regarding the interest of aircraft manufacturers in the 50-seat market, based on the Boeing and Airbus analysis reports, it can be affirmed that most airlines have no or little interest in aircraft with capacity smaller than 60 seats. The Canadian Bombardier believes the 50-seat jet market will be small in the coming years, but also believes that there may be potential for growth in demand due to emerging markets. However, there is apparently no change to the development of a new plane with 50 seats, mainly due to cost overruns of the CSeries program [17]. Because of the smaller AVIC (Aviation Industry Corporation of China), it is believed that there is little chance it wants to enter the regional jet segment because Bombardier and EMBRAER have already established themselves firmly in this market; but if AVIC wanted to risk an assault it would probably not threaten the market shares of the other manufacturers, winning just a small portion of the market.

Team 2 Report on 50-seat Regional Jet

The 50-seat jets "exploded" in the late 1990s, when they were ordered in copious quantities by airlines around the world. They enjoyed passengers' preference, had good range and reasonable operating costs. These jets were a suitable alternative to meet growing demand for fast and reliable regional air transport [10, 18]. The explosion in sales, however, faded out when sales plunged from the middle of 2000 decade on (Fig. **5.20**). The causes were mainly due to changes in the economic situation, with higher fuel prices making it unprofitable to use a jet of low demand and low distance routes. Thus, from the first decade of this century on, there was resurgence in demand for turboprop airplanes, concepts from the 1980s, like the ATR 42 and the Bombardier Q-400. Moreover, the growth of the regional segment led to a demand for higher-capacity aircraft. It is expected that in the coming decades, sales of airplanes with larger capacity will be considerably bigger than those of the 50-seat ones [19].

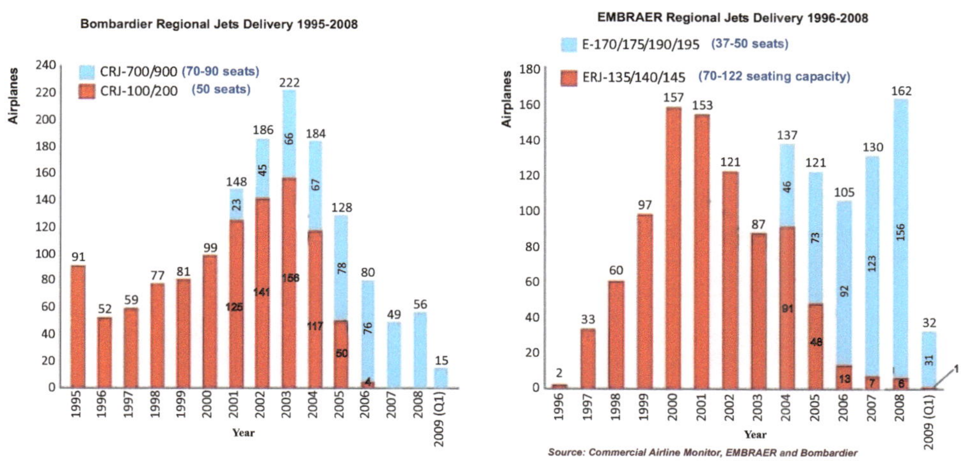

Fig. (5.20). Bombardier and EMBRAER jet deliveries [10, 18].

Currently, this market segment undergoes an ambiguous situation. With the aging of the regional jet fleet, companies start looking for a replacement, but there is a quite suitable alternative on the market. Although the turbo-propellers can be used in many of the routes served by jets before, there are some, notably the long-range, where only regional jets are suitable [19]. The growth in passenger numbers tends to generate demand for larger jets, but in some key markets such as the United States, such aircraft are barred by scope clauses (Table **5.9**) imposed by pilot associations [10].

Finally, a growing demand for regional aircraft in developing countries is expected, as regional transport is still incipient in these regions (Fig. **5.21**). It is expected however, that much of this demand is met by turboprops, as well as regional jets already used.

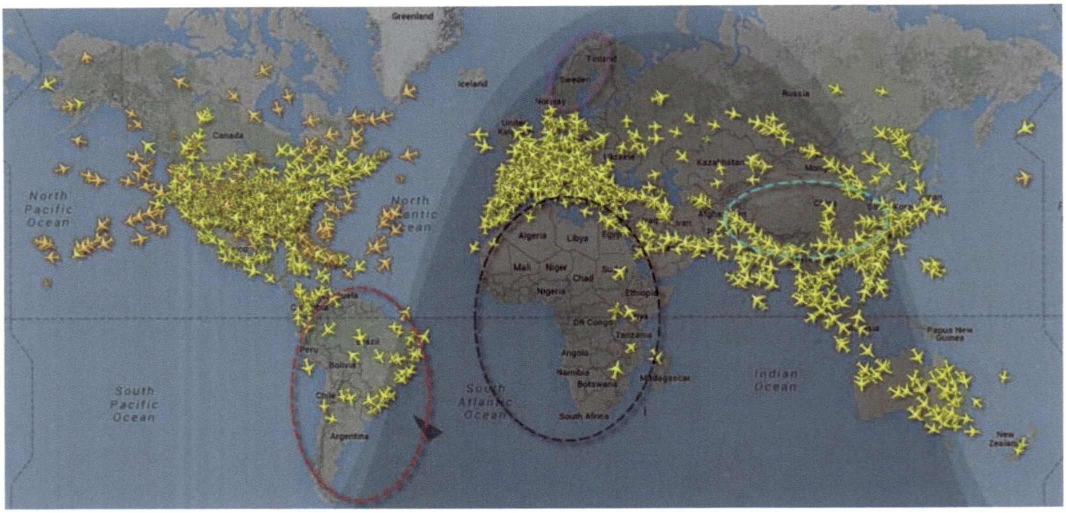

Fig. (5.21). Air traffic on May 2nd, 2015 at 18h00min Brasilia time. Highlight regions indicate potential for traffic growth (Courtesy Flightradar24.com).

Table 5.9. List of some scope clauses restricting regional airplanes operation by North-American airlines in 2009 [10].

Airline	Restrictions
American Airlines	• 50-70 seats a) 43 turboprops b) jets not allowed • Not allowed airplanes with capacity above 70 seats
Delta Airlines	• No limit for turboprops 70 seats • No limit for jets below 50 seats • Maximum 200 jets accommodating 50 to 70 passengers • Maximum 66 jets with capacity between 70 and 76 passengers • Airplanes seating more than 76 passengers not allowed
US Airways	• Maximum 250 jets below 44 seats • Maximum 336 jets with seating capacity between 44 and 86 passengers • Airplanes seating more than 86 passengers not allowed

Thus, the marketing of a new jet 50-set regional jet will not offer good business opportunities, because it is mainly dependent on the economic and financial situation of the United States, as this is the main potential market. If a jet able to compete in terms of DOC with turboprop were to be developed, it would probably have a good chance on the regional market. Elsewhere in the world, the demand for this jet class would be very low due to the need for larger capacity aircraft and/or lower cost per seat.

Reports of the leading manufacturers (Table **5.10**) estimate the demand for up to 50-seat airplanes in 300-400 units [20]. Turboprops will account for approximately 50% of this total. Thus, demand for jet-powered airplanes seating 50 passengers or less is estimated from 150 to 200 units. Therefore, Team No. 2 concluded the impracticality of a 50-seat airplane development to replace the ERJ 145 and CRJ-200 [19].

Table 5.10. Bombardier market outlook for the period ranging from 2011 to 2030 [20].

Passenger Capacity	Fleet in 2010	Deliveries	Retirements	Fleet in 2030
20-59	3,600	300	2,500	1,400
60-99	2,200	5,800	1,200	6,800
100-149	5,200	7,000	3,000	9,200
Total →	11,000	13,100	6,700	17,400

FINANCIAL ANALYSIS

Reasoning

Any design team is normally required to work with a limited amount of funds and time, which could dictate various aspects of the design process. For example, innovations which could lead to a spiraling budget might be shelved. Also, in case of highly competitive markets, the ability to get the airplane ready in the prescribed term is very crucial. The design team must ensure that cost and time over-runs are minimized to the extent possible.

The analysis of the economic viability of a product development program involves calculating financial parameters of investment to conclude its viability. This analysis is usually initiated after market research. The cost estimated for the program will establish the purchase price of the product, which will make the program viable and cover the costs involved in development and manufacturing.

Definitions

In this activity, key financial indicators relating the program to the final product are defined, such as the product cost, cash flow, break-even point, the Net Present Value (NPV), the internal rate of return (IRR), and the payback method (amortization). This analysis of the economic and financial viability performed during the program planning is the initial reference to the following phases in the development of the product itself. It is one of the most important criteria for maintaining the program.

There is a need for a periodic analysis review throughout the program. This is because during the planning activity only preliminary information is available. Thus, along the initial phases of the program, eventual market and technological changes can affect the program. With the progress of the program, the envisaged conditions are getting closer to the actual conditions of the product at launch time. At this point, the certainty concerning the desired product characteristics increases. Issues like product receptivity and role in the market, the market itself (competition, latest trends, economic changes, *etc*.), and volume of sales become clearer. Thus, the economic and financial feasibility analysis can be refined and confronted with the first plan for learning effects regarding the predictive capacity at the beginning of a product development program. This review of the economic and financial viability occurs at the end of each phase of product development, sometimes coupled with the Product Review (Critical Design Review). Reviews can also occur at any time when major modifications of the product or the administration of the program so demand it, to verify that the product will remain financially viable.

Mechanisms

The main element that justifies the existence of a company is profit-making. For investors, however, it is not enough that the project has a positive outcome. To be an attractive development project, it is necessary that the amount of profit generated exceeds the one that the company could get with other investments, for example, by investing money in the financial market. Therefore, the essence of the economic and financial evaluation is to measure the project's return on comparable terms with other investments.

The first step that should be taken to carry out the economic analysis is the preparation of cash flow, *i.e.* the definition of the flow of cash inflows and outflows during the life cycle planned for the product.

Cash flow

Cash flow is a key management tool in making business decisions. Its objectives are the collection and organization of data and the generation of subsidies for the financial analysis of performance and the achievement of budget forecasts. The three main components of cash flow are the following:

1. Investment in New Products

This corresponds to the expenses required to generate long-term benefits. It is the amount of money spent on the specification, development, preparation and production of the product. The determination of the investment spent should take into consideration the following factors:

- *The kind of product development*: depending on the design, investment can be large or small. For example, in the case of a product which should generate only incremental gains over an existing one, the investment is smaller than that of radical concepts. This is so, because the necessary products and processes are derived or adapted, hybrid or with minor modifications in relation to what already exists. Radical or completely innovative projects involve the creation of a whole new product, or significant product changes, therefore requiring innovative technologies, big modifications of existing processes, new materials, purchase of new equipment, new tooling, *etc*.
- *The availability of resources*: this refers to expenses to acquire resources, such as manpower, machines, equipment, vehicles, appliances, buildings and other items of that nature;
- *Payment obligations*: royalties, patents, laboratories, and licensing;
- *Surveys and analyzes*: market surveys, professional training, and consulting;
- *The working capital*: there is a necessity for working capital, including its use in unexpected situations.

One way to calculate the necessary investment involves creating specific working sheets for each program, which would contain all carried payments and expenses. The biggest challenge is to compute the cost for personnel, mainly for team members who divide their time between various programs. One should also clearly define the time when the costs and revenues will be calculated. Generally, this time is at the end of the pilot batch approval. The product leaving the assembly line can then be marketed, starting the two other components of cash flow: revenues and production expenses.

2. Revenues

Revenues correspond to estimated sales of products and by-products to be produced. To calculate them, factors such as price and demand of end products must be considered.

- *Product Purchase price*: This value will depend on the market in which to sell the product and the profit expected by the manufacturer. The higher the price, the lower the market share. Studies of the variation of these two factors to find a good compromise between profitability and market share are mandatory.
- *Demand*: This value will depend on the product (products with high added value generally have a lower sale volume), the market and the market share that the product means to achieve, the sale price, and the locational analysis.

To calculate the revenues, one must estimate the amount of demand for the products, and then multiply it by the estimated street price. In addition to the sales revenue generated, other factors must be taken into consideration, such as governmental subsidies, financing, and residual value of the investment.

3. Production Costs and Expenses

It must be ensured that the money is spent directly and indirectly on the production and marketing of the product. Costs are the expenses on goods or services used to produce other goods. Each enterprise, personal or business, involves two types of costs: recurring and non-recurring. Isolated costs, often called startup costs are non-recurring. Costs that occur on a regular schedule are listed on a budget as recurring costs and should be considered in the manufacture of series of aircraft.

The main costs are:

- Raw materials, packages, auxiliary materials.
- Direct manpower.
- Consumption of electric power, water and fuel.
- Maintenance, insurance, rentals, diverse.

Expenses consist of goods or services used to generate revenues. The main expenses are:

- Sale expenses, financial and administrative;
- Salaries of administrative staff;
- Taxes and fees.

Costs and production expenses must be differentiated, which is a task that is often difficult. For example, spending on a production that aims to produce a prototype part is investment. However, the cost of the same operation in an identical part, after releasing the pilot batch, which will be marketed, should already be recognized as a direct cost, to be accounted to that product. After the start of serial production, when some prototypes are no longer used, some companies sell them at a discount to customers. This should be considered in the preparation of cost sheets.

The interval for the calculation of cash flow depends on the length of the product life cycle. An airliner, in general, is conceived to be 15 to 20 years in operation and, therefore, the calculations are performed on a yearly basis. These calculated values are summed up to obtain a final value of the rate of return on investment as shown in Fig. (**5.22**).

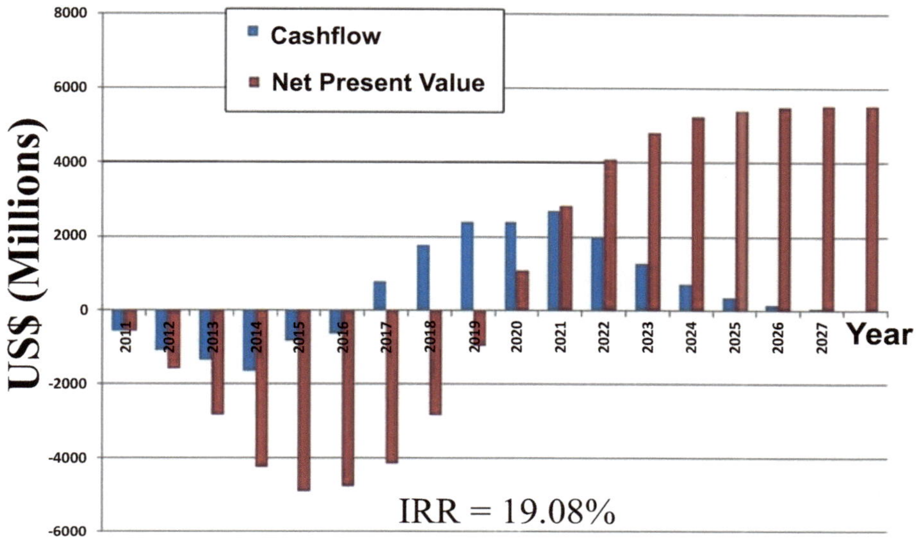

Fig. (5.22). Example of cash flow for the development and production of an airliner.

Financial Indicators

Fig. (**5.22**) shows an estimation of the cash flow over time (years) of the product life cycle. To conclude whether a project is economically feasible or not, it is necessary to evaluate and compare it to other investments available to company owners. This calculation should consider that money has a value dependent on time, that is, receiving US$ 500 today represents a different value to receiving the same amount next year. Therefore, the use of financial ratios and parameters calculated with cash flow data allows comparisons of project financial performance. Three of the financial indicators most commonly used in product development projects are:

Net Present Value (NPV)

This method of investment analysis determines the present value of future payments. This method consists of a simple mathematical and financial formula in which the value of investments and the current and future cash flows are converted to an equivalent value in the current date by a conversion rate. The reason for this conversion is that the purchasing value of money changes over time. The conversion rate used in this method is the Minimum Attractiveness Rate (MAR).

Equation 5.1 shows the formula for the calculation of the NPV.

$$NPV = \sum_{t=0}^{n} \frac{FC_t}{(1+i)^t} \begin{cases} \text{t = time (years or months)} \\ \text{n = project time} \\ \text{i = minimum acceptable rate of return (MAR)} \\ \text{FC = Cash flow} \end{cases} \quad \textbf{(5.1)}$$

The net present value of an investment project has the following possible results:

- *Greater than zero*: means that the investment is economically attractive because the present value of inflow capital is higher than the present value of expenses.
- *Equal to zero*: the investment is indifferent because the present value of cash inflows equals the present value of cash outflows.
- *Less than zero:* Indicates that the investment is not economically attractive because the present value of cash inflows is less than the present value of cash outflows.

The project presenting the highest NPV is the most attractive from an investment point-of-view.

Example: The management of a given company is considering the installation of new equipment. The investment proposition contemplates an initial expense of US$ 10,000.00 to achieve a yearly cost reduction of US$ 1,000.00 for 10 years. Considering that the minimum attractiveness rate is 10% per year, the management must know whether the investment is feasible.

Solution:

Utilizing **Eq. 5.1** leads to:

$$FC(0) = +10000,00; \;\; FC(1 \rightarrow 10) = -1000,00; \;\; \text{and } \; i = 10/100.$$

Resulting in a NPV of US$ -38,55.43, thus indicating that the investment is not feasible.

The inverse problem finds out the minimum cost reduction value that makes the investment indifferent. The following MATLAB® code performs this task:

```
function vpl()
clc
clear all
n=11;
i=10/100;
FCi=-10000;
FCstart=2000;
[solucao, valor]=fsolve(@resvpl,FCstart,[],FCi,n,i);
fprintf('\n Valor da reducao de custo para empate do investimento = $ %7.2f
\n',solucao)
fprintf('\n Valor Present Liquido (VLP) = $ %7.2f \n',valor)
function vplval=resvpl(x,FCi,n,i)
FC(1)=FCi;
FC(2:n)=x;
for j=1:n
t(j)=j-1;
end
for j=1:n
vp(j)=FC(j)/((1+i)^t(j));
end
vplval=sum(vp);
```

The NPV becomes zero for a cost reduction of US$ 1,627.45 in a 10-year period.

Internal Rate of Return - IRR

It establishes the economic rate needed to equalize the value of an investment in its future returns. It refers to the rate of return that must be provided by the project so that it equals its investment after a period. The IRR is calculated using the same formula described above, however equaling the NPV to zero and using the IRR conversion rate as unknown.

Later ITR is compared with MAR established by the company to verify the project performance. Three scenarios arise:

- IRR > MAR: means that the investment is economically attractive.
- IRR = MAR: the investment is indifferent from the economic point-of-view.
- IRR < MAR: the investment is not attractive. Its return is overcome by others with a low-risk investment.

Among several investments, the best will be the one offering the highest IRR.

Payback

The payback is one of the simplest methods, explaining its widespread use. It consists essentially of determining the number of periods necessary to recoup the capital invested. With this assessment, the company's management, based on their time standards to recover the investment, the expected lifetime of the asset, associated risks and its financial position, decide to accept or reject the project.

Break-even Point

In economics and business, specifically cost accounting, the break-even point (BEP) is the point at which cost or expenses and revenue are equal: there is no net loss or gain, and one has "broken even." A profit or a loss has not been made, although opportunity costs have been "paid," and capital has received the risk-adjusted, expected return. It is shown graphically as the point where the total revenue and total cost curves meet. In the linear case the break-even point is equal to the fixed costs divided by the contribution margin per unit.

Recommendations for Feasibility Analysis

Each of the financial measures results in different information that can be used in a complementary way. The NPV is a method that provides a good sense of the amount that will be obtained with the program, that is, the value to be achieved, but it does not allow an easy comparison with other investments. This aspect is a great advantage of information obtained by the IRR, which provides an easily comparable metric. It is worth mentioning that the methods cited before depend on the following estimates:

- Product demand;
- Growth expectations;
- Selling price of the product that is accepted by the final consumer;
- Costs involved in the production of the product. The engagement of all parts of the organization, mainly of the marketing and sales departments, is essential.

There are projects that provide a good amount of money (NPV highly positive) and are also profitable (ITR higher than MAR), but the time to the return of the investment is long, meaning that the enterprise will face a long period expending money until profit is made. For this reason, for the analysis of these three indicators the following recommendations are made:

Premises for the Calculation of the Viability

The definition of the premises is the most strategic point to influence the viability analysis. The premises include the forecasts of the future demand; the price that will be stipulated; the resulting cost of the operation and basically the fees that will serve as reference in the future. It is not easy to foresee all that information and therefore it is considered premises for the analysis.

Viability Monitoring

The analysis of the economic viability is normally accomplished at the beginning of the product development and it is rarely revised. It makes no sense to calculate the investment again, because the expended money cannot be recovered. However, a simulation of all the analysis, adjusting the premises and verifying the indicators again, can supply a vision of the extent to which the company is accurate in its forecasts. In order to monitor the viability analysis, it is important to overturn decisions (for example, expenses) during the development for the acknowledgement whether that product/service is still viable, ahead of possible changes of the premises (*i.e.* competition launched a similar product first and the volumes of sales will therefore not be the same; financial crises; changes in the reference fees; *etc.*).

Consider Analysis with Possible Risks

When a feasibility analysis is performed, it is based on the belief that all the assumptions are correct. However, there are risks that cannot be foreseen. Basically, risks are classified into two categories: technological risks and market risks. The risks of the first category deal with issues associated with the probability of success (or failure) of technology and solutions adopted. This is more important to be examined in the case of innovations being incorporated into the product. The market risks consider the success or failure that a product could experience. Thus, it is mandatory to evaluate these risks during the feasibility analysis, as well as the assumptions that were made. For example, a given NPV will occur if associated with low risks.

What might happen if two development projects were to be compared? One might present a high NPV and the other could have a low NPV. What should be prioritized? The answer to this question could also depend on risk. If the probability of success of the second project were to be much higher than the first, in a balancing portfolio analysis of development projects, the latter might be prioritized.

Example of Financial Analysis

Any enterprise, personal or business, involves two types of costs: recurring and non-recurring. Isolated costs, often called startup costs are non-recurring. Costs that occur on a regular schedule are listed on a budget as recurring costs and should be considered in the aircraft serial manufacture.

In this section, the typical methodology for estimating the cost of a transport airplane program, and its viability is presented. Here, the same airplane specified in the previous section (market analysis) is used, a regional 50-seat jet. The analysis carried out by Team No. 1 [12] will be considered. It concludes that there is a market to be exploited with good business opportunities.

First, recurring and non-recurring costs are calculated and analyzed. Then, an estimate of cash flow and net present value of the program is calculated. Finally, the viability of the program is analyzed. The last four years were considered for aircraft development.

Non-recurring Costs

The cost of manpower was estimated using a weighted average of typical hour labor cost of an aircraft manufacturer and its partners considering a 30% partner in the non-recurring cost of the aircraft (Table **5.11**). The costs mentioned in Table **5.12** are considered for May 2015, with the calculation of the estimated inflation obtained from the Website: *http://www.usinflationcalculator.com.*

Table 5.11. Hourly cost of manpower [12].

Program share		**Manpower/h (US$)**
Aircraft manufacturer	70%	41.72
Partners	30%	83.44
Average		**54.24**

The total cost of labor was obtained by summing up the costs of each area of the aircraft development. For this estimate, working hours necessary for the development and learning of new technologies such as the use of composite structures developed by the partners and the use of welding by friction (Friction Stir Welding or FSW) were also considered. The total cost and the breakdown of working hours are shown in Table **5.13**.

Table 5.12. Workload for development activities [12].

Discipline /Activity	**Hours**	**Discipline /Activity**	**Hours**
Total – Management and administration	1,136,367	Ground testing	208.050
Preliminary design	27,983	System testing	111.933
Interior	229,950	Flight test	160.600

(Table 5.12) contd.....

Discipline /Activity	Hours	Discipline /Activity	Hours
Structure	279,833	Instrumentation	122.883
Electric/Electronic	365,000	Pilots	48.667
Mechanic	121,667	Prototypes	2.828.750
Hydraulic	60,833	Rigs	60.833
Propulsion	51,100	Prototypes/Body of proof	97.333
Total - Engineering	2.188.783	Prototype maintenance	585.217
Aerodynamics	135.050	Manufacturing tooling	526.817
Aeroelasticity	237.250	Methods and processes	784.750
Performance	76.650	Quality control	138.700
Structure	365.000	Total – product support	635,100
Interior	92.467	Service bulletin	19,467
Electric/Electronic	365.000	Spare parts	103,417
Mechanic	399.067	Operation manual	203,183
Hydraulic	97.333	Consumer service	6,083
Propulsion	121.667	Documentation	128,967
Certification	121.667	Technical support	77,867
Configuration control	62.050	Maintenance plan	96,117
Technical documentation	115.583	Total – working hours	**9.634.783**
Total – testing and validation	5,674,533	Average hourly cost of manpower (US$)	**54.24**
		TOTAL→(US$)→	**522,552,108.87**

Workload over time is shown in Table **5.13**:

Table 5.13. Manpower cost expenses over time (Product development) [12].

Year	Percentage	US$/Year
2015	25%	130,638,027.22
2016	35%	182,893,238.10
2017	30%	156,765,632.66
2018	10%	52,255,210.89

Table **5.14** shows the components of the infrastructure cost. It was considered that the company already commercializes a 50-seat airplane. The assembly line will be adjusted for the manufacturing of the new airplane. New tooling, tailoring of new production stations, and building adaptations were considered. Investment in new welding technology FSW (Friction stir Welding) is necessary. The schedule for modifications of the assembly line has a strong bias for the first year for this task, as can be observed in Table **5.15**. This table contains the planning for the assembly line update over time. The general cost composition and the expenses schedule for the aircraft development are provided in Tables **5.16** and **5.17** respectively.

Table 5.14. Infrastructure cost components [12].

Infrastructure	US$
Machines and equipment	17,880,000
FSW - machines/tooling/building	9,536,000
Prototypes	35,760,000
Assembly line rework	1,192,000
Computational resources	6,913,600
Control/acquisition instruments	596,000
Office supplies	596,000
Software	1,788,000
Diverse investments	596,000
Grand total →	**74,857,600**

Table 5.15. Distribution of expenses for infrastructure over time [12].

Year	Percentage	US$/Year
2015	55%	41,171,680
2016	25%	18,714,400
2017	15%	11,228,640
2018	5%	3,742,880

Table 5.16. General cost breakdown [12].

General Costs	US$
Communication	834,400.00
Instrumentation and flight testing	4,529,600.00
Tooling	2,980,000.00
Travel	5,006,400.00
Third-party Manpower from risk Partners	23,840,000.00
Third party manpower	27,416,000.00

(Table 5.16) contd.....

General Costs	US$
Fuel	4,872.900.00
Total →	**69,479,300.00**

Table 5.17. General cost spending over time [12].

Year	Distribution	US$/Year
2015	25%	17,369,825.00
2016	35%	24,317,755.00
2017	30%	20,843,790.00
2018	10%	6,947,930.00

The estimated non-recurring cost can now be seen in Table **5.18**. The cost of aircraft manufacturer is also indicated. In Fig. (**5.23**), the distribution over the four years of the initial investment can be observed in addition to the house of contribution a major contributor to the non-recurring cost.

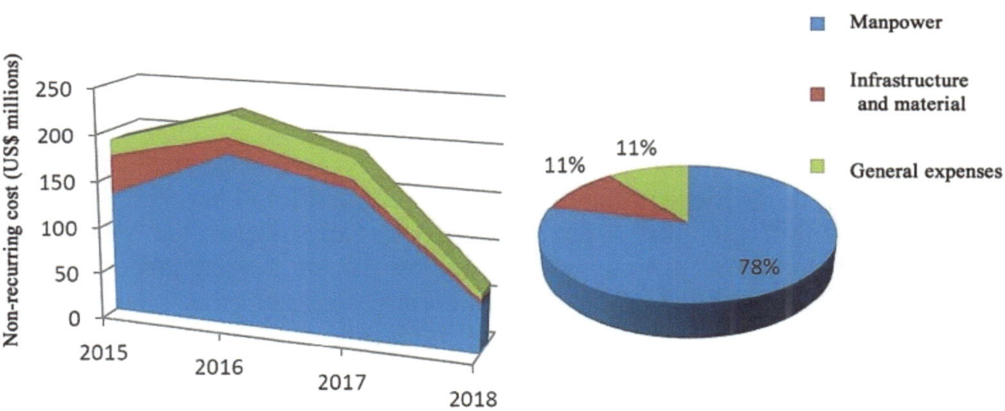

Fig. (5.23). Breakdown of non-recurring cost [12].

Table 5.18. Distribution of non-recurring costs along time (US$) [12].

Year	Manpower	Infrastructure and Material	General Expenses	Manufacturer (70%)	Manufacturer + Partners
2015	130.638.027	41,171,680	17.369.825	132,425,673	189.179.532
2016	182.893.238	18,714,400	24.317.755	158,147,775	225.925.393
2017	156.765.633	11,228,640	20.843.790	132,186,644	188.838.063

(Table 5.18) contd.....

Year	Manpower	Infrastructure and Material	General Expenses	Manufacturer (70%)	Manufacturer + Partners
2018	52.255.211	3,742,880	6.947.930	44,062	62.946.021
				TOTAL →	**666,889,009**

Recurring Cost

The recurring cost is dependent on the aircraft's life cycle, and is calculated for each aircraft. The recurring cost can be divided into: materials, labor, sales, process management and other miscellaneous costs. Note that besides work, other costs are fixed in time, since the paper presents a learning curve, with a cost that decreases with time, due to the acceleration of the manufacturing process.

Cost of materials can be divided into a few components. Using a simplified method, it is possible to determine the components from dimensionless parameters used by aircraft manufacturers, adjusted for inflation. The result can be seen in Table **5.19**.

In Table **5.19**, a column containing a complexity factor can be noted. This factor should be considered to fine-tune the dimensionless parameters. The undercarriage has a complexity factor of 1.2 because it is close to the wing, which requires a significant effort to design and integration with the structure of the wing and fuselage; the commands and flight controls have a complexity factor of 1.4, relatively high due to the choice of a full fly-by-wire system; Furthermore, the electrical systems present the 1.3 bias by conventional electrical systems substitutions (within the philosophy More Electrical Aircraft or MEA). The engines have a complexity factor of 1.1 due to use of geared turbofan (axial angular speed reduction) for higher fan efficiency. Such engine is heavier than conventional turbofan ones, making their integration into the aircraft more difficult. Finally, for the airplane structure, a complexity factor of 1.5 was set due to the use of composite materials, which usually have a more complex manufacturing process than metal structures.

Table 5.19. Recurring cost – Material (MTOW stands for Maximum Takeoff Weight) [12].

Components	US$/ Parameter	Parameter	Parameter Value	Complexity Factor	Cost (1000 US$)
Landing gear	8	kg of MTOW	22,010 kg	1.2	220
Flight controls	834	ft^2 of wing area	560 ft^2	1.4	654
Engines	2,000,000.00	unit	2 units	1.1	4400

(Table 5.19) contd.....

Components	US$/ Parameter	Parameter	Parameter Value	Complexity Factor	Cost (1000 US$)
Nacelles	11,920.00	Diameter in inches	63 in	1	751
Interior	19,072.00	passenger	50 pax	1	954
Electrical system	8,940.00	kVA	75 kVA	1.3	872
Electronics	953,600.00	Unit cost of an integrated assembly	1 unit	0.9	858
Structure	143	kg of MTOW	22.010 kg	1.5	4722
Fuel system	119	ft^2 of wing area	540 ft^2	1	64
TOTAL →					**13,496**

The calculation of the share of recurrent cost due to hand labor is done directly by the time required to produce the aircraft. To estimate the hourly charge per aircraft took up a 12% learning curve for the first aircraft and 2% in the learning factor. The average cost of labor is US$ 25 per hour. Using a forecasted 60% market share, we obtain the costs presented in Table **5.20**.

In addition to the costs previously discussed, the cost of sales, processing and other miscellaneous costs should be noted. These costs will be determined by a percentage of other recurring costs.

Table 5.20. Manpower in recurring cost [12].

Year	Deliveries (60% Market Share)	Working Hours per Unit	Manpower Cost per Unit (1000 US$)	Manpower Cost (1000 US$)
2019	6	36,714	918	5,507
2020	20	26,452	661	13,226
2021	44	23,363	584	25,700
2022	92	21,451	536	49,338
2023	94	20,218	505	47,511
2024	102	19,416	485	49,512
2025	94	18,899	472	44,413
2026	90	18,581	465	41,807
2027	84	18,389	460	38,617
2028	30	18,281	457	13,710

A good estimate for the cost of sale is taking it as 17% of the cost of materials and labor. Since the cost of processing, which includes support for process quality control management costs, can be estimated 8% of materials and labor costs. Finally, the various costs such as technical publications and training of the customer support team can be estimated as 5% of the cost of materials.

Table **5.21** compiles all recurring costs and provides an expense schedule to cover them. Fig. (**5.24**) shows the percentage of the recurring-cost components.

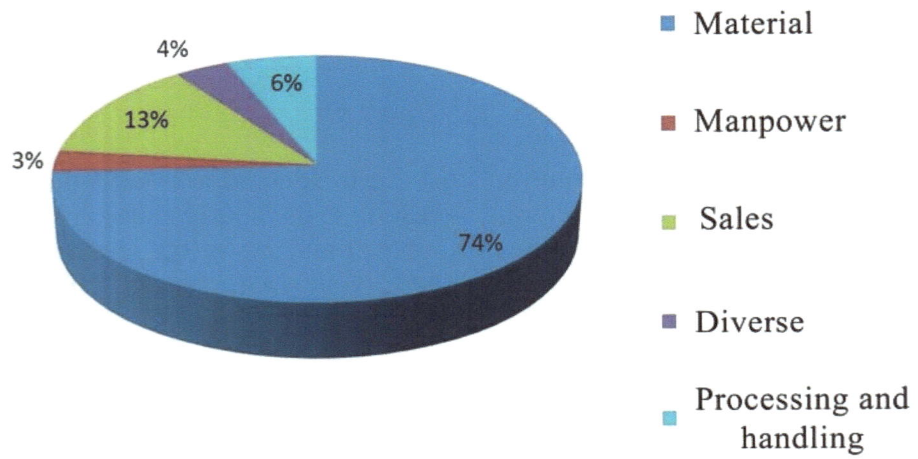

Fig. (5.24). Composition of recurring cost [12].

Table 5.21. Expenses schedule to cover the recurring costs [12].

Year	Deliveries	Material Cost	Manpower Cost	Cost of Sales*	General Cost**	Processing Cost***	Yearly Total
2019	6	81	6	15	4	7	112
2020	20	270	13	48	13	23	367
2021	44	594	26	105	30	50	804
2022	92	1,242	49	219	62	103	1,676
2023	94	1,269	48	224	63	105	1,709
2024	102	1,377	50	242	69	114	1,851
2025	94	1,269	44	223	63	105	1,705
2026	90	1,215	42	214	61	101	1,631
2027	84	1,134	39	199	57	94	1,522
2028	30	405	14	71	20	33	543

(Table 5.21) contd.....

Year	Deliveries	Material Cost	Manpower Cost	Cost of Sales*	General Cost**	Processing Cost***	Yearly Total
Total	656	8,853	329	1.561	443	735	11,921
* 17% of manpower + material cost ** 5% of material cost *** 8% of the manpower + material cost							

Based on Market studies, the share of 60% market has been defined by the program core team. From this number, it is then possible to determine a sales value of the aircraft based on the following points:

- Cost.
- Price competitiveness.
- Investment balance (*Break-even*).
- Internal rate of return.

After the price is defined, NPV can be calculated (Fig. **5.25**) and consequently the program's feasibility. A sales price of US$ 23 million is considered to be very competitive for the market share that was adopted. This price is US$ 500,000 lower than the competitor offering the lowest price. According to Fig. (**5.25**), the investment payback is achieved in the 5th production year, with 217 units sold. Considering that 656 airplanes will be manufactured, the break-even point is then obtained with just 33% of overall sales. The investment rate of return is 19.9% of the total amount invested over the project life cycle, including the recurring cost of each airplane. This provides an amount of US$ 2.5 billion in 2028.

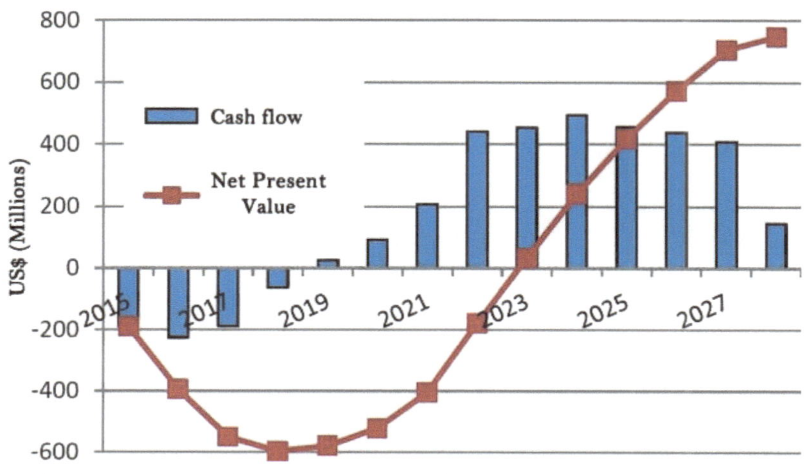

Fig. (5.25). Calculated cash flow of a 50-seat jet project [12].

Making use of the NPV method and considering a MAR of 10%, A IRR of 13.2% is achieved coupled with a US$ 746 million profit (in 2015 NPV). Thus, the Project is profitable and presents a *break-even* point that can be attained in relatively short time. If a very pessimistic market share is adopted, 30%, of the production of 328 airplanes provided 1% of IRR.

STRATEGY ANALYSIS

Overview

The pure competition model does not present a viable tool to assess an industry. Porter's Five Forces attempts to realistically assess potential levels of profitability, opportunity and risk based on five key factors within an industry. Industry structure and positioning within the industry are the basis for models of competitive strategy promoted by Michael Porter [21]. This model may be used as a tool to better develop a strategic advantage over competing firms within an industry in a competitive and healthy environment. It identifies five forces that determine the long-run profitability of a market or market segment. Fig. (**5.26**) shows those five forces and the most relevant factors concerning the four interaction factors between the forces.

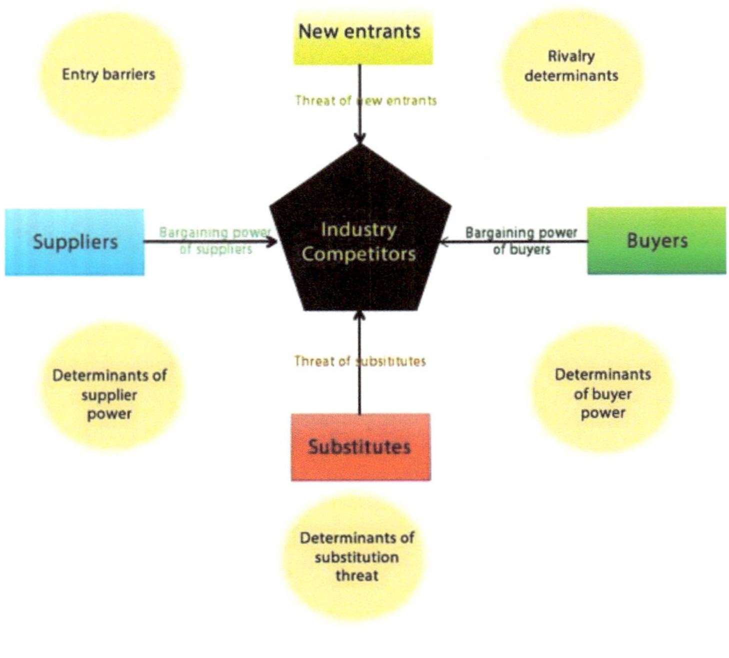

Fig. (5.26). Porter's Five Forces - Elements of Industry Structure [21].

Caution is advisable when using the concept of strategic analysis framework shown in Fig. (**5.26**). The elaboration of a list of forces in the competitive environment is not sufficient to obtain a strategic plan that works flawlessly. It is necessary to perform the analysis to identify the key driving factors that really define the industry. The Five Forces framework should be handled as sort of starting point checklist, and as a reminder of the many possible sources for what those key driving forces could be. To illustrate an application of Porter's Five Forces framework, the development of the 50-seat airliner is used again. The following sections contain the five determinants.

Barriers to Entry

In theories of competition in economics, a barrier to entry, or economic barrier to entry, is a cost that must be incurred by a new entrant into a market that the incumbents do not or have not had to incur. For illustration, the following items below apply to a development program of a 50-seat airliner, which was conceived in 2013 by undergraduate students [7, 19, 12]:

- Absolute cost advantages (low): There are designs that already have an important focus on cost reduction. Using the same technologies, new airplanes could hardly obtain an absolute cost advantage.
- Learning curve (high): Manufacturing learning curve is extremely dependent on company's previous experience. New competitors must first develop their own knowledge of manufacturing and learn from their own mistakes to improve their learning curves.
- Availability of suppliers (medium to high): If risk partners and suppliers are not involved in other aircraft projects, they will probably be seeking a participation in a new program of the competition.
- Government or other industrial development policy (high): Governments usually consider aeronautical industry as strategic. Thus, they provide funding and other resources for keeping it aloft. For example, Banco Nacional de Desenvolvimento Econômico e Social (BNDES), a Brazilian Development Bank, can provide financing for potential aircraft buyers at very attractive loan rates.
- Economies of scale (high): Non-recurring costs are very high in the aerospace industry. The highest probability for financial success is to sell many aircraft to spread this cost over the entire series of aircraft.
- Capital requirements (high): Companies usually count on governments, venture partners and/or security bonds to have sufficient funding for a project.
- Brand name (medium): Some important factors are the success of previous aircraft projects such as customer support, technological standard, a cost-effective product and financial situation.

- Switching costs (high): Operating one kind of aircraft is also creating a specific supply chain and developing specific knowledge in operation and maintenance, and change of this implies high cost. Likewise, inventory and tooling costs increase if different models of aircraft are operated. Finally, the high value and depreciation of the aircraft drive operators to keep using the same aircraft.
- Access to distribution (medium): New competitors are not expected to have problems to establish a supply chain with suppliers and partners. However, they will need to create a comprehensive distribution and support network if they want to compete for the worldwide market.
- Aggressive reaction (high): If players are powerful, they tend to fiercely defend their market shares. Therefore, their expected counter attack is high.
- Proprietary products (low): New competitors may have access to proprietary technologies through contracts with partners. This is high if new regulations for environment are put in practice in the coming years.

Threat of Substitutes

In this case, the threat of substitutes must be considered for the final client (the passenger) and not for the operator itself. In this situation, the main threats are other means of ground and sea transportation, besides virtual business meetings.

- Switching costs (low): Switching costs are very low, except for the case of virtual business meetings, which currently are not very user-friendly, requiring special knowledge and equipment.
- Buyer inclination to find alternatives (low): As airline fares are decreasing, passenger's inclination to fly in lieu of taking a bus or a train increases. On the other hand, the time spent on the procedures to take a plane and the distance of the airports favor other solutions when traveling shorter distances. Nearer airports, more options of flights at different times and simpler procedures may overcome this problem.
- Efficiency of available substitute products or services (high): automobiles are highly flexibility and present medium-to-low purchase prices and trip costs. However, they require considerable attention to traffic and are more prone to present unscheduled maintenance problems. Buses and trains offer acceptable trip costs but are slow when compared to airplanes. In addition, they may also pose difficulties if there are few departure times. Virtual business meetings (video conferences) offer the lowest costs regarding business travel. However, these meetings are in many cases much less effective than face-to-face meetings.

Supplier and Partner Power

As we use a partnership model instead of the traditional supplier model, most of the focus of this section is directed to partners.

- Partner concentration (high): In many aerospace areas there are few companies that are actuating and that detain know-how. This is the result of the high technological standards, confidential proprietary know-how and high investments that are needed to run state-of-art technology business.
- Importance of sales volume of partner (medium to high): Various products are customized and have high development and certification costs. As a result, partners need to find the proper balance between quantity and sale price to make profitable products. Generally, this balance tends to lead to higher sales volume.
- Differentiation of inputs (high): Supplied products are frequently unique and have high switching costs, so it is more difficult to negotiate with other possible partners. As an example, General Electric developed and offered an engine with small variations for three 70-seat airplanes: Bombardier CRJ-700, EMBRAER E170 and the doomed Fairchild-Dornier 728jet. The large-scale production of the core engine allowed for huge savings in manufacturing costs.
- Impact of inputs on cost or differentiation (medium to low): Supplies are usually customized. Thus, advantages obtained from cost or differentiation is agreed between the company and its partners and they established in contracts. After the deal is signed, all eventual differences from the contract imply penalties to the company that breaks the clauses.
- Switching costs of firms in the industry (high): Companies have difficulties to change partners. Eventually, there is no option for this.
- Presence of substitute inputs (low): Due to the high technological standards, confidential know-how and high investments needed, it is very difficult to develop new partners within companies that are not focused on the aeronautical market.
- Threat of forward integration (low): Each partner has its own core business and competencies. Each of these businesses is usually very different from each other, which makes forward integration very improbable.
- Cost relative to total purchases in industry (medium): Some of the supplied products, remarkably especially the engines, represent a great part of the direct costs of a new aircraft.

Buyer Power

- Bargaining leverage (medium to low): It is usually the company's choice whether to offer discounts or not. Some discounts may be offered according to the company's strategies, like entering a new regional market, finding a launch customer or selling a large quantity of aircraft.
- Buyer volume (high): Some of the contracts are for up to 10 aircraft. However, a major part of the sales comes from big contracts (for up to 100 firm orders and 100 options).
- Buyer information (medium): Buyers know, from press releases and other

sources, what the overall financial situation is and the number of aircraft delivered by the company. However, discount rates and other sensible information are kept secret.

- Brand name (low to medium): Most airlines, aircraft lessors and fractional ownership companies have well-established brand names in the air transport business. Thus, they usually do not care for the brand name of the aircraft manufacturer.
- Price sensitivity (high): Due to the type of product, buyers will usually make a technical choice when buying a new aircraft. If there is more than one aircraft that meets buyer's requirements, price will be an important selling point.
- Threat of backward integration (low): Airlines' core business is very different from those of aircraft manufacturers. Thus, just some overlapping of activities may occur like in maintenance and operations.
- Buyer concentration *vs*. industry (low): The concentration of aircraft operators is far lower than the concentration of aircraft producers.
- Substitutes available (high): There are substitutes available, and in some cases buying one aircraft or another may be a decision based on few details. This situation improves if the buyer already operates another aircraft from the manufacturer.

Rivalry

- Exit barriers (high): There is a high cost on abandoning a product. As the design costs are high, companies need to sell many aircraft in order to break-even. Also, as many equipment and tools are specially designed for a product, asset specificity is high.
- Industry concentration (very high): There are few players in the regional jet market. EMBRAER and Bombardier Aerospace hold together over 95% market share.
- Fixed costs (high): Since fixed costs are high, production must be maximized and this leads to a fight for market share.
- Perceived value added (medium): The main possibilities to add value are reducing operating costs and increasing technology, comfort and after sale services.
- Industry growth (low): Demand is growing at a small pace.
- Overcapacity status (medium): There is available capacity on industries.
- Product differences (low): Due to cost reduction focus and strong governmental regulation, products tend to be similar to each other in performance and other characteristics.
- Switching costs (very high): Operating one kind of aircraft is also creating a specific supply chain and developing specific knowledge in operation and maintenance, and changing implies high cost. Likewise, inventory and tooling

costs increase if different models of aircraft are operated. Finally, the high value and depreciation of the aircraft drive operators to keep using the same aircrafts.

- Brand identity (medium): Despite the fact that products from rivals are similar in many aspects, brand names and their implied values can be a selling point. Besides that, the family concept plays an important role in reinforcing a brand.
- Diversity of rivals (medium): Competitors are based in different countries and have different cultures and philosophies. However, the specificity of the product and of the market lead rivals to prize the same characteristics and selling points.

ANALYSIS OF COMPETITORS

Some Metrics

Competitor analysis in marketing and strategic planning is an assessment of the strengths and weaknesses of current and potential competitors. This kind of analysis provides both an offensive and defensive strategic context to identify opportunities and threats. Profiling coalesces all the relevant sources of competitor analysis into one framework in the support of efficient and effective strategy formulation, implementation, monitoring and adjustment.

Competitor analysis is an essential component of corporate strategy. It is argued that most firms do not conduct this type of analysis systematically enough. Instead, many enterprises operate on what is called "informal impressions, conjectures, and intuition gained through the bits of information about competitors every manager continually receives." As a result, traditional environmental scanning places many firms at risk of dangerous competitive blind spots due to a lack of embracing competitor analysis.

What is value? For a long time, the definition of value assumed different meanings with regards to industrial product. Some authors have attempted to quantify the concept of value. Johansson *et al.* [22, 23] proposes that the value can be expressed through the quality of the product Q, service *S*, selling price *SP* and lead time *LT*, according to the following relationship:

$$Value = \frac{Q \cdot S}{SP \cdot LT} \tag{5.2}$$

Some analysts propose that value must be defined by the ratio between its functionality and cost [23]:

$$Value = \frac{Function}{Cost} \tag{5.3}$$

Other definition is to consider value as the ratio between perceived benefits and perceived cost by the customer [23]:

$$Value = \frac{Perceived\ Benefits}{Perceived\ Price} \quad \textbf{(5.4)}$$

Another approach is known as value proposition. One of the many value proposition settings is as follows [24]:

> *"The unique value that your product or your company offers, encourages your customers to buy it."*

A value proposition should be short - some mention a limit of 10 words - highlight the competitive advantages of the product and its place in the market and among its competitors. Every product strategy should be summarized in a value proposition [24]. For instance, Fig. **(5.27)** lists some characteristics of business jets and luxury cars that are appreciated by customers.

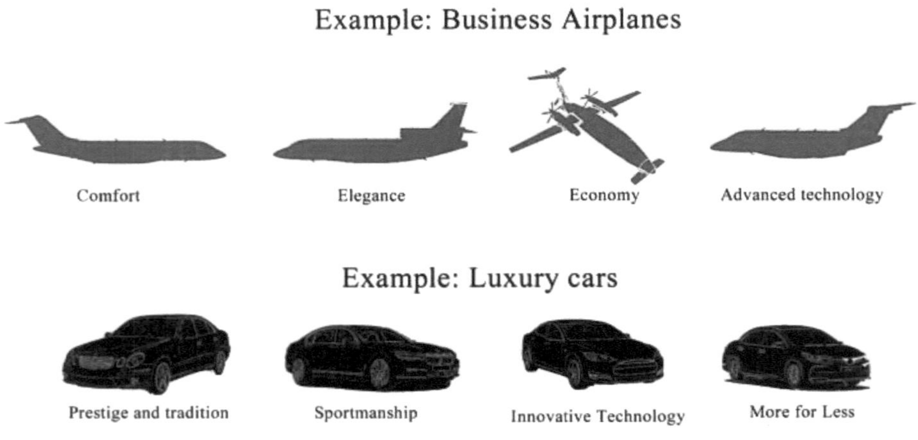

Fig. (5.27). Value proposition associated with business jets and luxury cars.

The Traditional Value Index (TVI) is widely used by the aeronautical industry (**Eq. 5.5**) [23]. It is easy to use, mathematically simple, and data can be easily obtained from technical reports and specialized publications. Fig. (**5.28**) displays the correlation between an index close related to TVI and the 2005 selling prices of business jets.

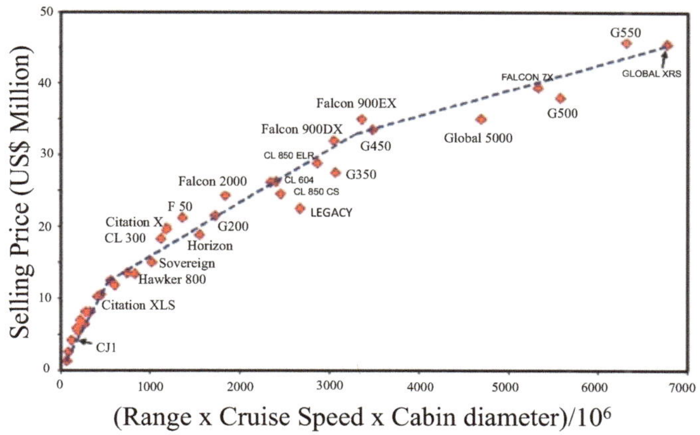

Fig. (5.28). An attempt to evaluate business jets and to find business oportunities.

$$TVI = \frac{Range \times Speed \times Cabin\,Volume}{Takeoff\ field\ length} \tag{5.5}$$

Regardless of the method, there are criteria that are easily measurable, and others are extremely subjective. The choice of criteria influences directly the product ranking. This presents big implications for business decisions because it directly influences marketing, market requirements, product definitions, management, and portfolio of products. Since an aircraft development program requires a considerable volume of investment, the customers' needs determine the product value. This approach will support financial return and boost the brand of the manufacturer. Aviation customers, airlines, military and private aircraft owners, have unique characteristics. This kind of customer is well informed about aircraft technical characteristics. He also exercises a methodical purchasing decision. Airplane buyers usually take months comparing numerous attributes of a variety of products before deciding. Some airlines joint efforts to order airplanes. Due to the higher number of airplanes being ordered, they can get bigger discounts.

Measuring Competition

The Herfindahl index (also known as Herfindahl–Hirschman Index, or HHI) is a measure of the size of firms in relation to the industry and an indicator of the amount of competition among them [25]. Named after economists Orris C. Herfindahl and Albert O. Hirschman, it is an economic concept widely applied in competition law, antitrust and technology management. It is defined as the sum of the squares of the market shares of the 50 largest firms (or summed over all the firms if there are fewer than 50) within the industry, where the market shares are expressed as fractions. The result is proportional to the average market share, weighted by market share. As such, it can range from 0 to 1.0, moving from a substantial number of very small firms to a single monopolistic producer. Increases in the Herfindahl index generally indicate a decrease in competition and an increase of market power, whereas decreases indicate the opposite. The major benefit of the Herfindahl index in relationship to such measures as the concentration ratio is that it gives more weight to larger firms. The measure is essentially equivalent to the Simpson diversity index used in ecology and to the inverse participation ratio (IPR) in physics [26].

For instance, two cases in which the six largest firms produce 90% of the goods in a market [26]:

Case 1: All six firms produce 15% each.

Case 2: One firm produces 80% while the other five produces 2% each.

We will assume that the remaining 10% of output is divided among 10 equally sized producers.

The six-firm concentration ratio would equal 90% for both case 1 and case 2. But the first case would promote significant competition, where the second case approaches monopoly. The Herfindahl index for these two situations makes the lack of competition in the second case strikingly clear:

Case 1: Herfindahl index = (0.152+0.152+0.152+0.152+0.152+0.152) + (0.012+0.012+0.012+0.012+0.012+0.012+0.012+0.012+0.012+0.012) = 0.136 (13.6%)

Case 2: Herfindahl index = 0.802 + 5 * 0.022 + 10 * 0.012 = 0.643 (64.3%)

This behavior rests on the fact that the market shares are squared prior to being summed, giving additional weight to firms with larger size [26].

The index involves taking the market share of the respective market competitors, squaring it, and adding them together (*e.g.* in the market for X, company A has 30%, B, C, D, E and F have 10% each and G through Z have 1% each). If the resulting figure is above a certain threshold, then economists consider the market to have a high concentration (*e.g.* market X's concentration is 0.142 or 14.2%). This threshold is 0.25 in the U.S., while the EU prefers to focus on the level of change, for instance that concern is raised if there is a 0.025 change when the index already shows a concentration of 0.1. So, in the present example, if in market X company B (with 10% market share) suddenly bought out the shares of company C (with 10% also) then this new market concentration would make the index jump to 0.162. Here it can be seen that it would not be relevant for merger law in the U.S. (being under 0.18) or in the European Union (because there is not a change over 0.025).

Mapping the Enemy

Most big companies have competitive intelligence departments. Competitive intelligence involves monitoring other players that operates in the same business, comparing their operation, technology, and products with its own. In addition, the intelligence department tries to riddle other players' next moves [27]. This approach relies heavily on benchmarking and comparisons that are performed using various indicators [27]. The result of the research will be a report, databases, and a set of organized information that was gathered from third parties and obtained by using software tools inside the company, the latter enabling that employees can also contribute with useful information. Reports must highlight areas where the company enjoys superiority over competitors and those in which it lags them. Strategy will then be guided by efforts to maintain advantages and close the gaps in areas where the rivals are running in front of the company [27]. Some aggressive practices may involve, for example, the leasing of an aircraft from a customer from the competition to gather data and information from it. However, such approach is not ethic and it and any illegal acts should not be practiced.

For decision making is mandatory the elaboration of alternative versions. Thus companies, government economists and planners will produce best, medium and worst-case versions of their forecasts [27]. Sensitivity analyses are a good form to carry out this and they help to explore the vulnerability of a project to environmental changes.

Aircraft manufacturers utilize several tools and information that also are available on the Internet, all that can provide useful information to map competitors. Fig. (**5.29**) shows air traffic provided by an online tool of two fierce competitors: Boeing 737 and Airbus A320. Pictures like this help to identify areas already crowded with airplanes and others that offer good sales opportunities.

Fig. (**5.30**) illustrates a comparative analysis of Phenom 100 competitors. Just a few parameters are compared in the illustration, but airplanes must be compared in all possible aspects to find out best business opportunities. Many aircraft manufacturers are steadily upgrading or changing their portfolio in face of market demands and new products developed by the competition.

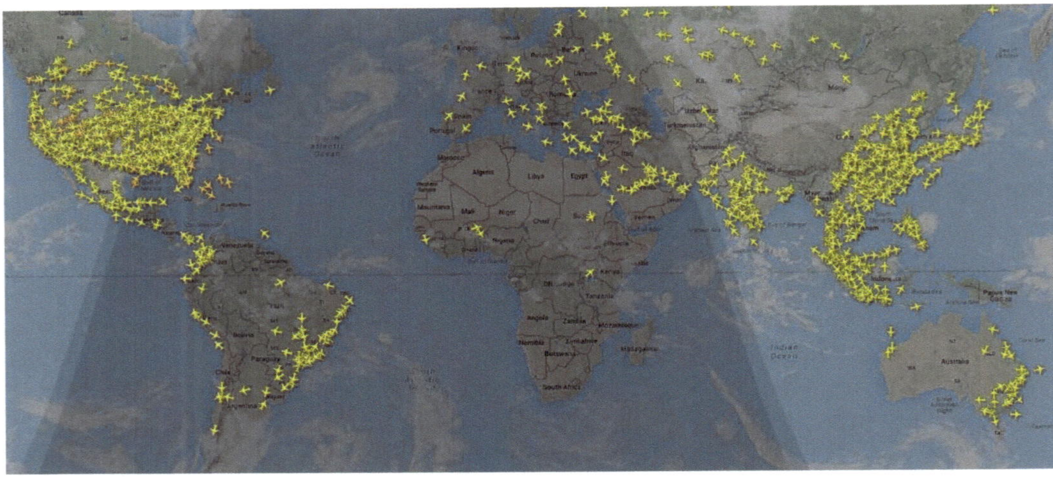

Fig. (5.29). Air traffic on May 8, 2015 considering only Boeing 737 and Airbus A320 (Courtesy Flightradar24.com).

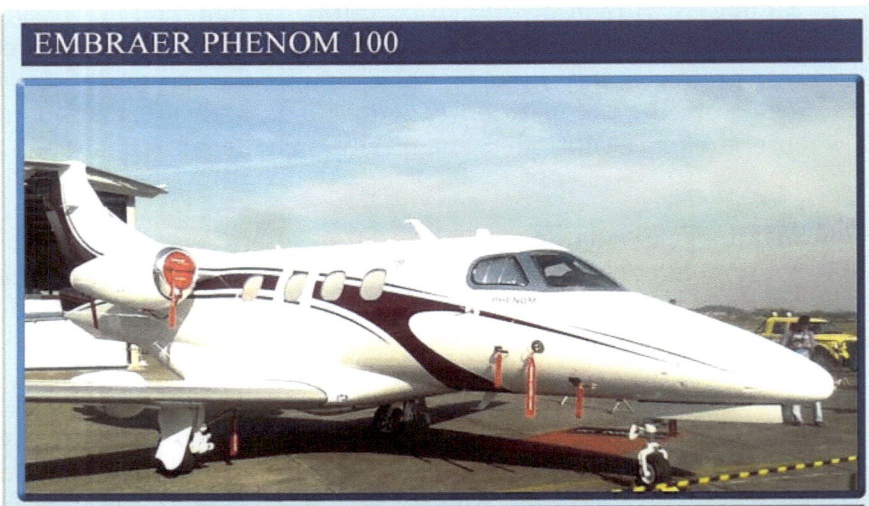

COMPETITIVE AIRCRAFT COMPARISON TABLE

Parameter	Phenom 100	Mustang	Eclipse 500
NBAA IFR Range (four occupants)	2,182 km	2,146 km	1,900 km
High-speed cruise	389 kt	340 kt	370 kt
Takeoff field length (MTOW, ISA, sea level)	1,061 m	958 m	715 m

Fig. (5.30). Comparative analysis encompassing some Phenom 100 competitors.

Another prominent issue for any line airplane is its interior layout (Fig. **5.31**). Several parameters are considered when designing the cabin layout: aisle width, seat width, seat-abreast, cabin height, seat pitch just for mention some of them. The number of seat abreast is a key figure in aircraft design. Market studies may suggest a value, but other considerations must be considered because larger fuselage sections will be translated into more drag and weight for the configuration. Fig. (**5.32**) displays a study involving two cabin cross sections obtained for specifying 5- and 6-seat abreast configurations.

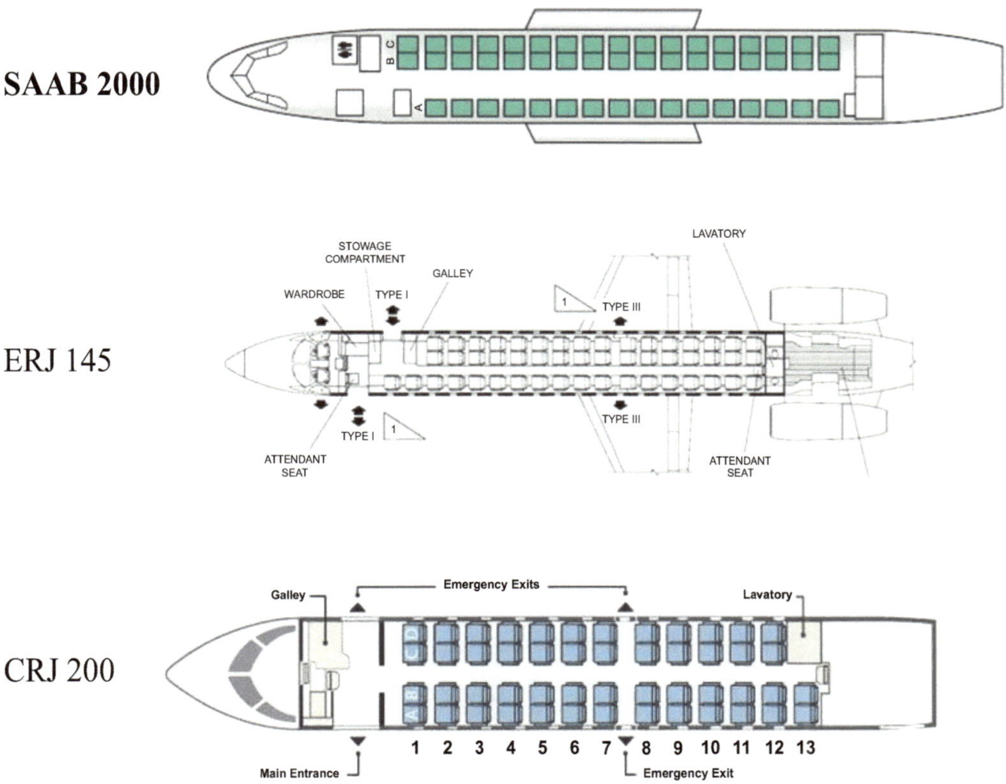

Fig. (5.31). Comparison of interior layout of similar airplanes.

The Gulfstream GIV-SP was an upgraded version of GIV. Later, it was re-designated G400. A short-ranged variant was developed based on the original GIV and designated G300. With the introduction of the G500/G550 (an upgrade to the GV model), the GIV received an upgrade based on the newly created G550. This created the G450 and its short-ranged variant the G350. G450 obtained FAA certification in August 2004. Indeed, the Gulfstream G450 is a cross between the G400 and the G550, designed using the G400 airframe with the G550 nose section grafted on. It has a Honeywell Primus Epic PlaneView avionics suit and a pair of Rolls-Royce Tay 611-8C engines. There were 291 Gulfstream G450 business jets in operation by August 2014. Large-cabin Gulfstream aircraft in operation by middle 2014 amounted 829 units. Comparisons of market share of some competitive products must also be elaborated in the feasibility phase. The chart of Fig. (**5.33**) represents the in-operation aircraft market share (as of June 2014) for the Gulfstream G450 (51%), Bombardier Challenger 605 (43%), and Dassault Falcon 900LX (6%). There are currently 572 total aircraft in operation of these three models.

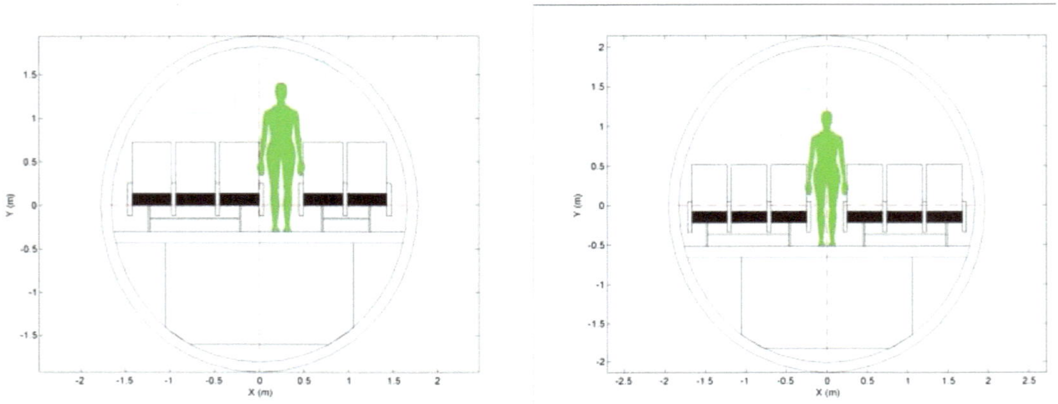

Fig. (5.32). Cross-section study with 5- and 6-seat abreast proposals.

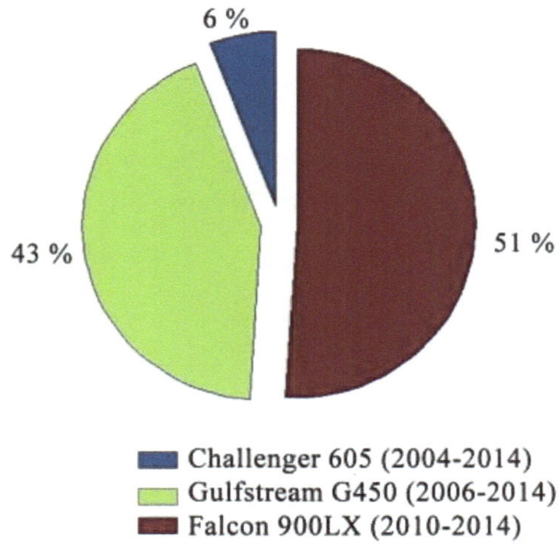

Fig. (5.33). Market share of Gulfstream G450 class (source: JETNET).

GAME THEORY

Introduction

Game theory is a decision-making tool based on the strategy. Specifically, it is the study of mathematical models of conflict and cooperation between intelligent rational decision-makers. Game theory application was recorded in ancient Babylon's Talmud to solve a marriage contract problem: a man has three wives whose marriage contracts specify that in the case of his death they receive 100, 200, and 300, respectively (Table **5.22**). He dies, leaving the estate E < 600. How should the estate be divided among the wives? The Mishna (religious law) stipulates the following division:

Table 5.22. Marriage contract problem.

		Debts		
		100	**200**	**300**
Earnings	**100**	33 1/3	33 1/3	33 1/3
	200	50	75	75
	300	50	100	150

The Talmud anticipates the modern theory of cooperative games. Each solution corresponds to the nucleolus of an appropriately defined game. Von Neumann and Morgenstern started the modern game theory after they published their 1944 book entitled *Theory of Games and Economic Behavior* [28]. They looked for a more effective way of solving certain kinds of economic problems to account for the presence of others who are making decisions in accordance with their own best wishes [29].

In a competitive environment, game theory provides a framework to analyze the impacts of competition on players' decisions. Lindstädt and Müller [30] describe their use of game theory as a technique to support managerial decisions by developing a range of outcomes based on decisions by reasonable actors. In a complex world, there must be a balance between simplifying a problem to make it manageable and retaining enough complexity to make it relevant. Managers must be aware of the assumptions that were used to find a solution, as the outcome is sensitive to the initial conditions [30]. A game has two or more players, each of whom is assumed to be rationally self-interested, seeking the highest possible benefit. The key requirements of a game theory analysis are:

- The structure of the game.
- The payoffs.

The structure of the game is the set of strategies available to each player. A strategy is a player's complete plan of action at each decision point to the end of the game. The payoffs available to each player for each strategy, given the other players' strategies, represent the benefit the player achieves at the completion of the game. Payoffs can be monetary or non-monetary. Time, utility, and happiness may be equally or more important than money. The payoff to use in the game theory analysis is dependent on the assumed objective function of the players.

A normal form game displays the strategies for each player, and the payoffs for each combination of the players' strategies, in a matrix where the first number in each cell represents the payoff for Player A, given Player B's strategy y, and the second number in each cell represents the payoff for Player B, given Player A's strategy. The maximum number of players in the games analyzed in was three.

Nash equilibrium is an approach to determine the outcome of games. It is a solution concept of a game involving two or more players, in which each player is assumed to know the equilibrium strategies of the other players, and no player has anything to gain by changing only his or her own strategy unilaterally [31]. If each player has chosen a strategy and no player can benefit by changing his or her strategy while the other players keep theirs unchanged, then the current set of strategy choices and the corresponding payoffs constitute Nash equilibrium.

Explained simply, Robert and Peter are in Nash equilibrium if Robert is taking the best decision he can, considering Peter's decision, and Peter is making the best decision he can, considering Robert's decision. Likewise, a group of players is in Nash equilibrium if each one is making the best decision that he or she can, taking into account the decisions of the others. However, Nash equilibrium does not necessarily mean the best cumulative payoff for all the players involved; in many cases all the players might improve their payoffs if they could somehow agree on strategies different from the Nash equilibrium (*e.g.* competing businesses forming a cartel in order to increase their profits).

nother example to better understand game theory:

- Two competing airlines.
- Prices set: compete in departure times.
- 70% of consumers prefer evening departure, 30% prefer morning departure.
- If the airlines choose the same departure times they share the market equally.
- Payoffs to the airlines are determined by their market shares.

Table **5.23** represents the pay-off matrix of the game. The first number in the parenthesis represents the pay-off of *Airline A*; and the second value the same for *Airline B*.

Table 5.23. Payoff matrix for the airline game.

		Airline B	
Airline A		**Morning**	**Evening**
	Morning	(15,15)	(30,70)
	Evening	(70,30)	(35,35)

The morning departure is a dominated strategy for *airline A* because if it does so, *Airline B* choses the evening departure. The same can be applied to *Airline B*, Thus, both airlines chose the evening departure.

Now suppose that *Airline A* has a frequent flyer program: when both airlines choose the same departure times *Airline A* gets 60% of the travelers. This changes the pay-off matrix. The pay-off matrix for this new environment is displayed in Table **5.24**. Now, if *Airline A* chooses the morning departure, the other airline will take the evening one. However, if *Airline A* chooses the evening departure scheme, *Airline B* will choose the same. Thus, *Airline B* has no dominated strategy. A morning departure is a dominated strategy for *Airline A*. *Airline B* knows this and takes the morning departure. The outcome for this game is the pay-off (70, 30).

Table 5.24. Payoff matrix considering a frequent flyer program.

		Airline B	
Airline A		**Morning**	**Evening**
	Morning	(18,12)	(30,70)
	Evening	(70,30)	(42,28)

Nash Equilibrium is not Optimization

An extension of Nash equilibrium can be employed to determine the expected flow of traffic in a network [32]. Consider the graph of Fig. (**5.34**). If it is assumed that there are *n* cars traveling from A to D, what is the expected distribution of traffic in the network?

This situation can be modeled as a game where every traveler has a choice of three paths or strategies, where each strategy is a route from A to D (ABD, ABCD, or ACD). The pay-off of each strategy is the travel time of each route. In the graph of Fig. (**5.34**), a car travelling *via* ABD experiences travel time of $\left(1+\frac{n_1}{100}+2\right)$, where n_1 is the number of cars traveling on edge AB. Thus, payoffs for any given strategy depend on the choices of the other players, as is usual. However, the goal in this case is to minimize travel time, not maximize it. Equilibrium will occur when the time on all paths is exactly the same [32]. When that happens, no single driver has any incentive to switch routes, since it can only add to his/her travel time. If, for example, 100 cars are travelling from A to D, then equilibrium will occur when 25 drivers travel *via* ABD, 50 *via* ABCD, and 25 *via* ACD. Every driver now has a total travel time of 3.75. Notice that this distribution is not, actually, socially optimal. If the 100 cars agreed that 50 travel *via* ABD and the other 50 through ACD, then travel time for any single car would actually be 3.5, being less than the time from the equilibrium solution of 3.75.

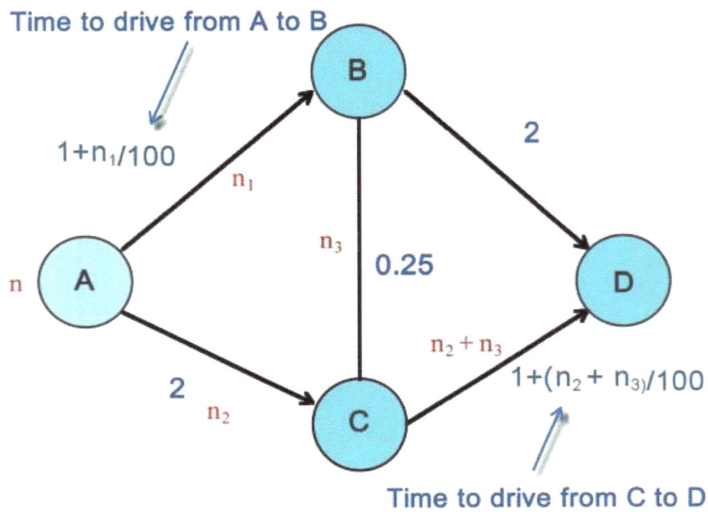

Fig. (5.34). This small traffic network can be solved by game theory.

Mixed Strategies

Mixed-strategy Nash equilibriums occur when a probability is assigned to each of the competitors' strategies. Mixed strategies can be used to determine unique Nash equilibriums when multiple pure strategy equilibriums exist; if there are no pure strategy equilibria, there must be unique mixed strategy equilibrium [33].

To exemplify a mixed-strategy game, let p de probability that Player B chooses X, so that $1-p$ is the probability that he chooses Y. In the same way, q is the probability that Player A chooses X. To obtain the mixed strategies, the q- and p-mixed options are calculated (Table **5.25**).

Table 5.25. Example of a mixed-strategy game.

		Player A		
Player B		X	Y	q-mixed
	X	(50, 50)	(80, 20)	***50q+80(1-q)***
	Y	(90, 10)	(20,80)	***90q+20(1-q)***
	p-mixed	***50p+10(1-p)***	***20p+80(1-p)***	

Fig. (**5.35**) Shows the payoffs for Player A if Player B chooses X. It becomes indifferent for Player A when Player B takes $p=0.70$. In this condition, Player A success rate is 38%.

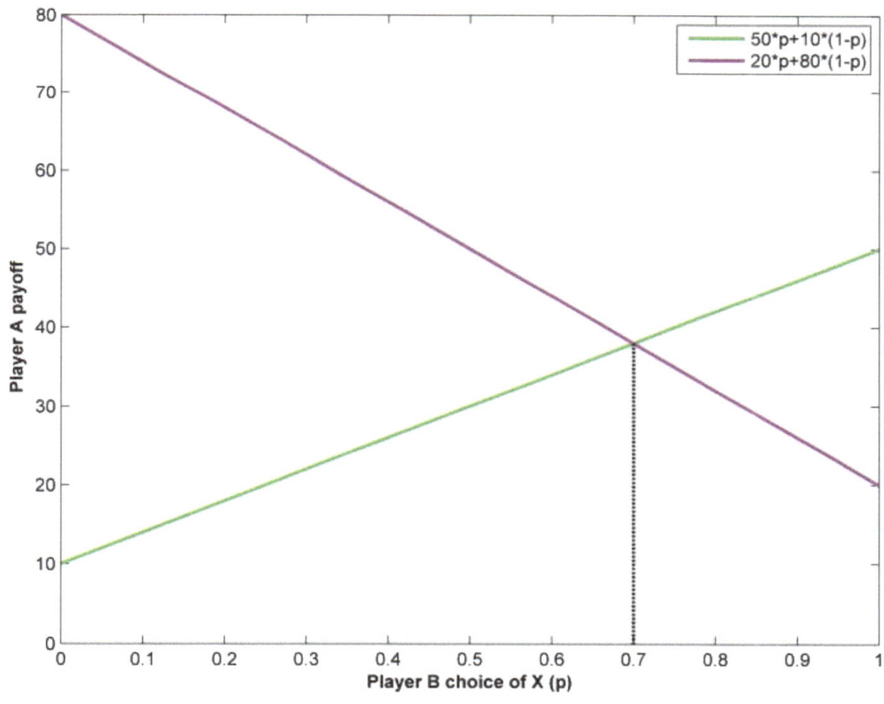

Fig. (5.35). Player B choice of p.

Fig. (**5.36**) Shows the payoffs for Player B if Player A chooses X. It becomes indifferent for Player B when Player A takes $q=0.60$. In this case, Player B success rate is 62%.

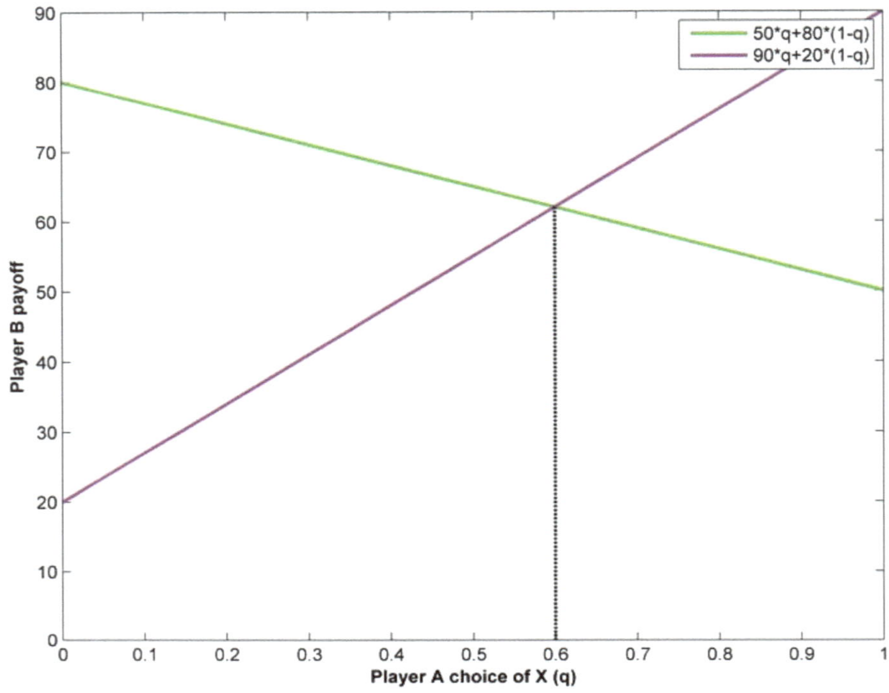

Fig. (5.36). Player A choice of q.

In the example described before, the pair (*p=0.70, q=0.60*) represents the mixed-strategy equilibrium. The Player B's payoff was 62 and the Player's A was 38. (Player B wins 62%, Player A 38%).

Reasons because the determination of the mixing probability is useful:

- In constant sum games, such as the example shown in this section, the opponent's indifferent situation is equivalent to minimizing the opponents' ability to recognize and exploit systematic patterns of behavior in player's choice.
- In constant sum games, keeping your opponent indifferent is equivalent to keeping yourself indifferent.
- The same objective works for finding mixed strategy equilibria in non□constant sum games as well, where players interests are not totally opposed to one another.

GAME THEORY APPLIED TO AIRCRAFT DESIGN

Introduction

To demonstrate the applicability of game theory as a decision-making tool for an aircraft program, the replacement strategy for a single-aisle 75-seat airliner is presented in this section. The methodology developed here aims to improve the objective analysis of product line decisions. A game involving the two largest small capacity airliners, EMBRAER and Bombardier, was then elaborated.

The analysis carried out in this Section has no direct relation to policies adopted by the two aircraft manufacturers or with the methodologies they use to analyze their market segment. It is shown here just for educational purposes. All data used here was obtained from the Internet, books and journals.

EMBRAER and Bombardier have existing in-production single-aisle aircraft below 130 seats. They share the market for 70-78 airplanes almost equally. The game offers both manufacturers four strategies:

1. Maintain their existing product lines, with incremental improvements over time,
2. Re-engine their existing 75-seat airliner, providing superior fuel burn improvement,
3. Develop new aircraft that offer considerable better fuel burn improvements, or
4. Exit the market segment.

The Game has two players and it is the base case that is compared to another game where regulations that obligate manufacturers to developed low-emission airplanes are in place. Their incentive to change strategy is to increase market share or prevent newcomers to gain access to their market segment.

Mixed strategies were not incorporated into the present analysis. Table **5.26** shows that the status quo is the competitive equilibrium. Both incumbents maintain their current aircraft, keeping their earnings splitting the market. The development of a new aircraft is strictly dominated by both players. This scenario provides a baseline against which scenarios explored in the next sections can be compared to understand their impacts.

There are several studies that positively link higher market share with profitability but many others have raised concerns about increasing market share at any cost [34]. It is a challenging task to establish the minimum market share that encourages the aircraft manufacturer to stay in certain market segment without introducing major improvements for their products. Most of them are backed by governments by direct and indirect subsidies, enabling manufacturers to stay aloft in face of increasing competition.

Airlines are conservative regarding costs and this prevents airlines from receiving a higher utility from aircraft that have a DOC advantage lower than 5% [35]. Therefore, incremental improvements generally do not result in market share increases as competitors generally match each other's incremental improvements, with some time lag. In the present work, the market share of each manufacturer is derived from the historical analysis carried out by the author.

Table 5.26. Aircraft development strategy game, market share.

		Manufacturer A		
		No move	**Re-engine**	**New**
Manufacturer B	**No move**	[~50,~50]	[35, 65]	[25, 75]
	Re-engine	[65, 35]	[~50,~50]	[40, 60]
	New	[75, 25]	[60, 40]	[~50,~50]

Development Cost for a New 75-Seat Airliner

Financial Analysis

A study about the development of a new 75-seat airliner was carried out by an undergraduate team of students [36]. Among several candidates, the team chose twinjet fitted with PW1700G geared turbofan, full digital fly-by-wire system, featuring a V-tail (Fig. **5.37**). Two configurations were considered in the final phase but the design team ultimately decided for the airliner with underwing-mounted engines [36]. This configuration was named ITA75ADV, which presents the characteristics shown in Table **5.27**. The direct operating cost (DOC) was estimated to be 14.50 US$/nm, the maximum takeoff weight (MTOW) 37,242 kg, and the empty weight 19,055 kg. Fig. (**5.38**) shows the distribution of the components of the recurring and non-recurring costs. Table **5.28** contains financial data of the program, which will cost US$ 1.76 billion.

Table 5.27. Some characteristics of ITA75ADV [36].

MTOW	Empty Weight	Max Fuel	Wing Aspect Ratio	DOC*
37,242 kg	19,055 kg	7,565 kg	9.35	13.86 US$/nm
* DOC for a 600-nm stage length, 75% load factor, Jet A1 price of US$ 3.26/gallon, 2014 dollar.				

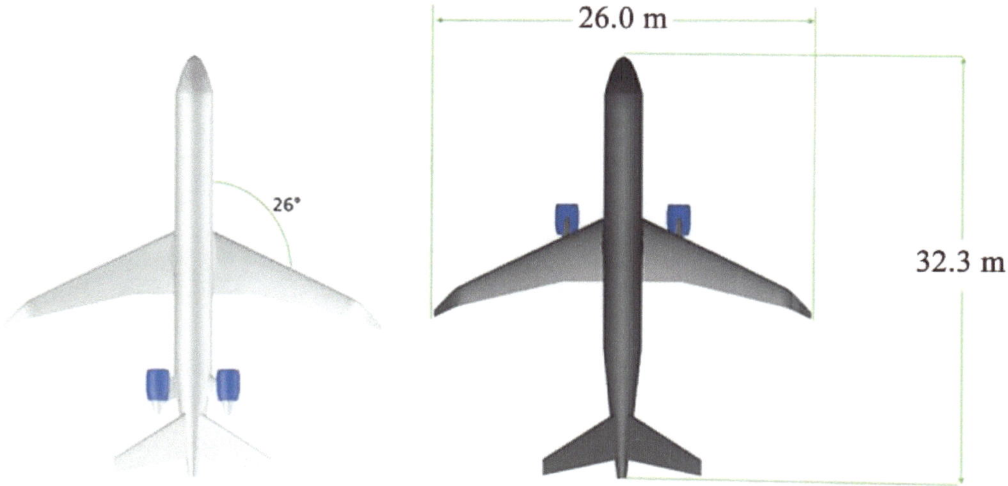

Fig. (5.37). Preset configurations considered for a definitive choice of a new-generation 75-seat airliner [36].

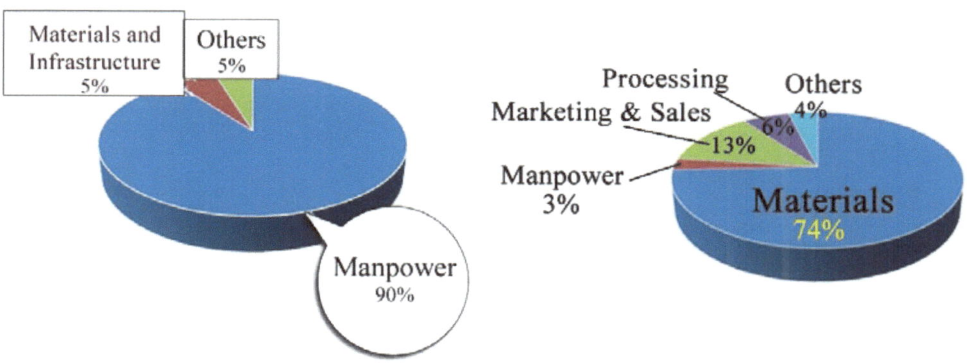

Fig. (5.38). Distribution of non-recurring (*Left*) and recurring (*Right*) costs for the new-generation 75-seat airliner [36].

Table 5.28. Financial picture of a new 75-seat aircraft program (2014 dollar) [36].

Program Cost (Million US$)	Manufacturing Cost Per Airplane (Million US$)	Profit Per Airplane (Million US$)	Breakeven (Years)
1,762	25.6	5.6	7.5

Fuel Price

In 2015, jet fuel consumption increased by an estimated 70,000 Barrel a day (4.7%) compared to the year before, according to U.S. Energy Information

Administration (EIA). Jet fuel price remained above US$ 3.00 per gallon in the 2011-14 period but experienced a sharp drop in 2015 (Fig. **5.39**). During the period shown in Fig. (**5.39**), the highest rate of increase took place in the July 2007-2008 timeframe, when jet fuel prices climbed 82%. Fuel became the greatest expense for the aviation industry in 2006 when it surpassed labor, the second largest airline cost component, as described in an IATA report from 2015 [37]. Thus, fuel costs eroded a larger share of industry revenue and exerted a greater impact on airline decisions and profit margins. As consequence, fuel costs also impact network structure and significantly alter the number of passengers that utilize the air transportation system. Fuel price increase has a deep social impact as demonstrated by many academic works [38].

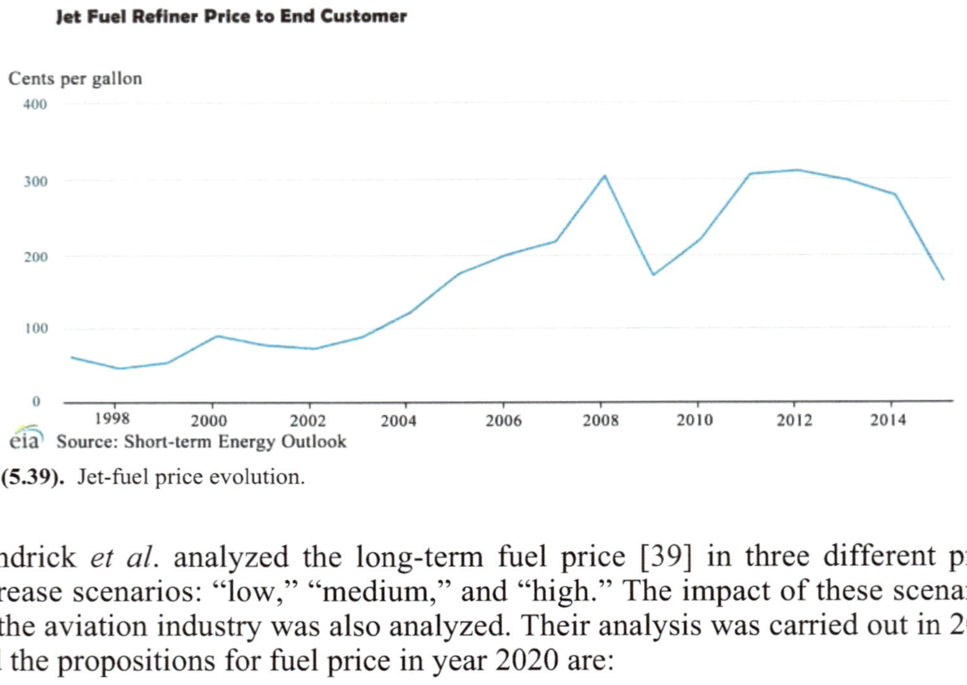

Fig. (5.39). Jet-fuel price evolution.

Hendrick *et al.* analyzed the long-term fuel price [39] in three different price increase scenarios: "low," "medium," and "high." The impact of these scenarios on the aviation industry was also analyzed. Their analysis was carried out in 2011 and the propositions for fuel price in year 2020 are:

1. Low-price scenario. From data extrapolated from US Bureau of Transportation Statistics data a price of US$ 1.33/gallon was estimated [39].
2. Medium-Price Scenario. The choice of the medium price, US$ 2.67/gal, which is twice the price from the low-price scenario. It also fits well to the historical maximum crude oil price at the height of the oil crisis following the Iran-Iraq war in the 1970s. For this fuel price estimation, it was assumed that rate of current price increases will diminish and will eventually flatten out to about the same as the slope of increase since 1991. In summary, this is the low-price scenario plus a constant [39].

3. High-Price Scenario. The estimated value for the high-price scenario represents a projection based on fuel cost data from Bureau of Transportation Statistics tabulated from 2002 to 2005. The estimated value, US$ 5.51/gal by 2020, is nearly 4 times higher than the 2011 fuel prices. This would occur in the event that 2011 world growth continues for several years and assuming that the growth only slows gradually. In addition, the projection asserted that global oil production reached a peak production in 2011 [39].

Fig. (**5.40**) displays the result of a direct operating cost estimation performed for the ITA75ADV airliner. The calculation considered two jet-fuel prices, US$ 1.05 and 2.67 (2014 dollar), a 154% increase. The resulting DOCs were US$ 7.85 and US$ 10.82, respectively. The participation of fuel in the calculated DOC rose from 25% to 46% for that price increase. Thus, as expected, the DOC is indeed very sensitive to fuel price.

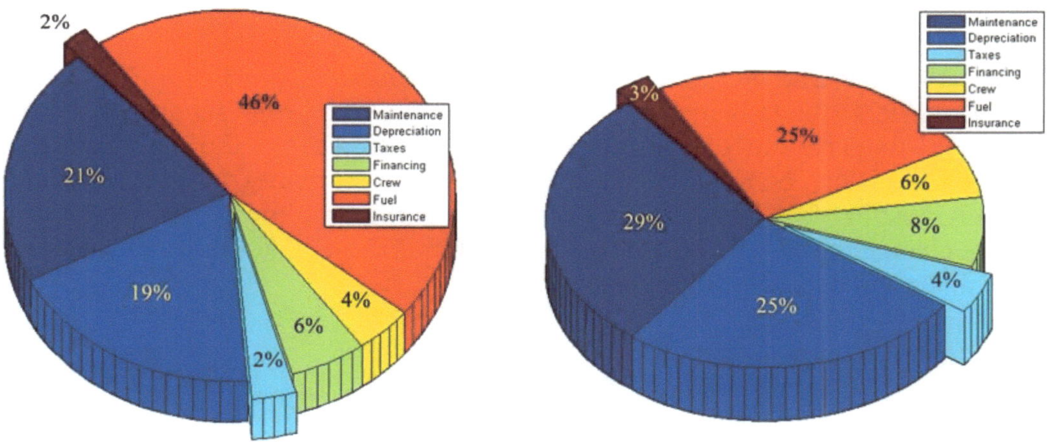

Fig. (5.40). DOC breakdown for the ITA75ADV considering two Jet A1 fuel prices [36].

Market and Revenue Estimation

EMBRAER forecasted a world demand for 6,250 new jets in the 70 to 130-seat segment over the next 20 years, representing a total market value of US$ 300 billion. According to EMBRAER, the Brazilian company had 60% of the market of jets below 120 seats in 2012 (Fig. **5.41**).

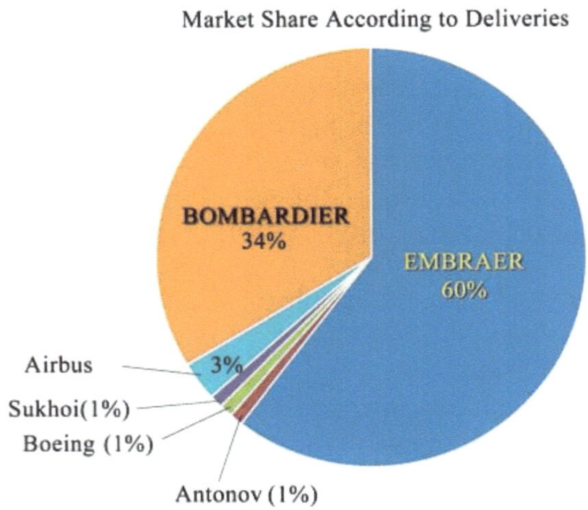

Fig. (5.41). Market share of jets with seating capacity between 70 and 120 passengers. Status: 2012 (Source: EMBRAER).

Table **5.29** shows the deliveries of the E-jets by October, 2015 [40]. The E175 airliner registers 332 deliveries of a total of 1158 airplanes, representing 28.7% of the whole E-Jets family. Considering the 60% market share of EMBRAER (Fig. **5.41**), this can be translated into 3,750 regional airplanes for that Brazilian company, leading to 1,076 E175 twinjets (considering that the 28.7% proportion will not change in the next 20 years). If we subtract the 166 airplanes in backlog, this number will be now 910 airplanes.

Table 5.29. E-jets orders and deliveries by October, 2015 [40].

Model	Firm Orders	Options	Deliveries	Firm Order Backlog
E-170	193	7	188	5
E-175	**477**	**332**	**311**	**166**
E-190	586	92	518	68
E-195	165	2	141	24
Total	**1421**	**433**	**1158**	**263**

Bombardier CRJ-700 presents a total of 341 units delivered by March 2015 (Table **5.30**), a figure very close to its rival, the EMBRAER E175 twinjet. Using a similar approach of that used to estimate the E175 demand in the next 20 years, a total of 996 CRJ-700 airplanes is expected to be sold in the envisaged timeframe.

Table 5.30. Bombardier CRJ-Series deliveries and orders by March, 2015.

	Total Order	Total Delivered	Backlog
CRJ 700 Series 701	334	325	9
CRJ 700 Series 705	16	16	0
CRJ 900	391	340	51
CRJ 1000	70	40	30
Total	811	721	90

Aircraft are rarely sold by their list prices. Usually, airlines obtain big discounts from manufacturers, noticeably when they place large orders. An analysis of Boeing and Airbus Annual Reports (2000-2009) demonstrated that revenues from commercial aircraft sales have never matched the list prices of the aircraft delivered in any one year [38]. The Airline Monitor (2004) reported average A320 and 737-800 sale prices of US$ 53.3 and US$ 49.4 million (2008 dollar), respectively [38]. This represents a 39 and 35% discount from list prices for the Boeing and Airbus airplanes, respectively. Considering that Bombardier and EMBRAER have a considerably lower sales volume than Airbus and Boeing, an average discount of 25% was considering in the present work,

The E175LR and the CRJ-700NG have an estimated list price of US$ 38.9 and 37.3 million, respectively [41]. Considering an average discount of 25%, we considered prices of US$ 28.18 and 27.98 million for E175 and CRJ-700, respectively. For the estimated market size, we have the sales amount:

- Bombardier receives US$ 27.87 billion in revenues and
- EMBRAER US$ 25.64 billion.

Next step is to evaluate the impact of the development of a new airplane on sales volume. In this highlight, Markish [42] demonstrated that there is no correlation between aircraft deliveries and sale price. Therefore, it was assumed here that aircraft orders evolve independently of sale prices, while the relative differences in competitor's sale price combined with lifecycle operating costs impacts market shares.

The adopted market-based pricing model assumes that the aircraft price balances the competitor aircraft's operating costs. It was assumed that current aircraft prices remain constant in real terms, but manufacturers are able to negotiate price increases proportional to reductions in lifecycle cost on the introduction of new aircraft with lower operating cost, as shown in Fig. (**5.42**). Assuming a basic bargaining game in which both parties have equal power, lifecycle operating cost reductions would be split evenly between the buyer and seller [38, 43]. Therefore, if a new aircraft with 25% fuel burn improvement yields an expected present value of US$ 22.8 million in lifecycle cost savings, it is assumed manufacturers would be able to increase sale price by US$11.4 million.

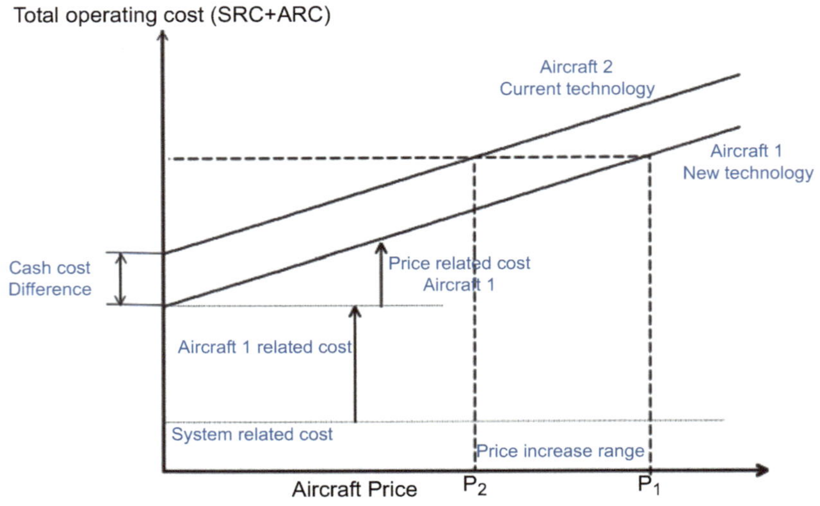

Fig. (5.42). Cost approach to price setting [43].

To apply the aircraft price methodology to the EMBRAER new airplane, the following conditions were considered:

- 6 trips a day with an average stage length of 500 nm.
- Utilization of 320 days each year.
- DOC of 9.8791 US$/nm, which is 15% better than that of the baseline airplane.
- Airplane operation of 10 years.
- Steady inflation rate of 2% a year

This furnishes a fuel saving bill of US$ 17 million over the envisaged operating time of the airplane. Thus, a price increase of US$ 8.5 million for the new 75-seat airplane was considered as outlined before.

The EMBRAER revenue for the new-airplane scenario will be then US$ 42.51 billion. If we consider the development cost (Table **5.27**), net earnings become US$ 40.75 billion. It is also assumed that this new airplane will impact Bombardier sales by 25% (see Table **5.25**). A similar approach was also adopted for Bombardier development of a new airplane.

Re-engining Programs

The Boeing 737-200 was fitted with two JT8-D small by-pass ratio turbofans. In 1984, it was replaced by the re-engined 737-300, which was quieter, larger and more economical aircraft and contained a host of new features and improvements. The new model featured many aerodynamic, structural, cockpit and cabin features developed for the new-generation Boeing 757 and 767. One of the redesign objectives was to have a high degree of commonality with the 737-200. This was to provide saving for airlines in maintenance, spares, tools for existing 737-200 operators. The 737-300 was designed to present similar flying qualities, cockpit arrangements and procedures to minimize training differences and permit a common type rating. The CFM-56 was chosen to equip the Boeing 737-300, the core of which is produced by GE and is virtually identical to the F101 as used in the Rockwell B-1. SNECMA produced the fan, IP compressor, low-pressure turbine, thrust reversers and all external accessories. However, the size of the engine had ground clearance issues. This was overcome by mounting the accessories on the lower sides to flatten the nacelle bottom and intake lip to give the "hamster pouch" look. The engines were moved forward and raised, level with the upper surface of the wing and tilted 5 degrees up which not only helped the ground clearance but also directed the exhaust downwards which reduced the effects of pylon overheating and gave some vectored thrust to boost take-off performance. The CFM56-3 proved to be almost 20% more efficient than the JT8D (specific fuel consumption).

Two sections were added to the basic -200 fuselage. Composite materials were used on all flight controls to reduce weight and aluminum alloys used in areas such as wing spars, keel beams and main landing gear beams which improved their strength by up to 12 percent thereby increasing service life. High lift characteristics were also enhanced by re-sequencing the slats and flaps. The leading edge slat radius was also increased which gave a 2.5kt reduction in V_{ref} over a -200 at the same weight. Other changes to the wing structure included strengthened materials and corrosion protection.

The Boeing 737-200 re-engine was responsible for the sales success of the 737 family that we see today. The fuel burn decreased 5.6% for the 737-300 over the 737-200 [44]. The 20% increase in efficient CFM56 over the JT8D was diluted by additional weight and other modifications introduced into the Boeing 737-300.

Weyman [44] suggests that the introduction of an improved aircraft version does not have a significant impact on aircraft values. He analyzed the aircraft value evolution in the 737-200 to -300 changeover. Looking at the values of two vintages of the replaced version - the oldest vintage and the vintage that would be

5 years old when the new variant was eventually introduced. Far from suffering a downfall, values of the 737-200 continued to appreciate after the announcement of the new model, even after the change in production occurred. Not until 1991 did values begin to fall, and this decrease was seen in the new -300 aircraft as well [44]. The downturn of the aviation industry in 1991 was the cause for airplanes' depreciation [44]. The introduction of the Boeing 747-400 appears to have the opposite effect, the data revealing a rapid fall-off in values of the replaced -200 at the time of introduction of the -400 version [44].

In order to apply the aircraft price methodology to the EMBRAER re-engined airplane, the following conditions were taken into account:

- 6 trips a day with an average stage length of 500 nm.
- Utilization of 320 days each year.
- DOC of 10.82 US$/nm, which is 5% better than that of the baseline airplane.
- Airplane operation of 10 years.
- Steady inflation rate of 2% a year

This furnishes a fuel saving bill of US$ 5.67 million over the envisaged operating time of the airplane. Thus, a price increase of US$ 2.835 million for the re-engined 75-seat airplane was considered as described before.

The re-engine program will cost 15% of that calculated for developing a new airplane. Thus, the EMBRAER revenue for the new-airplane scenario will be then US$ 32.85 billion. If we consider the development cost (Table **5.31**), net earnings become US$ 32.59 billion. It is also assumed that this new airplane will impact Bombardier sales by 15%. A similar approach was also adopted for Bombardier development of a re-engined airplane.

Table 5.31. Payoff matrix of the two-manufacturers game.

		EMBRAER		
		No Move	**Re-engine**	**New**
Bombardier	**No move**	[27.87/25.64]	[23.69/32.11]	[20.9/38.45]
	Re-engine	[34.12/21.8]	[29.97/27.54]	[26.95/33.27]
	New	[40.45/19.23]	[35.74/24.76]	[32.59/29.81]

The only possible outcome of this game is highlighted is the pair [32.59/29.81]: both manufacturers chosing to start a new aircraft development program. A simulation was also carried out to evaluate the impact of some variables on the payoff matrix. It was assumed that the EMBRAER market drops from 910 to 400 aircraft and the cost of launching a new aircraft program raises from US$ 1.762

billion to 3.8 billion. Table **5.32** shows the payoff matrix for this game, whose outcome is the pair [31.94/10.43], EMBRAER deciding for a re-engine program.

Table 5.32. Payoff matrix of the two-manufacturer game if EEMBRAER market and program cost for a new aircraft change.

		EMBRAER		
		No move	**Re-engine**	**New**
Bombardier	**No move**	[27.87/11.27]	[23.69/16.22]	[20.9/18.72]
	Re-engine	[31.49/9.581]	[29.67/11.65]	[20.9/18.72]
	New	[34.01/8.454]	[31.94/10.43]	[30.56/10.08]

CONCLUSION

An airplane feasibility study is not a well-organized, planned process, unless there is a client that sets the requirements. Usually there are not budget constraints and no strict timetable.

The Chapter describes some aircraft programs that resulted in disappointing sales, either by misunderstanding of market requirements or the establishment of inadequate technical requirements. Stating the problem properly is one of the design team`s most important tasks, because an elegant solution to the wrong problem is less than worthless. Problem stating is as important as problem solving. The problem must be stated in a clear, unambiguous manner.

Sometimes limited sales opportunity could be the engine behind the development of a new aircraft. This was the case of the EMBRAER ERJ 140 and Bombardier CRJ-440, which were sold in limited number and entered market just to avoid scope clauses established by pilot`s association.

The analysis of a 75-seat airplane project was only an initial step in using game theory to understand the impacts of competition, market conditions, and technological progress on large commercial aircraft manufacturer decisions. A number of simplifying assumptions have been made in the models presented to facilitate the analysis of a problem that quickly scales in complexity. To address this problem in a more embracing manner, a framework should be developed in which the technical and financial implications of strategic options are integrated into the multi-disciplinary aircraft design process.

While airplane efficiency improvements reduce airline operating costs, it is necessary to reorganize and rethink airplane operations to obtain further reductions. In order to meet environmental goals, efficiency may not be enough and new aircraft and engine technology are required. In addition, improving the efficiency of energy use will lead to a reduction in energy consumption. Energy efficiency lowers the implicit price of energy, potentially leading to greater use. As a greater share of the world's population gains access to affordable air transportation in developing countries, aviation's environmental damage will continue to grow. To face the world's climate change challenge without limiting the economic enabling effects of air transportation by suppressing demand, aircraft technology will need to be improved. The incentives for manufacturers to stand still will need to be overcome. Future feasibility analysis should take this into account.

REFERENCES

[1] M. Hepperle, "The Sonic Cruiser – A Concept Analysis", *International Symposium Aviation Technologies of the XXI Century: New Aircraft Concepts and Flight Simulation,* 2002 Aviation Salon ILA, Berlin

[2] D. Collingridge, *The Social Control of Technology* St. Martin Press: New York, 1980.

[3] J. Richard Smith, *Focke-Wulf Fw 200* Profile Aircraft, Profile Books Ltd, 1982.

[4] Transport Canada, "Bombardier CRJ Series", *Government of Canada, Transport Canada,* 2016. https://www.tc.gc.ca/eng/civilaviation/standards/commerce-4059.htm#_Toc324504230

[5] S. Ackert, "Basics of Aircraft Market Analysis", *Aircraft Monitor,* 2012. http://www.aircraftmonitor.com/uploads/1/5/9/9/15993320/basics_of_aircraft_market_analysis___v1.pdf

[6] L.G. Fine, *SWOT Analysis.* 1st ed. CreateSpace Independent Publishing Platform, 2009.

[7] B. Mattos, "Especificação Para Projeto de uma Aeronave de 50 Assentos", *Material de Aula da Disciplina PRJ-22, Instituto tecnológico de Aeronáutica, São José dos, Campos (Curitiba),* 2013.

[8] K. Majcher, "Parting Ways", *Aviation Week Network,* 2011. http://aviationweek.com/ awin/parting-ways

[9] Airfleets.net, *Production List,* 2014. http://www.airfleets.net/listing/index.php?file=listing

[10] M. Kownatzki, T. Hoyland, and A. Watterson, *The 50-Seat Jet: A Plane with No Future. Think again!* Oliver Wyman Aviation, Aerospace&Defense, 2013.

[11] F.A. Admiistration, *FAA Aerospace Forecast Fiscal Years 2013-2033.* Federal Aviation Administration: Washington, DC, 2012.

[12] G. Bravo, "Projeto Conceitual de Aeronaves", *Report No 1, Instituto Tecnológico de Aeronáutica, São José dos Campos, May,* 2013.

[13] Japan Aircraft Development Corporation, *"Worldwide Market Forecast for Commercial Air Transport 2009-2028,"* June 2009.

[14] Japan Aircraft Development Corporation, *"Worldwide Market Forecast for Commercial Air Transport 2012-2033,"* June 2013.

[15] Secretaria da Aviação Civil – Presidência da República, *Governo Anuncia Programa de Investimentos em Aeroportos,* 2012. http://www.aviacaocivil.gov.br/noticias/2012/12/governo-anuncia-programa-de-investimento-em-aeroportos

[16] B. Aerospace, *Commercial Market Forecast 2012-2031, Canada*, 2012.

[17] The Globe and Mail, *CSeries Numbers Still don't Add Up,* 2013. http://www.theglobeandmail.com/report-on-business/c-series-numbers-still-dont-add-up/article14390594/

[18] S. Silva Paulo Cesar, "Commercial Aviation Update", *EMBRAER*

[19] Equipe 2, "Projeto Conceitual de Aeronaves – Análise Mercadológica e Financeira", *Report No 1, Instituto Tecnológico de Aeronáutica, São José dos Campos,* May, 2013.

[20] Bombardier Aerospace, *Commercial Market Forecast 2011-2030, Canada*, 2011.

[21] M. Porter, *Competitive Advantage* The Free Press: New York, 1985.

[22] H.J. Johansson, and P. McHugh, *A. John Pendlebury, and William A. Wheeler III, Business Process Reengineering: Breakpoint Strategies for Market Dominance.* John Wiley & Sons: New York, 1993.

[23] T.D. Dowen, *"A Multi-Attribute Value Assessment Methodfor the Early Product Development Phase"*, PhD Thesis, Massaschsetts Institute of Technology, 2005.

[24] R. Duermeyer, *Value Proposition,* 2011. http://homebusiness.about.com/od/glossary/g/def_valueProp.htm

[25] C. Liston-Hayes, and A. Pilkington, "Inventive Concentration: An Analysis of Fuel Cell Patents", *Sci. Public Policy,* vol. 31, no. 1, pp. 15-25, 2004. [http://dx.doi.org/10.3152/147154304781780190]

[26] Wikipedia, *Herfindahl index.* https://en.wikipedia.org/wiki/Herfindahl_index

[27] C. Murphy, *Competitive Intelligence – Gathering, Analysing and Putting it to Work.* Gower Publishing Company: Burlington, 2005.

[28] von Neumann and Oskar Morgenstern, *Theory of Games and Economic Behavior.* Pricenton University Press, 1944.

[29] M. Davis, *Game Theory: A Non-Technical Intorduction.* Dover Books: New York, 1977.

[30] H. Lindstädt, and J. Müller, "Making Game Theory Work for Managers", *McKinsey&Company,* 2010. https://www.ibu.kit.edu/rd_download/McKQ_Lindstaedt_Mueller_final.pdf

[31] D. Avinash, S. Skeath, and D. Reiley, *Games of Strategy.* 3rd ed. W.W. Norton & Company, 2009.

[32] Wikipedia, *Nash Equilibrium.* https://en.wikipedia.org/wiki/Nash_equilibrium

[33] D. Easley, and J. Kleinberg, *Networks, Crowds, and Markets: Reasoning about a Highly Connected World.* Cambridge University Press, 2010. [http://dx.doi.org/10.1017/CBO9780511761942]

[34] B. Wernerfelt, "The Relation between Market Share and Profitability", *J. Bus. Strategy,* vol. 6, no. Iss: 4, pp. 67-74, 1986. [http://dx.doi.org/10.1108/eb039133]

[35] Vikrant and Vaze Cynthia Barnhar, *Modeling Airline Frequency Competition for airport Congestion Mitigation,* 2011. http://web.mit.edu/vikrantv/www/doc/TS.pdf

[36] Team No Class 2015, "Projeto Conceitual da Nova Aeronave E-175", *Final Report, Instituto Tecnológico de Aeronáutica, São José dos Campos,* November, 2014.

[37] IATA, "Economic Performance of the Airline Industry", *IATA 2015 mid-year Report,* 2015.

[38] K.D. Morrison, S. Sgouridis, and R.J. Hansman, "Game Theory Analysis of Aircraft Manufacturers Innovation Strategies in the Face of Increasing Airline Fuel Costs", *Report No. ICAT-2011-4,* June 2011.

[39] Robert Hendricks, Nathan Lowery, David Daggett, and Peter Anast, "Future Fuel Scenarios and Their Potential Impact to Aviation", *NASA/TM-2011-214042,* 2011.

[40] EMBRAER, "Delivers 21 Commercial and 30 Executive Jets in 3Q15", *EMBRAER Press Release,* October 15, 2015.

[41] Leeham News and Comment, *More Odds and Ends: Aircraft List Prices, Airline Break-even,* 2012.

http://leehamnews.com/2012/02/14/more-odds-and-ends-aircraft-list-prices-airline-break-even/

[42] J. Markish, *"Valuation Techniques for Commercial Aircraft Program Design"*, Master of Science Thesis: Massachusetts Institute of Technology, 2002.

[43] D. Ferreri, *Marketing and management in the high-technology sector: strategies and tactics in the commercial airplane industry.* Praeger: Westport, Conn, 2003.

[44] O. Wyman, *To Re-Engine or Not to Re-Engine: That is the Question,* 2010. http://speednews.com/article/6950

CHAPTER 6

Environmental Aspects on Airplane Design

Abstract: Airplane design consists of putting together several thousand parts to ultimately fulfill a set of requirements defined principally by airlines, manufacturers, and certification authorities. From the traditional perspective of an airline, an interesting airplane is one that can generate the highest revenue with minimum operating cost – a maximum profit airplane. However, the airline industry is constantly broadening its consideration of what constitutes a nice-to-buy airplane. In recent times, not only economics, but also environmental considerations, are taking part in fleet-planning considerations. Following this trend induced by environmentally-aware passengers, and noise and pollution-related charges, airplane conceptual design methodologies are being expanded to incorporate methodologies for preliminary assessment of airplane noise and emissions. This chapter presents some methodologies for assessing airplane noise and emissions during the conceptual design phases.

Keywords: Aircraft conceptual design, Airframe noise, Emissions, Engine noise, Environmental issues, Multi-disciplinary design and optimization.

AIRPLANE NOISE

Historical Aspects

The introduction of jet airplanes into operations in the beginning of the 1950s was greeted with enthusiasm as it was expected to reduce traveling times between countries and continents. A decade later, one serious shortcoming of jet airplanes was causing a commotion with communities living near or beside busy, international airports: airplane noise.

Noise is formally defined as a sound that annoys. It wasn't different with airplanes: disturbed communities prompted governments to act against airplane noise, be it by enforcing manufacturers to design quieter airplanes or by reducing and shutting down airplane operations close to populated areas.

The first attempt to create a standard for aircraft noise evaluation was made at a conference in London, in 1966, which was barely successful. However, three years later, the United States Federal Aviation Authority (FAA) issued a Notice of

Bento S. de Mattos, José A. T. G. Fregnani & Paulo Eduardo C. S. Magalhães

Proposed Rule-Making (NPRM) concerning airplane noise certification (NPRM 69-1). Meanwhile, the International Civil Aviation Organization (ICAO) constituted a committee to investigate and propose regulations concerning aircraft noise.

Following NPRM 69-1, the FAA issued in 1971 the first version of the Part 36 of its aviation regulations (14CFR36) [1]. The first version of the 14CFR36 set a maximum of 108 EPNdB for noise either at fly-over, sideline or approach, which was about 10 EPNdB lower than the noise produced by jet airplanes in operation back then. As such noise level was applied to airplanes which were certified and went into operation even before 1969, it forced manufacturers to improve their on-going projects, like Lockheed L-1011 Tristar and Douglas DC-10, or even redesign parts of airplanes just certified like the Boeing B-747.

As the airplane noise levels were still considered unacceptable and certification authorities believed there was room for improvement, regulations were reviewed to set more strict limits on airplane noise. As a result, a limit of 97.1 EPNdB was set as the maximum allowable noise produced by an airplane. This second step in the legislation, named Stage 2, also introduced the effect of weight in the noise limit, to correct a distortion created by the single limit of 108 EPNdB of Stage 1, which was applied to both the Boeing B-747 Jumbo Jet and the Learjet series 20 business jet.

To further reduce the noise produced by airplanes, a so-called Stage 3 was created for airplanes certified after October 1977. Although Stage 2 addressed the weight issue on noise limits, it was then believed that noise levels were still biased as airplanes with similar weights and performances, operating from the same airports, but with different number of engines, were required to meet the same noise levels. In a typical situation, a three-engine DC-10 could meet the same noise levels of a four-engine Boeing B-747, which forced the B-747, equipped with the same engine model of the DC-10, to have a much quieter airframe. Therefore, as it reduced the maximum allowable noise level, Stage 3 also introduced the number of engines as a parameter for airplane noise limits.

More recently, the FAA started requiring what is called the Stage 4 of airplane noise certification. The reference noise levels are the same of Stage 3, but during certification, the airplane must have a minimum margin of 2 EPNdB in each of the measuring conditions and a cumulative margin of 10 EPNdB when the three measuring points are considered together. Meanwhile, standards for a stage 5 on noise level limits are already being discussed as well as a ban on the operation on the operation of aircraft certified to stage 3 standards.

Muraro developed of a numerical tool for the external noise estimation of airliners [2]. Here, only the noise generated by installed turbofan engines was modeled.

The tool was based on several methods described in a batch of NASA TM-X reports. Each of those reports addressed some specific component of the engine such as inlet, fan [3], core [4], turbine, and nozzle [5]. The MATLAB® platform was chosen to house the code under consideration. The ability of the code to correctly predict the noise signature was evaluated by the confrontation with the ESDU methodology [6, 7] and a similar work developed in the University of Berlin [8].

Bertsch *et al.in situ.* from the German DLR developed a tool for the design of aircraft with low-noise characteristics [9]. The main of their work objective is not the prediction of aircraft noise for an observer positioned on ground but a comparative noise evaluation among aircraft. The tool is target to the conceptual design phase, where they believe only a few key parameters are fixed so that geometry modifications are still feasible [9]. According to them, many aircraft design concepts can be directly evaluated and compared in a multidisciplinary design process. Some configurations can be selected for deeper investigation with high fidelity methods or wind tunnel tests.

Henderson developed a multi-disciplinary design framework encompassing environmental aspects to design and optimize aircraft according to environmental constraints [10]. The environmental metrics considered in the framework include fuel burn, landing-takeoff nitrogen oxides and fuel burn per distance flown. The engine model adopted by Henderson considers some component maps. Indeed, his performance analysis in the off-design envelope begins with the selection of proper component maps for turbomachinery components only. It is therefore assumed that the ducts and nozzles have fixed losses, as defined at the cycle design point, and the pressure ratio and efficiency of the combustor are also held constant. The generic component maps are scaled to fit the cycle reference point. These maps then define the operating points of the components at all off-design conditions within the engine operating envelope. Concerning applications, additional airplane concepts such as the design of short-range large aircraft are also considered in some simulations.

There are many researches that explore the feasibility of integrating noise and emissions as optimization objectives at the aircraft conceptual design phase, thereby allowing a quantitative analysis of the trade-offs between environmental performance and operating cost [11 - 13].

Noise Metrics

Noise, like sound, is a pressure fluctuation in a medium, which travels in all directions at a characteristic speed and with decreasing intensity. Noise is therefore described by its intensity, frequency, human reaction, and sound duration. To have a proper assessment of noise, all these aspects must be considered. The FAA, later followed by ICAO, developed a metric for quantifying airplane noise considering all those aspects [14].

The first aspect to be addressed is intensity, with a lower threshold being established as a reference. As noise depends on human reaction, hearing threshold (20 μPa) is set as the reference point for the definition of sound pressure level, SPL, as shown in Eq. **6.1**:

$$SPL(dB) = 10 \cdot log_{10} \frac{p^2}{p_{ref}^2} \quad \textbf{(6.1)}$$

Pressure levels depend on frequency. A standard set of frequencies is then defined for noise assessment. These frequencies are chosen based on average human hearing limits, from 50 Hz to 10 kHz, divided into 1/3-octave bands.

Human response to noise shows greater sensitivity to frequencies in the 1 Hz to 4 kHz range and therefore an estimation of perceived overall sound pressure level must account for this greater sensitivity. Another key aspect of noise assessment is the annoyance it causes in human beings. This subjective aspect of human reaction was addressed in researches conducted in the late 1950s. A subjective scale was created to convert pressure levels into noisiness, which is the term used to express human annoyance towards noise. This subjective scale, which considers both the frequency and level of the noise at each frequency, is shown in Fig. (**6.1**).

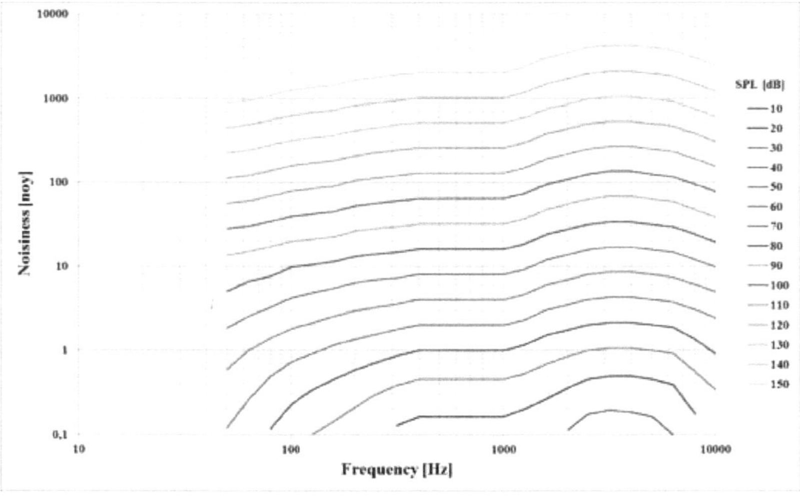

Fig. (6.1). Noisiness subjective scale.

The noisiness is then converted into Perceived Noise Level, PNL, using Eq. **6.2**:

$$PNL = 40.0 + \frac{10}{log_{10}2} \cdot log_{10}N \quad \textbf{(6.2)}$$

where N is the perceived noisiness, calculated through Eq. **6.3**, where n(i) is the noisiness at each of the 1/3-octave bands and n_{max} is the maximum of these noisiness' values:

$$N = 0.85 \cdot n_{max} + 0.15 \cdot \sum_{i=1}^{24} n(i) \quad \textbf{(6.3)}$$

In addition to the overall frequency content of noise, it was realized that discrete tones protruding in the frequency spectrum created greater subjective impact. To allow for this effect, an additional tone correction must be applied. This additional correction depends on how much the tone exceeds the noise in the neighboring frequencies. When this correction is applied to the PNL, it originates the PNLT (tone-corrected PNL). The tone correction, in terms of protruding noise levels is shown in Fig. (**6.2**).

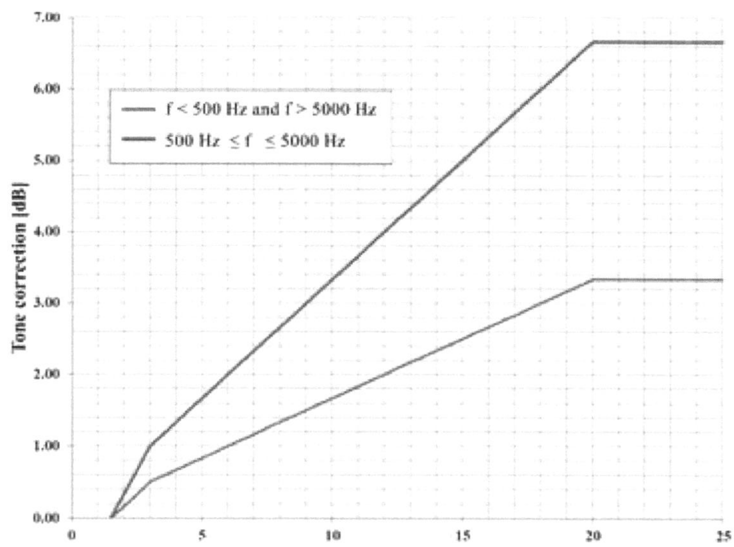

Fig. (6.2). Tone correction.

A final correction must be made to the measured sound pressure levels to account for the duration of the noise event. This is achieved by integrating the PNLT levels (at 0.5 second intervals) over a period where noise is above a threshold of

10 PNdB below the peak level observed during the complete event, as shown in Fig. (**6.3**). The resulting number is termed Effective Perceived Noise Level, EPNL, measured in EPNdB.

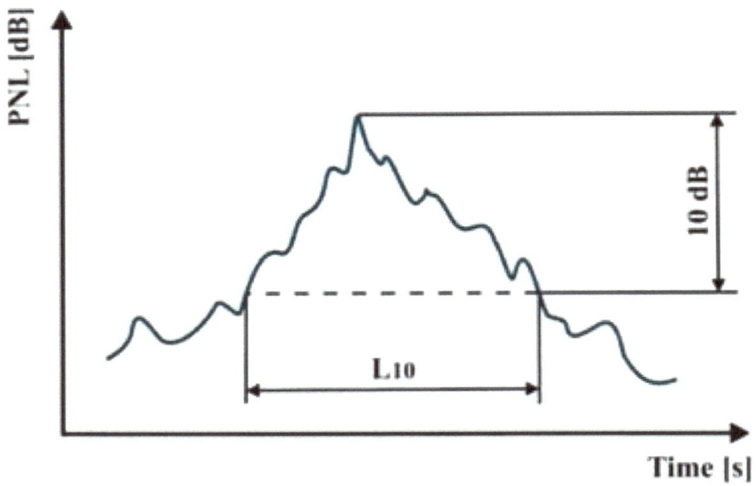

Fig. (6.3). Duration correction (EPNdB).

Certification Aspects

For type certification purposes, airplane noise must be assessed under defined conditions. The Federal Aviation Administration defines three noise measuring points as shown in Fig. (**6.4**):

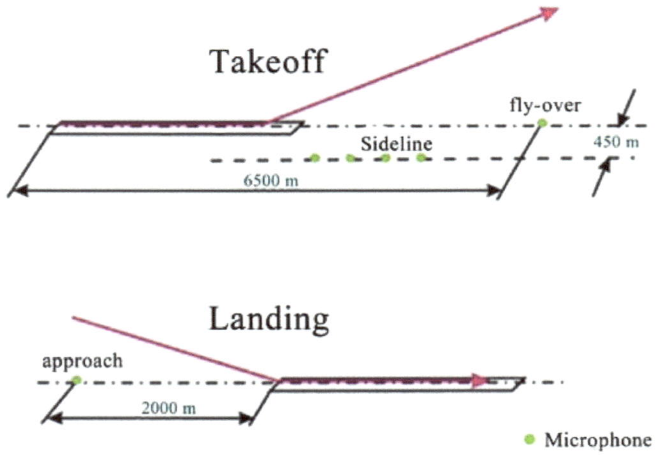

Fig. (6.4). Noise measuring points for airplane certification.

During takeoff, noise is assessed at two points: the fly-over point, laying 6500m ahead of the brake-release point, under the airplane flight-path, and the sideline point, located 450m to the side of the projection of the flight path on the ground. Noise is measured during the approach to land at a point 2000m before the touchdown point, under the airplane trajectory.

Noise measurement locations are defined to allow evaluation of various aspects of airplane noise. The fly-over measuring location is expected to assess the airplane performance impact on the noise it generates whereas the sideline noise addresses the noise generated by the engine while operating at full throttle. The approach noise measurement tackles the noise produced by the airframe – at this flight phase, engines are throttled back and their effect on the overall noise is usually less marked than during takeoff.

Figs. (**6.5** and **6.6**) show the airplane noise limits set by 14CFR36 for Stage 3 certification.

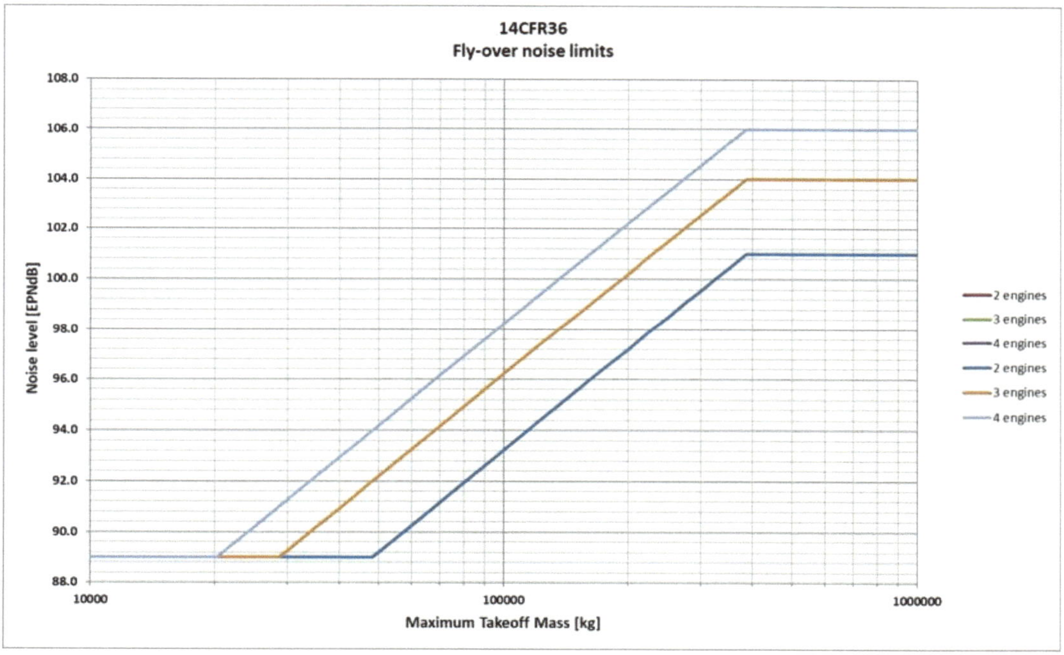

Fig. (6.5). 14CFR36 Noise limits – Fly-over.

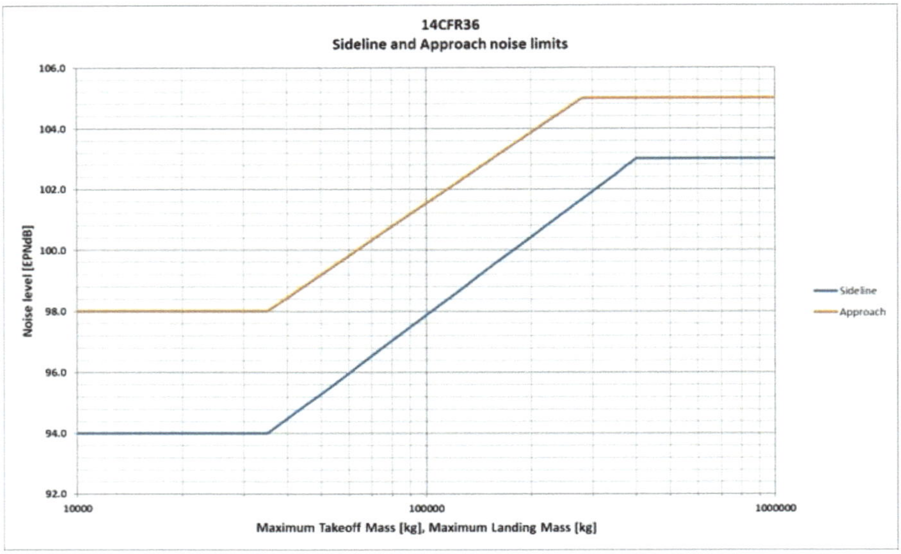

Fig. (6.6). 14CFR36 Noise limits – Sideline and Approach.

Over the years, considerable attention has been given to reduce airplane noise signature, not only to meet the certification standards, but also as a competitive advantage. A historical trend of airplane noise, considering the fly-over measurement condition, is shown in Fig. **(6.7)** for turbojet and turbofan-powered airliners.

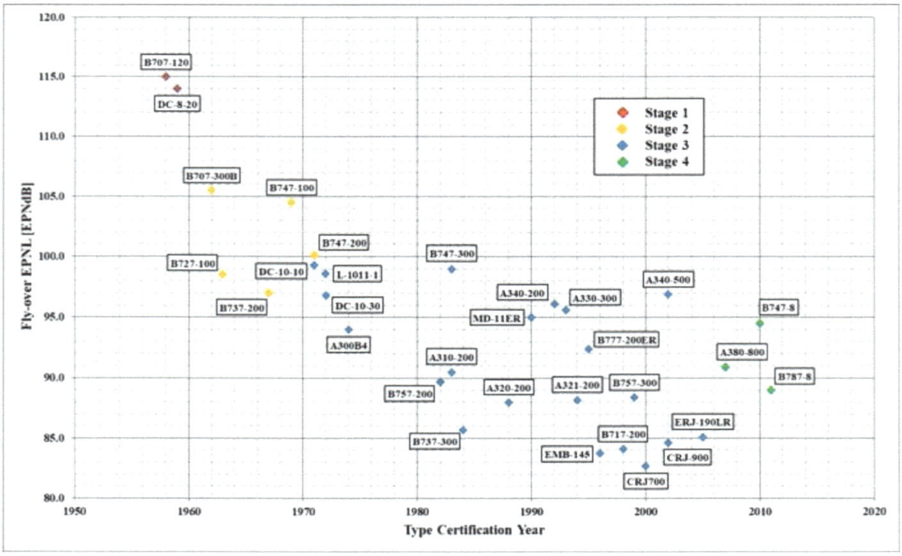

Fig. (6.7). Timeline of airliner fly-over noise.

Noise Sources

Airplane noise sources are shown in Fig. (**6.8**) [15].

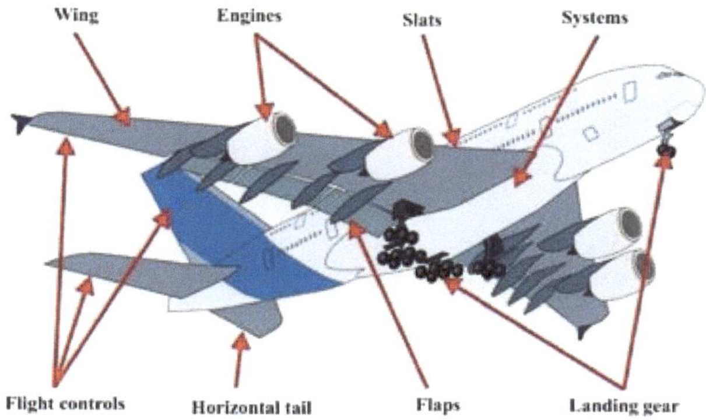

Fig. (6.8). Airplane noise sources.

Airplane noise sources are normally divided into two basic groups: engine noise and airframe-generated noise. Each of these two groups is further divided into its components as shown in Fig. (**6.9**). The noise of each of these components can be analyzed according to its origins as follows. Fan and compressor noise originates essentially from pressure fluctuations and interactions due to the air flow over rotating components. They are composed of:

- Noise emitted from the fan or compressor inlet duct:
    - Broadband noise;
    - Discrete-tone noise;
    - Combination tone noise;
- Noise emitted from the fan discharge duct:
    - Broadband noise;
    - Discrete-tone noise.

Engine core noise originates from:

- The combustion process;
- Flow around internal obstructions;
- Scrubbing of the duct walls;
- Local temperature fluctuations;
- Flow through the turbine;
- Turbine blade and stator interactions.

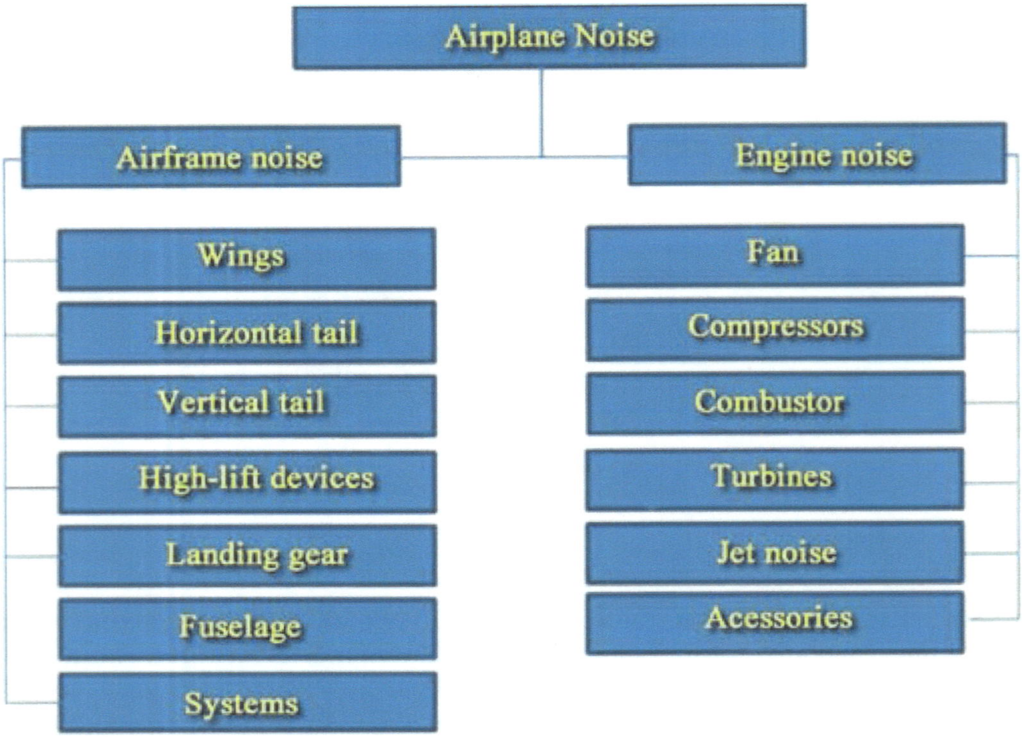

Fig. (6.9). Airplane noise breakdown.

Turbine noise is treated separately due to its distinctively high frequencies. It is like compressor noise, consisting of broadband and discrete tone noises, which are related to the relative tip speed of the turbine's last stage, the primary mass flow and the local speed of sound at the turbine exit.

Jet noise, by far the most evident form of engine noise, originates from the turbulence created by the jet mixing with the surrounding air. The acoustic power for a jet is proportional to the eighth-power of jet velocity (V_j^8) [5].

The introduction of jet engines on commercial service triggered the concerns with airplane noise and, for some time, engines were regarded as the most critical noise source. As engines evolved, their noise reduced to the point of being comparable to airframe-generated noise. A typical engine noise breakdown is shown in Fig. (**6.10**).

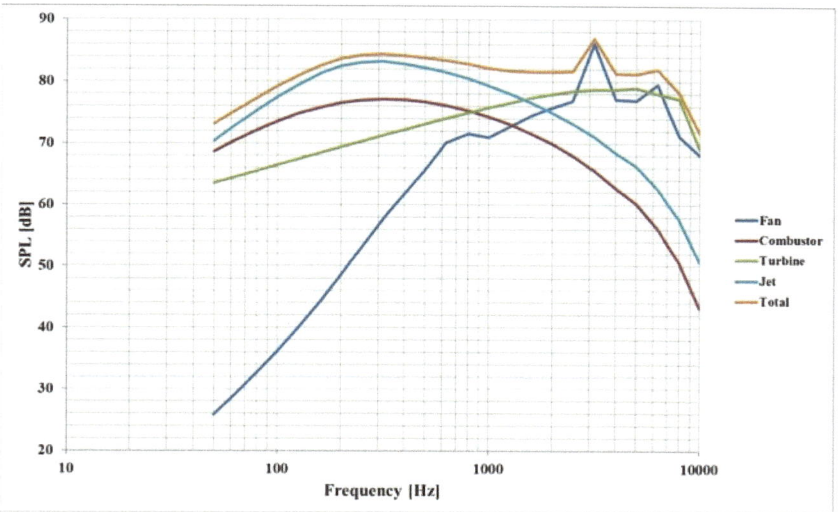

Fig. (6.10). Typical engine noise breakdown (full throttle, θ=120deg, 200m, 80m/s).

Airframe noise is caused by airflow over airplane surfaces (Fig. **6.11**). It depends on the configuration (takeoff, landing and cruise) and, for each configuration, it represents the limit below which further improvements in engine noise do not lead to overall improvement in airplane noise.

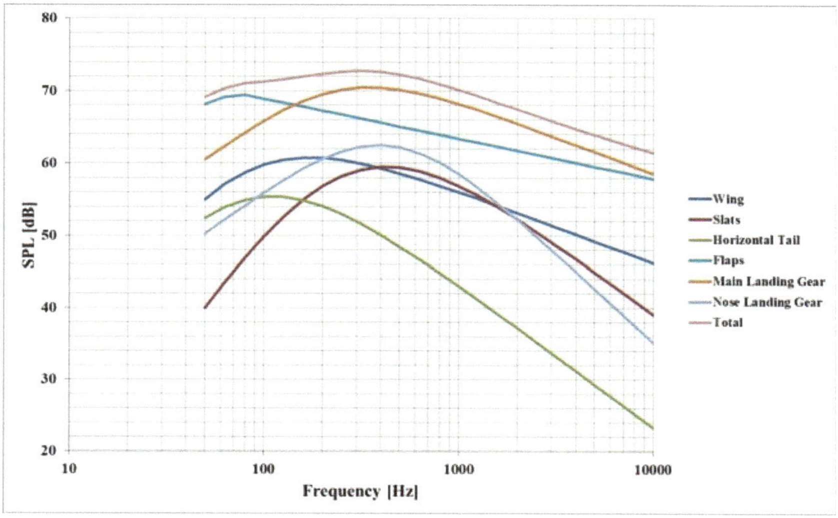

Fig. (6.11). Typical airframe noise breakdown (landing, θ=120deg, 200m, 80m/s).

Noise Modelling for Airplane Design

Airplane engine models are usually classified into three types [16]:

- Amplitude frequency (type-1) models, where SPL(F) = f(r, F, Θ, Π, Config.);
- Frequency correction (type-2) models, where SPL_Σ = f(r, Θ, Π, Config.);
- Noise-power-distance (type-3) models, where SPL_Σ = f(r, Π, Config.).

Although being the most complex models, type-1 models are the foundation for constructing a basic preliminary model of any aircraft type. They consist of a spectral analysis of the general acoustic field around the aircraft and the contributions of the component noise sources to the general acoustic field. They consider the distance from the airplane to the receiver (r), the frequency (F) and directivity (Θ) of the sound (referred to the airplane x-axis), the engine throttle setting (Π), and airplane configuration.

Type-2 models are derived by applying a frequency correction to the type-1 models based on a directivity pattern. Type-3 models, usually obtained from flight tests, consist of an integration of the noise over the acoustic field, *i.e.*, directivity integration. It is the simplest model as it is intended to enable estimations of local or regional influences of aircraft noise. A type-1 model for predicting airplane noise follows the structure defined in Eq. **6.4**:

$$SPL_\Sigma(F) = 10 \cdot log_{10}\left[\sum_i 10^{0.1 \cdot SPL_i(F)}\right] \quad \textbf{(6.4)}$$

where SPLi, the contribution of each noise source, is given by Eq. **6.5**:

$$SPL_i(F) = SPL(F) - \Delta SPL_\Theta - \Delta SPL_F - \Delta SPL_V - \Delta SPL_{int} - 20 \cdot \frac{r}{r_0} - \Delta SPL_{atm} + \Delta SPL_{gnd} \quad \textbf{(6.5)}$$

where:

- SPL(F) is the sound pressure level for a particular frequency band, normalized to a reference distance r_0 (=1 m);
- ΔSPL_Θ is the correction for directivity of sound radiation;
- ΔSPL_F is the spectral correction;
- ΔSPL_V is the correction for airplane speed, usually in terms of Mach number;
- ΔSPL_{int} is the correction for interference of elements;
- ΔSPL_{atm} is the correction for sound absorption in the atmosphere;
- r is the distance from the airplane to the receiver;
- ΔSPL_{gnd} is the ground reinforcement or attenuation due to absorption and reflection.

Models for predicting each of these components can be found in available extensive literature. Typically, models follow the structure defined by Eq. **6.5** in that they:

- Enable pressure level calculation at a reference distance from the source (1 m);
- Present directivity, spectral, and speed corrections;
- Present a method for accounting for atmospheric absorption.

Atmospheric absorption is a key aspect to be considered when evaluating airplane noise. Although several models are available, the one proposed by Ruijgrok is presents a good balance between fidelity and complexity [16].

The change in sound pressure level due to atmospheric absorption is determined using Eq. **6.6**:

$$\Delta SPL\_atm=(\alpha \cdot r)/100 \quad \textbf{(6.6)}$$

where α is the absorption's coefficient, which is a function of air temperature and humidity.

Ground absorption and reflection and element interference may be ignored at first on the basis that computing their effects would unnecessarily increase the complexity of conceptual studies.

When certification levels are considered as a target, all the sound pressure levels are calculated at the receiver at the standard temperature (25°C) and humidity (70%) for the standard field elevation (sea level).

AIRPLANE EMISSIONS

Historical Aspects

Modern airliners are powered by turbofan or turboprop engines burning kerosene. Kerosene is a mixture of hydrocarbons obtained from the refining of petroleum. This mixture contains a large variety of carbon chain molecules, generally with chain lengths of nine to sixteen atoms, as is the case with JET A-1, which is produced to internationally standardized specifications for use in civil aviation [17]. When a turbofan engine is in operation, fuel is injected in the combustion chamber, where it is mixed with flowing compressed air and ignited. Combustion takes place under conditions of high temperature and pressure, with the fuel burn further rising the temperature of the pressurized mixture. The hot, compressed mixture is partially expanded in the turbine section to drive the compressor and fan and then further expanded in the nozzle to propel the airplane. To fly efficiently, airplanes require engines with a high thrust-to-weight ratio, therefore imposing limitations on the designs that can be used in aviation.

In ideal conditions, kerosene undergoes complete combustion to produce carbon dioxide (CO_2) and water vapor (H_2O), Eq. **6.7**:

$$C_nH_m + O_2 \rightarrow CO_2 + H_2O \tag{6.7}$$

However, kerosene contains sulfur components originating from imperfect distillation and from additives used to improve fuel properties. In the real process, despite large quantities of ambient air (essentially N_2 and O_2) passing through the engine, combustion is not complete, and several by-products result (soot, unburned hydrocarbons) that contribute to acid rain and global warming, among other side effects. The real combustion process may then be more accurately described by Eq. **6.8**:

$$C_nH_m + S + O_2 + N_2 \rightarrow CO_2 + H_2O + O_2 + N_2 + NO_x + UHC + CO + C_{soot} + SO_2 \tag{6.8}$$

The complete combustion of any fuel requires an adequate amount of air. The ratio of the fuel quantity to the amount of air required for complete combustion is termed the stoichiometric fuel-to-air ratio. If more air is fed into the combustion process, the mixture is considered lean whereas if the fuel-to-air ratio is greater than the stoichiometric, the mixture is termed rich.

For air-breathing engines, instead of fuel-to-air ratio, the equivalence ratio, ϕ, is normally used. It is the ratio of the actual combustion fuel-to-air ratio to the stoichiometric ratio, where $\phi<1$ represents lean mixtures and $\phi>1$ represents rich mixtures. The equivalence ratio association to engine operation and emissions is shown in Fig. (**6.12**).

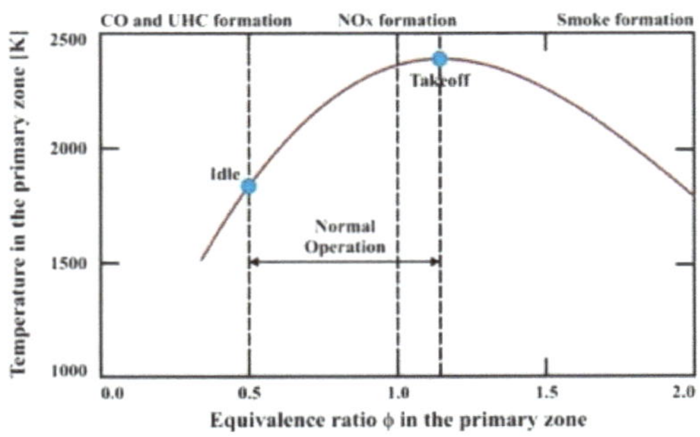

Fig. (6.12). Equivalence ratio and engine operation.

Airplane engines are required to operate under very efficient conditions. This leads to combustion products during cruise amounting to only 8.5% of the total mass flow leaving the engine, of which only around 0.4% in volume terms are residuals of the non-ideal combustion, as shown in Fig. (**6.13**).

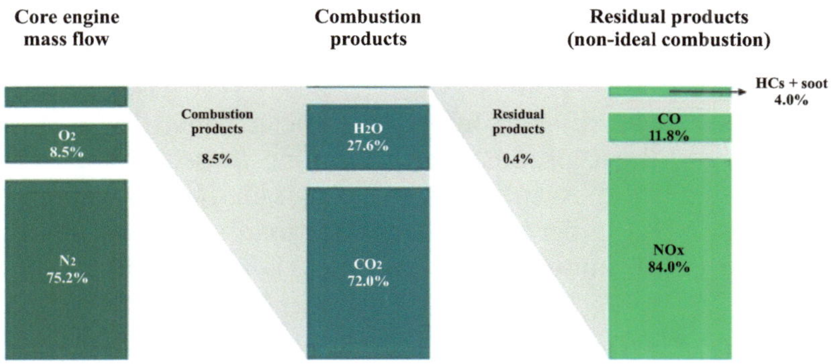

Fig. (6.13). Emissions and engine efficiency.

Airplane engine emissions, like other anthropogenic sources, are likely to change the atmospheric properties through three types of processes [18]:

- Emission of radiatively active substances, like CO_2 and water vapor, which contribute directly to the worsening of the atmospheric Greenhouse Effect;
- Emission of chemical species that produce or destroy radiatively active substances, like NO_X, which modifies O_3 concentration;
- Emission of substances that trigger the production of aerosols or lead to changes in the cloud cover (*e.g.* contrails).

To assess the aviation emissions impact in the atmosphere, the metric considered is termed radiative forcing (RF). Radiative forcing is the global, annual mean radiative imbalance to the Earth's climate system caused by human activities. It is a means of predicting changes to the global mean surface temperature, *i.e.*, a positive RF means global warming. The first estimates made in 1992 indicated that, at that time, radiative forcing of climate change due to aircraft emissions was +0.05W/m^2. This corresponded to 3.5% of the total anthropogenic radiative forcing, considering the baseline as +1.4W/m^2, which is the estimate for a pre-industrial atmosphere. Projections made in 1999 by the IPCC, based on several scenarios for economic grow and technological developments in the engine technology (Henderson & Wicrkama, 1999), forecasted that the radiative forcing of aircraft emissions would increase to +0.11 W/m^2 (about 5% of the anthropogenic total) by 2015. For 2050, the aviation RF was estimated to increase to +0.13 to +0.28 W/m^2 depending on more optimistic (or pessimist) scenarios for the industrialized nations' GDP growth and engine technological improvements.

Engine Emissions

Overview

As it was the case with noise, a practical standard is required to assess emissions modeling suitability. This standard is found in the certification procedures defined by ICAO in the annex 16 to its aviation convention [19, 20].

Engine emissions can be divided into two basic groups: those proportional to engine fuel burn and those proportional to engine thrust setting. The fuel-burn proportional emissions are essentially carbon dioxide (CO_2), water vapor (H_2O), and sulfur oxides (SO_X), whereas those proportional to thrust setting comprise carbon monoxide (CO), unburnt hydrocarbons (UHC), nitrogen oxides (NO_X), soot, and smoke.

Thrust-setting-proportional emissions can be further divided into two groups: those emissions whose production increase with thrust setting increase (NO_X, soot, smoke), reaching a maximum at full thrust, and those whose production decrease with thrust setting increase (CO, UHC), which reach a maximum at idle thrust.

Carbon Dioxide

Carbon dioxide is a greenhouse gas that occurs naturally in the environment and the single most important waste product of industrialized economies. It is produced in the engine at a rate of approximately 3,155 grams per kilogram of fuel burnt in the engine.

CO_2 is not the strongest greenhouse gas, but it is relatively abundant and has a very long life in the atmosphere, having, therefore, a leading importance in the global climate system. It is also one of the key pollutants addressed in the Kyoto Protocol.

Water Vapor

Like CO_2, water vapor (H_2O) is emitted in direct proportion to the quantity of kerosene burnt in the engine, at a rate of 1,240 grams per kilogram of fuel burnt. It is a powerful greenhouse gas, playing a critical role in the Earth's natural greenhouse effect. The lower part of the atmosphere is relatively humid because of natural hydrological processes.

The amount of water vapor emitted by airplane engines is very small compared with ambient concentrations. Most of these emissions is released in the troposphere and is rapidly transformed into precipitation in a timescale of weeks.

However, a small proportion of water vapor is emitted in the lower stratosphere where it can accumulate. In the middle and upper parts of the stratosphere, where the air is extremely dry, the introduction of water is therefore likely to increase atmospheric warming.

Sulfur Oxides

Sulfur oxides are produced in the engine because of the oxidation of sulfur-containing compounds either already present in the fuel (remains of the refining process) or added in low quantities in order to improve fuel properties. Emissions of sulfur oxides are therefore directly dependent on fuel quality.

Most of the sulfur present in the fuel is emitted in the form of sulfur dioxide (SO_2), which is acknowledged as an important local air pollutant. However, some oxidation to sulfur trioxide (SO_3) and gaseous sulfuric acid (H_2SO_4) occurs within the engine and in the exhaust plume.

Although thrust setting plays a key role in the production of sulfur oxides, as the overall amount of SO_2 emissions is very small in comparison with ambient concentrations, it is usually treated as a fuel-burn proportional emission. The importance of airplane-derived SO_2 is the formation of sulfate particles, which have several environmental effects including being nuclei for the formation of condensation trails (contrails), Fig. (**6.14**).

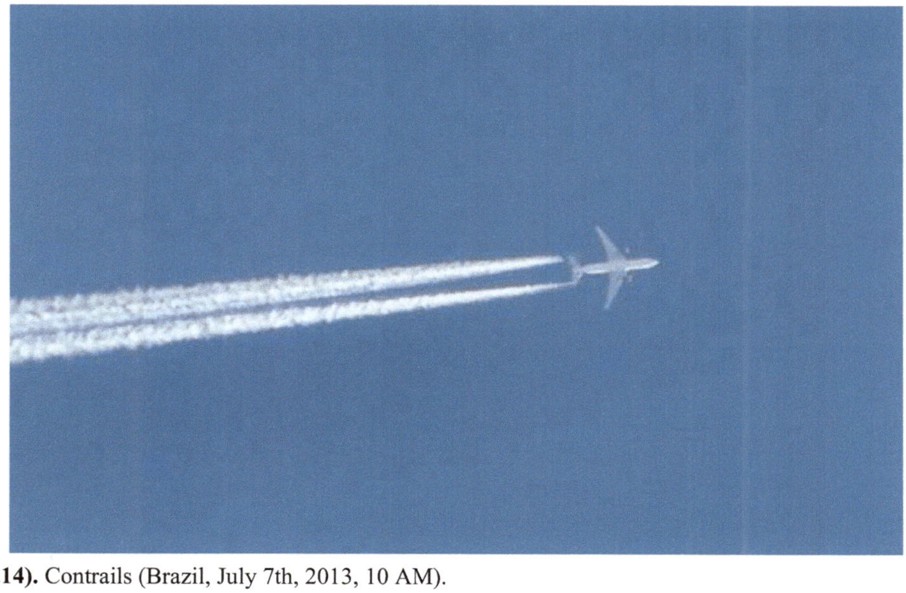

Fig. (6.14). Contrails (Brazil, July 7th, 2013, 10 AM).

Nitrogen Oxides

Nitrogen oxides comprise nitric oxide (NO) and nitrogen dioxide (NO_2). Their formation in the engine is a complex function of combustion temperature, pressure and combustor design. In general, nitrogen oxides are formed by the oxidation of atmospheric nitrogen in the high temperature conditions occurring in the combustor, with a small amount of NO_X being originated from nitrogen content of the fuel. Most of the nitrogen oxide content emitted is in the form of NO, but this is rapidly converted to NO_2 in the atmosphere. The amount of engine-emitted NO_2 is termed "primary NO_2".

The production of NO_X in the engine is unavoidable, but it can be minimized through better combustor design. However, the trend in NO_X emissions shows an increase, not a decrease, as engine design and fuel efficiency are improved. Higher fuel burn efficiency is routinely obtained through higher pressure ratios in the compressors, which lead to higher pressures and temperatures in the combustor, increasing NO_X formation.

Unburned Hydrocarbons

Hydrocarbon emissions consist of unburned molecules of hydrocarbons (UHC) that pass through the combustor and leave the engine through the nozzle with the rest of the mass flow. These molecules are both molecules originally present in the kerosene which escaped the flame zones and lighter hydrocarbon molecules formed during the complex chemical reactions occurring inside the engine.

Particles

Particulate matter tends to be very small, with diameter ranging from 3 nm to 4 μm. They may be non-volatile or volatile.

- Non-volatile particles are essentially carbonaceous material (soot) formed in the primary zone of the combustor due to incomplete combustion and tend to be burned out in further combustion, although some small amount manage to escape the engine in the exhaust plume. Soot particles' size range from 30 nm to 60 nm.
- Volatile particles are mostly sulfates, although some other organic material is also present when the exhaust plume is analyzed. Sulfates are formed mostly in the exhaust plume (and sometimes in the engine itself) as a result of the oxidation of sulfur-containing compounds added to the fuel. These volatile particles are roughly one or two orders of magnitude more abundant than soot and are classified as airplane-emitted aerosols.

Soot and sulfates have a small direct effect on climate by absorbing or scattering solar radiation. They also work as cloud condensation nuclei in the formation of condensation trails (contrails) and cirrus clouds.

Other Emissions

Many other substances are emitted by airplanes in small quantities in addition to the ones mentioned before. These include carbon monoxide (CO), hydroxyl radicals (OH), nitrous acid (HONO) and nitric acid (HNO_3).

Emissions Tradeoff

The basic engine emissions tradeoff relates fuel-burn-proportional and thrust-setting-proportional emissions through burning process efficiency. Essentially, for a given combustor design, the higher the pressure ratio, the higher the combustion pressure and temperature, the larger the amount of thrust-setting-proportional emissions (*i.e.* NO_X) produced, and the smaller the amount of fuel-burnt proportional emissions (CO_2, H_2O, SO_2). In other words, the more efficient the engine operation is, the smaller the amount of fuel-burnt-proportional emissions produced and the larger the amount of thrust-setting-proportional emissions produced.

Certification Aspects

The International Civil Aviation Organization has defined a set of conditions for the assessment of local emissions, termed Landing-Takeoff (LTO) cycle, which covers NO_X, CO, UHC, and smoke emissions. These conditions, summarized here, are detailed in the volume II (Emissions) of the Annex 16 (Environmental Protection) to the Convention on International Civil Aviation.

The LTO cycle considers the airplane engine operating at the takeoff, climb, approach and taxi (idle) settings. These settings are defined as a percentage of the rated engine thrust ($F\infty$): 100% $F\infty$ (takeoff), 85% $F\infty$ (climb), 30% $F\infty$ (approach) and 7% $F\infty$ (idle). The engine is supposed to operate at each setting for a definite time as follows: 42 s (takeoff), 132 s (climb), 240 s (approach) and 1,560 s (idle/taxi). LTO cycle is shown in Fig. (**6.15**).

Based on the LTO cycle, the ICAO Committee on Aviation Environmental Protection (CAEP) sets forth the limits for engine certification. These limits consider the total pollutant emission (D_p) parameterized by the total reference engine thrust ($F\infty$) which enables the comparison of engines of different sizes.

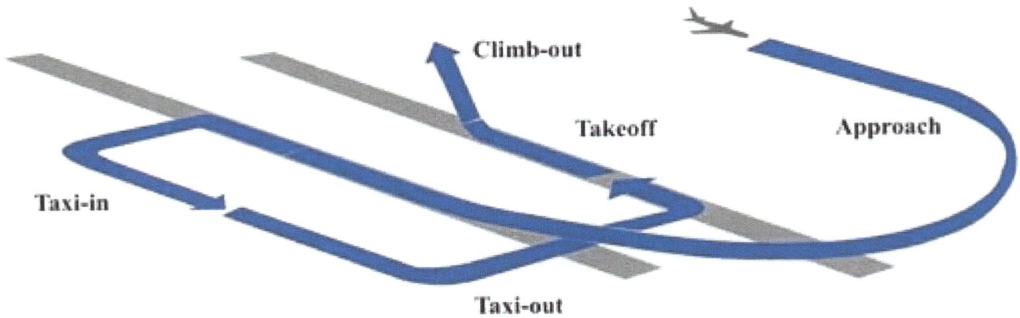

Fig. (6.15). LTO-cycle for emissions' evaluation.

Starting in 1983, with the first smoke standards, and 1986, with the initial standards for gaseous emissions, the limits on engine emissions based on the LTO cycle have become stricter over the years. These limits, which define different acceptable levels, are named CAEP-1, CAEP-2, *etc*., after the committee meetings at which they were defined (1st meeting, 2nd meeting, and so forth). For engines certificated after 2007 (CAEP-4), the limit for unburnt hydrocarbons (UHC) is $Dp/F\infty = 19.6$ g/kN whereas for carbon monoxide (CO), the limit is set at $Dp/F\infty = 118.0$ g/kN. For nitrous oxides, the limits vary according to the rated takeoff thrust ($F\infty$) and the overall pressure ratio (OPR).

Present day certification levels are set only for the LTO cycle, although ICAO is pursuing other methodologies and limits to cover the en-route phase of flight. Nevertheless, improvements in the emissions for the LTO cycle (mainly NO_X) are likely to generate improvements in the en-route phase as well. A timeline of LTO NO_X per passenger, per nautical mile, for common airliners is presented in Fig. (**6.16**).

Emissions Modelling for Airplane Design

Emissions' modeling consists of defining suitable models for estimating the emissions index (EI) for each pollutant. Emissions' prediction models can be classified into four types: correlation models, semi-empirical models, multi-reactor models, and high-fidelity flow-field simulations.

Correlation models are the simplest type of models, using correlations between recorded variations of emissions and critical engine operating parameters. They can be used to predict emissions at various operating conditions, despite not taking into consideration chemical and physical phenomena occurring inside the combustion chamber.

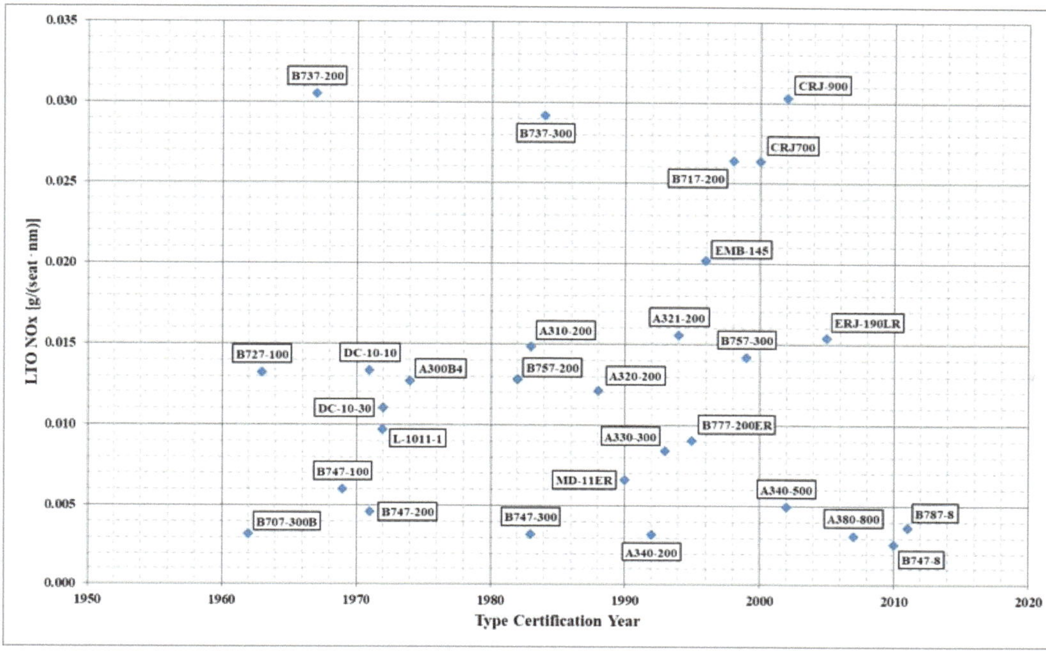

Fig. (6.16). LTO-NO_X evolution.

Semi-empirical models are obtained by considering the combustion chamber as a single thermochemical reactor. This model is characterized by average performance parameters based on engine cycle performance and experimentally gathered data on key parameters such as residence times, kinetic times and primary zone temperatures. Although the model can also be used to predict other emissions like CO, the experimental data required is usually very difficult to obtain.

Multi-reactor models simulate the combustion chamber by considering it as a network of thermochemical reactors, where turbulent flow is sufficiently idealized so that typical rates of mixing can be prescribed parametrically and the time-dependent chemistry of pollutant formation computed exactly. The main disadvantage of these models is the higher computational demand when compared to empirical and semi-empirical models. These models show, however, an improvement over the previous two because it offers better insight into the effects of using other fuels, deviations of air properties, and the use of water injection.

Finally, high-fidelity flow-field simulations use numerical solution techniques for the governing flow equations in a domain representative of the combustor geometry. The models used in these simulations require detailed kinetic mechanisms, large eddy simulations and complex three-dimensional geometry considerations, resulting in an intensive, complex and expensive computer use. The main advantage of these simulations is their accuracy, not requiring any reference data for calibration purposes.

Empirical (correlation) models are normally chosen for use in conceptual design based on the tradeoff of fidelity *versus* computational burden.

Models for Emissions Proportional to Fuel Consumption

Fuel-consumption proportional emissions are simply defined in terms of a constant EI. The emissions usually considered are the more common: CO_2, H_2O and SO_2. The following indexes are considered for these emissions (Table **6.1**):

Table 6.1. Emissions indexes.

Emissions	EI (g/kg fuel)
CO_2	3,155
H_2O	1,240
SO_2	0.8

Models for NO_X emissions

For NO_X emissions, several models have been proposed, from which a summary is presented. NO_X formation is a function of stoichiometric flame temperature in the combustor. A first approximation to its emission index is then given by Eq. **6.9**:

$$EI_{NO_x} = A \cdot e^{\left(\frac{T_{st}}{B}\right)} \qquad \textbf{(6.9)}$$

where T_{st} is the stoichiometric flame temperature and A and B are constants. This method is based on the so-called Lipfert models, developed by F.W. Lipfert in 1972 [21]. Lipfert showed that a good correlation exists between turbine inlet temperature, TIT, which is a function of flame temperature, and the NO_X formation. Lipfert models indicate that reductions in the stoichiometric flame temperature lead to reduction in NO_X formation. However, stoichiometric flame temperature is not a parameter readily obtained from engine performance models, which usually deal with pressure and temperature ratios at entry and exit of components. This is, therefore, the main disadvantage of Lipfert models. An evolution of the Lipfert models is represented by Eq. **6.10**:

$$EI_{NO_x} = 0.00036 \cdot \sqrt{p_3 \cdot e^{\left(\frac{T_3}{200}\right)}} \quad \textbf{(6.10)}$$

where p_3 and T_3 are the total pressure and total temperature at the entry of the combustor.

A semi-empirical model, derived from ICAO emissions database is given by Eq. **6.11**:

$$EI_{NO_x} = \frac{A \cdot p_3{}^{1.25} \cdot V_C \cdot e^{0.01 \cdot T_{st}}}{m \cdot T_{pz}} \quad \textbf{(6.11)}$$

In eq. 6.11, V_C is the volume of the combustion chamber, T_{st} is a function of total temperature at the entry of the combustion chamber, $m^{\cdot}$ is the mass flow through the combustion chamber and T_{pz} is the combustor primary zone temperature.

A model was proposed at NASA for advanced combustor technology consistent with entry into service from 2015 onwards. This model is described by Eq. **6.12**:

$$EI_{NO_x} = a \cdot (p_3)^{0.35} \cdot e^{\left(\frac{T_3 - 459.67}{300}\right)} \cdot \left(\frac{f_a}{\Delta\phi}\right)^{2.4} \quad \textbf{(6.12)}$$

where f_a is the combustor fuel-to-air ratio, $\Delta\phi$ is the combustor cooling air percentage and a is a function of $\Delta\phi$ and combustor technology level.

The models proposed so far are either too simple or require information not readily available during airplane conceptual design phase. An interesting compromise between simplicity and fidelity for emissions estimate is embodied in Eq. **6.13**:

$$EI_{NO_x} = 4.194 \cdot T_4 \cdot \left(\frac{p_3}{439}\right)^{0.37} \cdot e^{\left(\frac{T_3 - 1471}{345}\right)} \quad \textbf{(6.13)}$$

where T_4 is the total temperature at the combustor exit. EI_{NOx} is given in g/kg fuel.

CONCLUSIONS

The methodologies for noise and emission modeling described in the present Chapter is sound and they are so not time consuming to run on a desktop PC. However, the integration of the methodologies with an airplane model requires a deeper intrusion in the engine model. Contrary to this, the airframe noise calculation is something easier, but demands the proper design of the landing gear system.

Noise and emission were set as objectives in many works presented in conferences and journals. However, a more reasonable approach would be to handle them as constraints.

For twin-engine airplanes with conventional or "T"-tail configurations, the resulting noise optimized designs should present the following characteristics:

- Higher empty weight;
- Higher maximum takeoff weight;
- Larger, more powerful engines;
- Larger, less swept and more elongated wings;
- Takeoff flap setting with a smaller deflection to improve climb-out characteristics;
- Landing flap setting with a larger deflection to reduce approach speed;
- Smaller, less elongated horizontal tail;
- Larger, more elongated vertical tail, with a larger rudder deflection, to account for the higher thrust asymmetry in case of an engine failure.

Expected trends for NO_X-optimized designs are the following:

- Reduced engine size;
- Reduced overall pressure ratio of the engine;
- Reduced turbine exhaust temperature;
- Higher empty weight;
- Higher takeoff weight;
- Larger, slightly more swept and less elongated wings;
- Smaller flap deflection for takeoff and landing;
- Engines placed farther from fuselage;
- Less tapered, less elongated and less swept horizontal tail;
- More tapered, more elongated and less swept vertical tail.

REFERENCES

[1] Federal Aviation Administration, *14CFR36 Noise standards: Aircraft type and airworthiness certification.* FAA: Washington, 2013.

[2] D.A. Muraro, and B.S. Mattos, "Estimation of Noise of Installed Turbofan Engines", *Brazilian Symposium on Aerospace Eng. & Applications, São José dos Campos,* 2009.

[3] M.F. Heideman, *Interim Prediction Method for Fan and Compressor Source Noise.* NASA Lewis Research Center: Cleveland, 1979.

[4] R. G. Huff, B. J. Clark, and R. G. Dorsch, "Interim Prediction Method for Low Frequency Core

Engine Noise", *NASA Lewis Research center,* 1974.

[5] J.R. Stone, *Interim Prediction Method for Jet Noise.* NASA Lewis Research Center, 1974.

[6] ESDU, *Airframe Noise prediction - 90023.* IHS Group: London, UK, 2003.

[7] ESDU, *An introduction to aircraft noise - 02020.* IHS Group: London, UK, 2002.

[8] M. Schmid, *Entwicklung eines Programmmoduls zur Prognose des Lärms von Strahltriebwerken im Flugzeugvorentwurf.* Institut für Luft- und Raumfahrt der Technischen Universität Berlin: Berlin, 2001.

[9] L. Bertsch, W. Dobrzynski, and S. Guérin, "Tool Development for Low-Noise Aircraft Design", *J. Aircr.,* vol. 47, no. 2, pp. 694-699, 2010. [http://dx.doi.org/10.2514/1.43188]

[10] R. Henderson, *"Multidisciplinary Design Optimization of Airframe and Engine for Emissions Reduction"*, University of Toronto, PhD Thesis, Toronto, 2010.

[11] N. Antoine, *"Aircraft Optimization for Minimal Environment Impact"*, Satnford University. PhD Thesis, Stanford, 2004.

[12] B. Mattos, and P.C. Magalhães, "Conceptual Optimal Design of Airliners with Noise Constraints", *50th AIAA Aerospace Sciences Meeting including the New Horizons Forum and Aerospace Exposition, Nashville,* 2012 [http://dx.doi.org/10.2514/6.2012-338]

[13] L.T. Leifsson, *Multidisciplinary Design Optimization of Low-Noise Transport Aircraft.* Department of Aerospace and Ocean Engineering, Virginia Polytechnic Institute and State University: Blacksburg, 2005.

[14] International Civil Aviation Organization, "Annex 16: Environmental Protection, Aircraft Noise", *ICAO Convention on International Civil Aviation,* 2008 Montreal

[15] M. Smith, *Aircraft Noise.* Cambridge University Press: Cambridge, U. K., 1989. [http://dx.doi.org/10.1017/CBO9780511584527]

[16] G.J. Ruijgrok, *Elements of Aviation Acoustics.* Delft University Press: Delft, 1993.

[17] Wikipedia, The Free Encyclopedia, "Jet Fuel", https://en.wikipedia.org/wiki/Jet_fuel

[18] IPCC, "Potential Climate Change from Aviation", *Intergovernmental Panel on Climate Change,* 2009.

[19] International Civil Aviation Organization, "Annex 16: Environmental Protection - Aircraft Engine Emissions", *ICAO Civil Aviation Convention,* 2008 Montreal.

[20] IPCC, "Aircraft Technology and its Relations to Emissions", *Intergovernmental Panel on Climate Change,* 1999.

[21] F.W. Lipfert, "Correlation of Gas Turbine Emissions Data", *ASME 1972 International Gas Turbine and Fluids Engineering Conference and Products Show,* 1972 San Francisco. [http://dx.doi.org/10.1115/72-GT-60]

CHAPTER 7

An Innovative Approach for Optimal Airplane Design Encompassing an Airline Network

Abstract: A Multi-disciplinary design and optimization platform for transport airplane with environmental considerations is developed. Instead of employing the usual optimization approach that minimizes the averaged direct operational cost in a set of stage lengths, an enhanced multi-disciplinary methodology involving a considerable detailed airplane model is presented here. In the past, the suitability of the product for a realistic airline network has not been entirely considered, and even disconnected from airline real needs. Increased computer power, sophisticated surrogate models, and new optimization techniques make possible to optimize the complete system with aircraft inserted in an air transport network including complex mission analyzes. In this context, a sophisticated airplane design framework with multi-disciplinary approach encompassing several aeronautical disciplines including noise and emissions was elaborated for the design of optimal airplane configurations that are suited for a desired airline network. Artificial neural network is used as a surrogate model to calculate the airplane aerodynamics with a high-fidelity approach, to perform a realistic mission analysis enabling operation aspects to properly be considered in the optimization task. The simultaneous minimization of total network direct operational costs and maximization of Total Network Yield is performed to optimize fifteen aircraft design variables, encompassing airframe and engine definition. The MOGA-II genetic algorithm, available in the modeFrontier® Integrated Optimization Environment is employed in the present design simulations

Keywords: Aerial network, Aircraft conceptual design, Applied aerodynamics, Artificial neural network, Evolutionary computation, Multi-disciplinary design and optimization, Propulsion, Stability and control.

INTRODUCTION

The commercial air transport business is characterized by low operational margins and fierce competition among airlines. According to Doganis [1], the average world airlines profit margins have been very small since the 80s, varying from -4% to 3%. Data from the U.S. Department of Transportation (DoT) confirm this (Fig. **7.1**).

Bento S. de Mattos, José A. T. G. Fregnani & Paulo Eduardo C. S. Magalhães

Besides pointing to a volatile market, U.S. Department of Transportation statistics reveals a major shift in operations of the North-American airline industry in the first half of the 2000s. Table **7.1** shows a comparison of airline performance for two years: 2000 and 2005. These data are very useful to analyze the change in efficiency and profitability of both network airlines and low-cost carriers. At the end of 2005, the legacy or network airlines reduced their capacity (measured by ASMs), by 11.2 percent since 2000, while four network carriers, United Airlines, US Airways (twice), Delta Air Lines and Northwest Airlines, filed for bankruptcy [2]. During the same period, low-cost carriers increased capacity 61.1 percent and accounted for nearly one-fifth of all passenger revenue-miles for the year ending 2005 [2]. A single low-cost carrier, ATA Airlines, filed for bankruptcy, ceasing operations in 2008. In 2017, Southwest airlines, the largest low-cost airline, recorded a fleet of 727 airplanes and a net income in the first quarter of US$ 321 million [3].

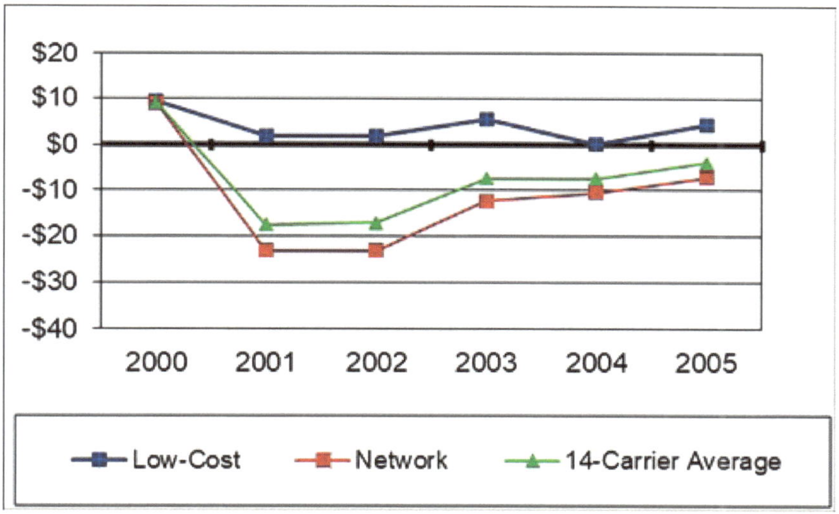

Fig. (7.1). Operating profit or loss per enplanement of the U.S. airlines (Source: Bureau of Transportation Statistics, Form 41 Airline Financial Data and T-100 Segment Data).

The impact of efficient fleet management, including operation, and the choice of right airplanes to the assigned networks is crucial for the survival of airlines. In this context, the efficient aircraft flight path management is also a major topic that has been explored by airlines, and the supported by aeronautical industry, with focus on operational costs reduction. Besides efficient operations, the design of aircraft has been more and more influenced by customers' needs and therefore the coupling of the operational and design disciplines has been demonstrated necessary.

Table 7.1. Bottom-line statistics for the U.S. aviation sector.

	Network Carriers	**Low-cost Carriers**
Full time equivalent employees	**-33.3%**	**+22.4%**
2000	423,040	55,242
2005	282,321	67,240
Number of aircraft	**-15.2%**	**+41.9%**
2000	3,358	602
2005	2,847	854
Mainline pax revenue (excluding RJ activity)	**- US$ 12.6 billion**	**+ US$ 4.8 billion**
2000	US$ 77.2 billion	US$ 10.2 billion
2005	US$ 64.6 billion	US$ 15 billion
Operating expense (excluding fuel & regional contract operations)	**- US$ 13.5 billion**	**US$ 3.9 billion**
2000	US$ 54.2 billion	US$ 7.6 billion
2005	US$ 37.7 billion	US$ 11.5 billion

(Courtesy: U.S. Department of Transportation, Bureau of Transportation Statistics)

Typically, the conceptual design of commercial transport airplanes is determined by academia and aircraft manufacturers through optimization of averaged direct operational cost in each set of stage length (range), which is chosen by the project team. Considerations about the suitability of the product into a realistic airline network are usually not properly considered. The outdated approach of conducting surveys among airlines to incorporate some needs into the design gave way to the practice to allocate airline representatives in the aircraft development program council. However, different airlines present different requirements for the airplanes they are intending to purchase and just some of the them seating in the program council may not be enough to elaborate right requirements. Besides this, many tools used in aircraft design in the conceptual phase are very limited, modeling the aeronautical disciplines taken into consideration with low fidelity. Sometimes the design framework that are employed with the objectives and constraints adopted may not be adequate. Specifically, studies to determine airline needs for its aerial network are carried out by groups in airlines, which present a distinct profile regarding the ones which belong to aircraft manufacturers. The teams simplify and perform optimizations focused on subsystems, ignoring the high degree of dependency that exists between airplane and network, resulting in the inefficiency of the system. However, it is possible to optimize the complete system, aircraft and network at once, in a more effective manner, thus optimizing the aircraft or group of aircraft that can operate inside a typical network of major airline. This must be carried out with a detailed description of the optimized configuration, not just representing the airplane with a few parameters such as MTOW, OEW, T/W, without a precise and concise performance calculation.

The conceptual design of an aircraft is nowadays carried out using Multidisciplinary Design Optimization (MDO) frameworks. A great deal of computational analyses is required to obtain optimum configurations to satisfy many objectives and design constraints. Disciplines such as aerodynamics, propulsion, flight mechanics, structures and aeroelasticity, among others, are frequently considered in the optimization framework to obtain more realistic geometries of flight vehicles in addition to mission analysis into the network. Nowadays, many design variables may be employed and advanced optimization algorithms enable that complex models of the aeronautical disciplines should be considered. Empirical formulae (*i.e.* the Class-I and Class-II methods [4] for drag and weight estimation), may be used for modeling and provide faster results with reasonable accuracy. In addition, surrogate models have been frequently adopted with the objective to provide better accuracies and at the same time reducing the computational time of complex and heavy calculations in MDO frameworks. For example, neural network analysis enables huge reductions in computational costs in aerodynamic simulations. Several optimization models have been used in such frameworks. Due to the non-linear nature of the objective functions and constraints of this kind of problem, gradient methods are difficult to converge to global minima and therefore, more robust solutions have been tried. Besides the integration of disciplines under gradient methods is a serious drawback.

The airplane designed in the optimization of such kind of framework shall therefore be considerably more complex than that adopted by Taylor [5, 6], where the airplane was optimized considering single objective cost functions. A new methodology is needed to be developed to optimize multi objective variables related to the airplane design, considering the airline network. Some of the airplane characteristics to be optimized that are listed: geometry variables (fuselage cross-section dimensions like aisle width and cabin height, wing aspect ratio, wing taper ratio, wing sweepback angle, wing airfoil geometry, tail characteristics, winglet geometric definition, *etc.…*), topological variables (low or high wing; wing structural layout, engines placed at rear fuselage or under the wing, “T” or conventional tail, *etc...*), configuration variables (shape of the fuselage cross-section, seating abreast, number of aisles, number of engines, *etc.…*), engine variables (by-pass ratio, overall pressure ratio, fan pressure ratio, turbine inlet temperature, fan diameter, *etc...*), environmental constraints (noise and engine emissions) and design constraints (FAR regulations; maximum cruise speed, flutter speed, flight qualities, *etc.…*). In addition, considering the complex network theory [3], the main indicators reflecting the statistical features of air transport network structure may be included in the framework such as the degree of nodes, average degree, average path length, density, clustering coefficient, *etc*. Airports characteristics in the network may be included in the mission profile computation. Information such as noise levels constraints for operating airplanes, runway length, elevation and environmental conditions could be set as fixed parameters in the framework.

Genetic Algorithm is a method that mimics the evolution of living beings and operate on populations applying the principle of survival of the fittest. This enables the reproduction of the population in such a way that solutions that comply with objectives and obey constraints are generated. It has been demonstrated to work with acceptable levels of robustness on multi-objective/multivariable problems, aiming to reduce the number of qualitative decisions required and with the increasing the number of design variables [7 - 9]. At each generation, a new set of approximations is created by the process of selecting individuals according to their level of fitness in the problem domain and breeding them together using operators borrowed from natural genetics. This process leads to the evolution of populations of individuals that are better suited to their environment than the individuals that they were created from (just as in natural adaptation). Individuals are encoded as strings (chromosomes) composed over some alphabet(s), so that the genotypes (chromosome values) are uniquely mapped onto the decision variable (phenotypic) domain. The genetic characteristics of an individual are stored in a chromosome, which is represented by the set of chosen Design Parameters.

The GA methods differ substantially from more traditional search and optimization methods as follows:

1. Ability to generate population with parallel processing.
2. Does not require derivative information or other auxiliary knowledge. Only the objective function and corresponding fitness levels are needed.
3. Uses probabilistic transition rules, not deterministic ones.
4. Works on an encoding of the parameter set rather than the parameter set itself.
5. Allows the use of continuous, discrete, and integer design variables in the same optimization process. This feature is especially interesting on aircraft design and sizing need to be integrated with network parameters in a single optimization process.
6. Has no requirement for objective functions and constraints to be continuous and no gradient calculations is involved in the optimization process.

It is important to note that GA methods provide several potential solutions to a given problem and the choice of final solution is left to the user. In cases where a problem does not have one individual solution, for example a family of Pareto-optimal solutions, (as is the case in multi-objective optimization) GA methods are potentially useful for identifying these alternative solutions simultaneously. Genetic algorithms are now of generalized use in optimization problems, including aircraft design and air transport networks [5, 6, 10 - 13]. However, one drawback is that stochastic algorithms in general can have difficulty obeying equality constraints. In addition, GA is sensitive to the initial population used. Wide diversity of feasible solutions is what it is usually wanted.

The first generations of Multi Objective Generic Algorithms (MOGA) [7, 14] had its efficiency ruled by its inherent operators (crossover, mutation and selection) and the use of elitism, *i.e.*, the best organism from the current generation to carry over to the next. The direction of improvement was always evaluated by comparing the fitness of the individual from generation t with the fitness of its parents belonging to generation $t-1$. The new individual is then created by moving in a randomly weighted direction that lies within the ones individuated by the given individual and his parents. In MOGA algorithms, the user constraints lead always to objective function penalization and allow concurrent evaluation of independent individuals [7].

In latter developments Deb [15] proposed the Non-Dominated Sorting Genetic Algorithm (NSGA) as an improvement of previous versions. In this method, a fast-non-dominated sorting procedure is used on a modified elitism rule: the solution adopts an Elitism-preserving approach, storing all non-dominated solutions discovered so far, beginning from the initial population, enhancing the convergence properties towards the true Pareto-optimal set. In addition, the constraint handling method does not use penalty parameters. Therefore, this algorithm implements a modified definition of dominance to solve constrained multi-objective problems more efficiently [15]. The main advantage of using this method on network and aircraft multi-objective design optimization problem is a faster convergence on complex modeling using both continuous and discrete variables.

MDO for aircraft design may vary in single level and multilevel optimization. In single level approach, both disciplinary and system design variables are determined by the system optimizer, while in the second one system each discipline has its own optimizer. In addition, simultaneous analysis and design (SAND) or nested analysis design analysis (NAND) may be chosen, per the size and complexity of the problem. In SAND both disciplinary design and state variables are determined by the optimizer, while in NAND only disciplinary design variables are determined [16]. Multilevel optimization and NAND approaches are more suited for aircraft design tasks that encompasses aerial network optimization.

Many forms of approximation methods were developed to model disciplines to enhance the speed of the optimization when heavy computations are required. Recently surrogate models (such as Kriging interpolation and artificial neural networks), have been providing satisfactory results replacing heavy aerodynamic and structural modeling [17]. The mission investigation integrated to aircraft design was proposed by the first time by Isikveren [18], where the optimization range and fuel consumption with semi-empirical formulations applied on aircraft design variables. Cavalcanti [19] and Cabral [11] proposed a multi-objective optimization of wing planform carried out by the minimization of the block time and block fuel for a given mission. Henderson developed an environmental design framework to design and optimize aircraft for specific environmental metrics [20]. Since then MDO is proposed to be used to optimize aircraft by simultaneously considering airframe, engine and mission design. However, the research on integration of detailed airplanes with a network saw considerable development in the last ten years due to the increase of computational power and development of robust optimization solvers which are capable to handle multivariable, multi-objective functions and submitted to non-linear constraints.

Recent studies show that the direct coupling of aircraft design and airline fleet-route allocation frequently use mixed-integer, nonlinear programming (MINLP) formulation, a suitable solution *via* a decomposition approach [21, 22]. It is worth to mention that most of the researches are until now directed to the identification of aircraft characteristics that reduce direct operational costs. Some studies worthy to be mentioned in this domain are reported in the remaining paragraphs of this section.

Roth and Crossley [23] employed genetic algorithms for aircraft conceptual design in a specific mission combined with gradient based method, providing the first insight for using this methodology in such kind of problem. Some years later, Crossley *et al* [24]. suggested a problem formulation and a solution approach for a 50-seater aircraft design and mission requirements posed as a combinatorial multi-objective optimization problem using a two-branch tournament Genetic Algorithm. This new method proposes a search through the design space, incorporating discrete, integer, and continuous variables and generates a range of designs that represent the best tradeoffs or compromises among engineering objectives.

Taylor and Weck [5] presented the first investigation of the benefits of optimizing an integrated air transportation network and vehicle design, concurrently defined. A case study presented focuses on design an air transportation network for overnight package delivery on two turn around hubs configuration connecting seven cities. By concurrently optimizing both the vehicle (simplified model base on Breguet Range equation) and network for a selected few cities with fixed demand, it was obtained a minimum of a ten percent improvement in operational costs over that obtained by optimizing the network design using a set of pre-defined aircrafts. This was accomplished by embedding a linear programming solver in the perturbation step of simulated annealing to solve for the considerable number of linear constraints imposed by the capacity and demand requirements of the network.

Bower and Kroo [10] presented a methodology to design one or more aircraft to satisfy demand on a given route network. The objectives were to minimize direct operating costs and emissions (CO_2 and NO_X). In their work, a hierarchical decomposition was used with discipline-specific optimization algorithms using simplistic models. A modified version of the NSGA-II multi-objective genetic algorithm is implemented in the system level aircraft design subspace. The CPLEX integer solver was proposed to be used in the fleet assignment subspace. Results were presented for a test problem that involves designing a single aisle commercial aircraft for a route network consisting of four cities and eight route segments, using eighteen design variables. Under this scope, Mane and Crossley [21] presented an approach to couple the uncertain aircraft assignment problem of fractional operations and the aircraft design problem of aircraft manufacturers. The stochastic characteristic of the problem is considered to influence the aircraft design that directly improves operations and identifies operating strategies that influence, and take advantage of, the characteristics of the new aircraft.

Roy *et al.* [25, 26] proposed a sophisticated algorithm combining branch and bound, Efficient Global Optimization, Kriging Partial Least Squares, and gradient-based optimization to solve Mixed Integer Non-Linear Programming problem with 100's of integer design variables, 1000's of continuous design variables. The algorithm was applied to a network with 8 nodes using a sophisticated module of for aircraft design and allocation problem with the nineteen allocation variables and solving a thousand-variable aircraft design optimization problem using CFD simulation.

Davendralingam and Crossley [27] proposed a unifying conceptual framework on concurrently design aircraft and the operational network by incorporating established passenger demand models. A conceptual scenario involving six city pairs is formulated and solved to exhibit the methodology employed and reflexivity of demand. In subsequent studies [28] these authors present a concurrent engineering strategy for an airline that wishes to investigate the impact that aircraft design choices and target market capture decisions have on tradeoffs between expected profit and risk in serving demand itineraries and impact of economic risks.

Hwang *et al.* [29] propose a concurrent optimization encompassing aircraft design, mission profiles, and the allocation of aircraft to routes in an airline network. To enable this, a gradient-based optimization approach was adopted with a parallel computational framework, which boost the computation of derivatives in the multidisciplinary analysis. A surrogate model for the CFD analysis is re-trained in each optimization iteration given the new set of shape design variables. The resulting optimization problem contains over 6,000 design variables and 23,000 constraints, and it is solved in approximately 10 hours on a machine with 128 processors. The optimization revealed a 27% increase in airline profit when comparing the allocation-mission-design optimization to allocation only optimization.

Cabral *et al.* [11] presented a computational tool for the conceptual design of families of aircraft for a given mission using the MDO framework. Twenty design variables were employed and four disciplines, using Class-I modeling. Expanding this methodology Siqueira *et al.* [13] developed a methodology for aircraft optimal conceptual design employing advanced turbofan engine and airplane models. Wing and engine position in the configuration, number of engines, tail configuration, wing and horizontal tail geometries are adopted as design variables.

METHODOLOGY

Overview

A MDO framework for airliner that best fits into an airline network with passenger demands is described here. The network chosen by the authors to demonstrate the features of the framework is a regional one in Brazil encompassing 5 cities connected through 16 routes with fixed demand. In fact, it is an improvement of the methodology proposed by Bower and Kroo [10], mainly due to the detailed airplane configuration that is considered in the optimization process and to the fidelity of some aeronautical disciplines, noticeable performance calculation, noise calculation according to ICAO rules, and aerodynamic analysis, the latter performed with a ANN surrogate model featuring a high accuracy for the aerodynamic coefficients [30]. The full MDO flow proposed to solve the complete optimization of the aircraft and network system is shown in Fig. (**7.2**), in a multilevel-NAND approach, using two design frameworks (aircraft and network).

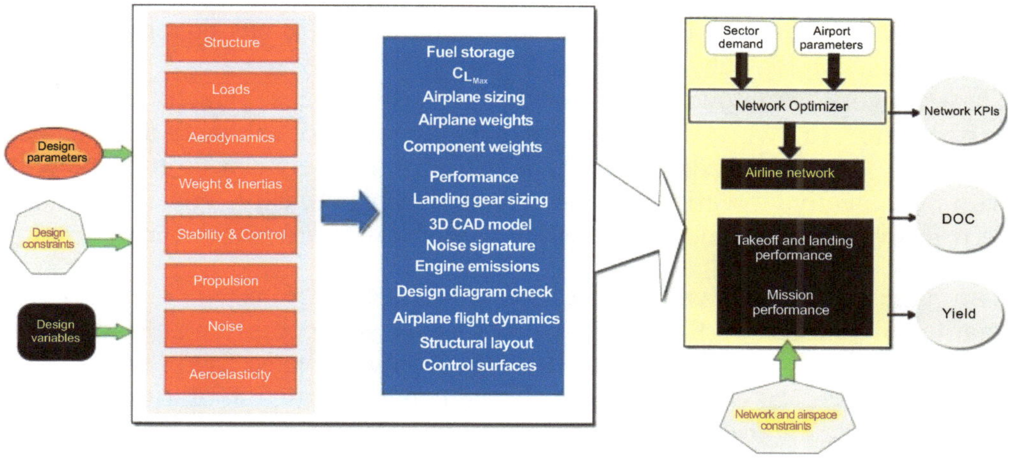

Fig. (7.2). Aircraft and Network features employed in the optimization framework.

A requirement check is performed after the aircraft weight is calculated and before the computation of the network characteristics presented by the configuration. This is carried out to ensure that the design produced in the aircraft framework is compliant with performance, stability, and certification requirements.

Many aeronautical disciplines are present in the airplane module and they are sufficient to properly represent the complete set of characteristics involved in the design of an aircraft. In this study, however, three disciplines in the aircraft framework are developed in detailed models with focus to support the inclusion of network characteristics in the optimization cycle: Aerodynamics, Propulsion and Weight Estimation. In addition, the network framework is introduced to the optimization cycle considering two more disciplines (takeoff/landing performance and mission analysis). Also, the air transport network, airport characteristics and correspondent route demands are provided as fixed parameters in the network framework. This eliminates the need for the development of the network optimizer turning the problem into a single level optimization type.

The MDO framework has two design cycles:

1. The aircraft framework, in which the disciplines related to the aircraft design are integrated (in this study aerodynamics, propulsion and weight estimation) providing the necessary input variables for the mission calculation (such as drag, thrust and weights) in each calculation cycle, based on fixed and design parameters. The reference aircraft adopted in design framework has the

geometric characteristics of a Regional Jet, equipped with high by pass turbo fan engines, low wings and capable to accommodate 78 passengers in a single class with 32" pitch between seats.

2. The Network Framework, in which the disciplines related to mission performance (in which the performance model is developed) and network calculations. A design diagram check is performed between both frameworks with the objective to verify that the current design is feasible considering some certification aspects, before proceeding the network framework calculations.

The airplane module was validated against a series of airplanes and, besides other crucial features, it can perform sizing of tail surfaces to comply with stability and control requirements [31]. The network cycle is only activated for a given airplane if it passes a series of constraints such as fuel storage, noise footprint, sufficient thrust at cruise condition, and others. Two objective functions are considered: network yield (YIELD) and network Direct Operational Cost (NDOC). A genetic algorithm was chosen as optimizer due to its robustness and ability in dealing with global minima or maxima in poor-known search space.

Airplanes are described by the following variables (some of them were kept fixed in the present optimization simulation) with respective boundaries:

1. Wing reference area [72 - 130 m^2]
2. Wing aspect ratio [7.5 - 10]
3. Wing taper ratio [0.25 - 0.50]
4. Wing quarter-chord sweepback angle [15 - 35°]
5. Incidence angle of the break station [0 - 1°]
6. Twist angle [from -5 to -1 degrees]
7. Location of break station – fraction of semispan [0.32 – 0.40]
8. Engine by-pass ratio [4.5 - 6.5]
9. Engine fan diameter [1.28 - 2 m]
10. Engine fan pressure ratio [1.2 - 1.8]
11. Engine overall pressure ratio (compressor + fan) [22 - 32]
12. Engine turbine inlet temperature [1350 – 1500 K]
13. Maximum range with typical passenger payload [1,600 nm for all airplanes]
14. Service ceiling [41,000 ft for all airplanes]
15. Maximum operational Mach number [0.82 for all airplanes]
16. Passenger seating at 32" pitch between two consecutive seats [70 -130]
17. Seat rows [4, 5]
18. Fuselage height-to-width ratio [1 - 1.15]
19. Number of aisles [1 for all airplanes]
20. Horizontal tail aspect ratio [4, 5]
21. Vertical tail aspect ratio [0.80 - 1.2]

22. Engine location (underwing configuration or at rear fuselage)

The MDO framework was elaborated by using the modeFrontier® integration platform [32]. Fig. (**7.3**) displays the workflow of the framework. Basically, there are two MATLAB® nodes where the airplane and network characteristics are calculated. Constraints adopted in this simulation are the following:

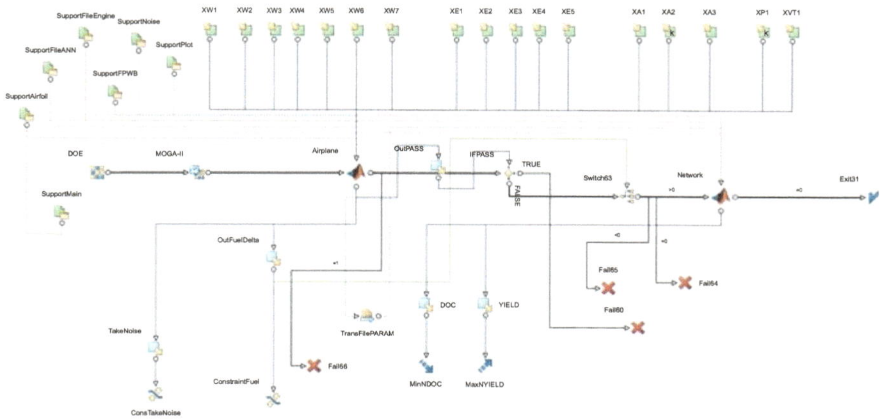

Fig. (7.3). MDO workflow elaborated with modeFrontier®.

1. Level of fly-over noise [12].
2. Fuel storage - all mission fuel must be accommodated in the wing fuel tanks.
3. Performance and certification requirements: rate of climb at initial cruise altitude, available thrust to power the airplane at desired service ceiling, climb in 2nd segment, missed approach, takeoff and landing field lengths, and others.
4. Airplane stall must begin in the inner wing.
5. Longitudinal flight quality level 3.
6. Divergence Mach number must be higher than MMO at given lift coefficient.
7. Static margin (this is an iterative process for tail sizing and wing positioning).
8. Critical angles and clearance boundaries for landing gear design.

Other parameters that were adopted in the present design simulations are shown in Table **7.2**.

Table 7.2. Some parameters adopted in the present design simulation.

Symbol	Parameters	Value
DISA	Isa Deviation [ºC]	10
RROC	Residual rate of Climb [ft/min]	300
BuffMGN	Buffet Margin (g)	1.3

(Table 7.2) contd.....

Symbol	Parameters	Value
ALTA	Altitude of cruise to alternate destination [ft]	25,000
Ct	Time Related Cost ($/min)	25
Cf	Fuel Related Cost ($/kg)	1
SPDLIM	Speed Limit Below 10,000 ft [KCAS]	250
ALTD	Alternate Airport distance [nm]	200
HOLDT	Holding time [min]	45
MAXFUEL	Maximum Fuel Capacity (kg)	9,400
Maxalt	Maximum Certified Altitude (ft)	41,000
MMO/VMO	Maximum Cruise Speed (Mach/CAS)	0.82/340
Range	Range with typical payload [nm]	1,600
TAKEOFL	Takeoff field length (TOW, ISA, sea level) [m]	2,000
LANDFL	Landing field length (MLW, ISA, sea level) [m]	1,500
PAXM	Passenger weight with luggage [kg]	100
AisleW	Aisle width [m]	0.50
SeatW	Seat width [m]	0.46
PCABH	Minimum Pax cabin height [m]	2 m
IR	Incidence at wing root (degree)	2°
MMO	Maximum operating Mach number	0.82

Reference Airplane

A reference airplane that was chosen for comparative purposes has its characteristics shown in Table **7.3** and Fig. (**7.4**) provides a picture of the configuration. The airliner presents a maximum range with 74 passengers of 1,600 nm cruising at 41,000 ft.

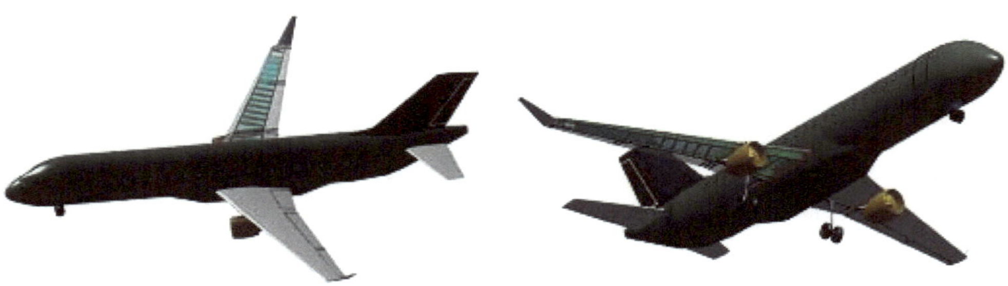

Fig. (7.4). Reference Aircraft (regional aircraft capable of accommodating 78 passengers in a single class).

Table 7.3. General view of the baseline airplane.

Pax (32" pitch)	**Seating abreast**	**Wing area [m²]**	**Wing Aspect ratio**	**Wing sweepback angle**	**Twist angle**
74	4	76	8.6	23.5 degrees	-3°
Engine Bypass ratio	**Engine overall pressure ratio**	**Turbine inlet temperature [K]**	**Maximum thrust @ takeoff (Single engine) [lbf]**	**MTOW [kg]**	**OEW [kg]**
5	28.5	1405	14,400	33,188	19,106
Fly-over noise [EPNdB]	**NDOC [US$/nm]**	**Network Yield [US$/nm pax]**	**Height of Pax cabin**	**Fuselage width [m]**	**Fuselage height [m]**
82.7	5.8265	0.00470	2 m	2.91	3.18

The wing reference airfoils were obtained with another optimization framework (Fig. **7.5**) where a mixed strategy encompassing inverse design with a full potential code was employed [33]. Only the break and tip airfoils were optimized, the 13.5%-thick root airfoil was kept unchanged during the optimization process. Other wing parameters were also employed as optimization variables. This framework was developed with modeFrontier® and made use of the same ANN surrogate modeling for the aerodynamic coefficient calculation that was employed in the present work [30]. The aerodynamic calculation with ANNs is considerably fast and eased the computation of the divergence Mach number at several lift coefficients, a way to guarantee excellent off-design characteristics.

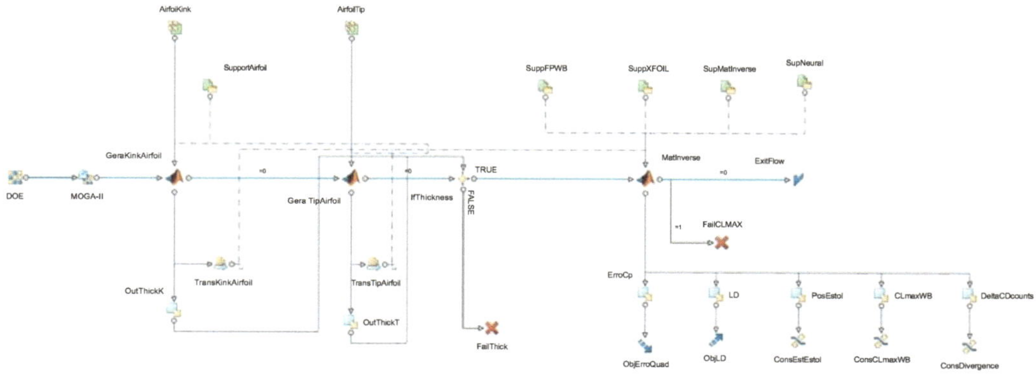

Fig. (7.5). Aerodynamic framework for the wing design involving airfoil design.

Fig. (**7.6**) shows the outstanding aerodynamic characteristics of the optimized airplane configuration. Lift coefficient and the Mach number plus the aerodynamic efficiency are displayed there for Mach numbers ranging from 0.62 to 0.85 (the top speed for which the ANNs were trained). An important consideration about the *ML/D* variation is its "flat" behavior against a broad range of Mach numbers. This is a highly desirable characteristic because it allows the airline to operate the airplane without performance degradation for distinct flight profiles, encompassing many weights and cruise altitude. Fig. (**7.7**) contains some pressure coefficient distributions for stations along the wing semispan. This was the design point and the *Cp* distribution strongly resembles an isentropic recompression. To assure a good off-design behavior as seen in Fig. (**7.6**), the drag coefficient increase from a subsonic condition was constrained for some lift coefficients.

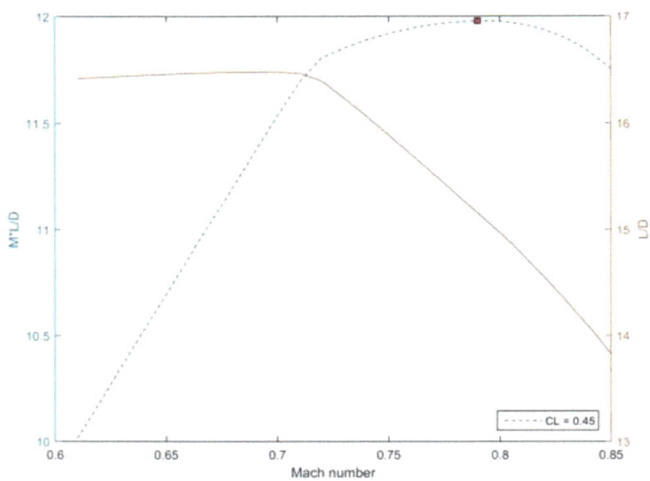

Fig. (7.6). *ML/D* and *L/D* for the reference airplane.

Network Fixed Parameters

The proposed air transport network for a hypothetic regional airline consists of 5 airports interconnected by 16 routes (Fig. **7.8**). There is one hub, assumed to be São Paulo International Airport/Guarulhos (SBGR), from where all the aircraft are originally stocked. It is assumed that the airline has a 10% market share and transport passengers only. Actual airway distances, extracted from the Brazilian High Altitude Enroute Charts (ERC) [34], are considered for the route connections between main airports, assuming direct routing from the most used departure runway to the first enroute waypoint and the most used arrival runway to the last enroute waypoint. Table **7.4** shows the considered route connections and respective route distances. The airport data used in the mission analysis computations, extracted from the Brazilian Aeronautical Information Publication (AIP) [27], are: airport coordinates (Latitude, Longitude), average field elevation, reference temperature (average temperature of the highest temperatures of the hottest month of the year) and the most likely used runway length data (Takeoff Run Available, Landing Distance Available). Table **7.5** shows the airport data. Average delays on each airport are considered by the model proposed by Newell [35] as function of runway configuration and capacity: for departure delays, which occur on ground, 10 minutes for airports with two or more active runways (for SBGR, SBGL and SBBR) and 5 minutes for airports with 1 active runway (for SBPA and SBSV). For arrival delays, associated with terminal holdings and enroute speed reductions, are assumed to be 5 minutes on airports with two or more active runways and 3 minutes for airports with one active runway. Route passenger demand per day and route average load factors are listed in Table **7.6**. Airline operational parameters assumed in this study are listed in Table **7.7**.

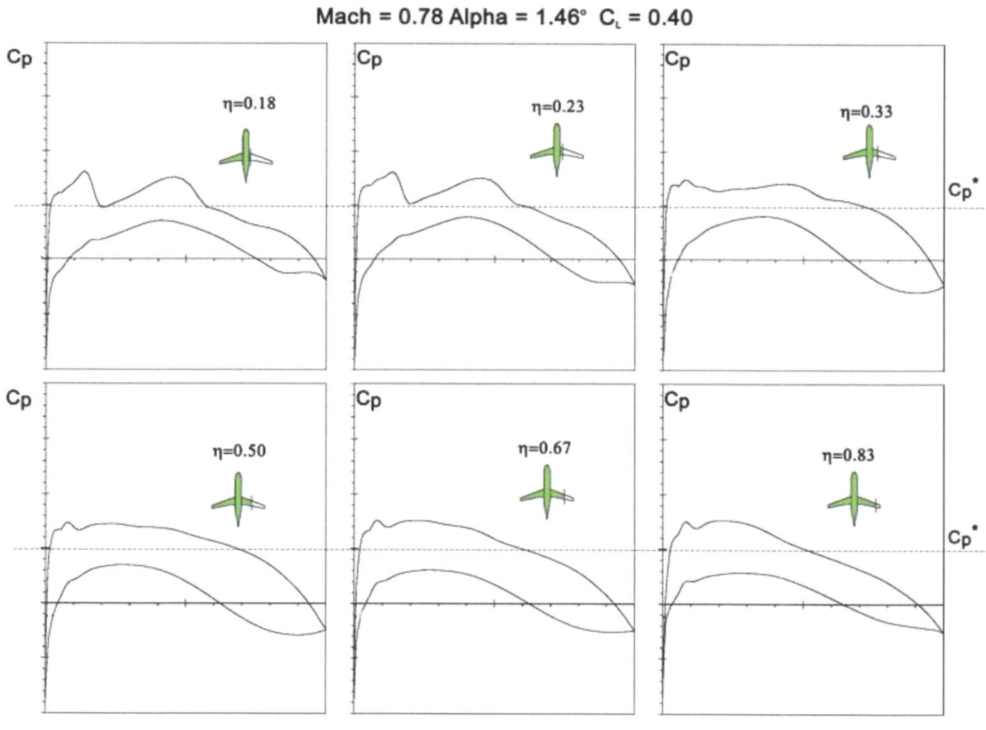

Fig. (7.7). Pressure distributions for the reference airplane at Mach number of 0.78 and lift coefficient of 0.40. Obtained with a full potential code with viscous and non-isentropic corrections.

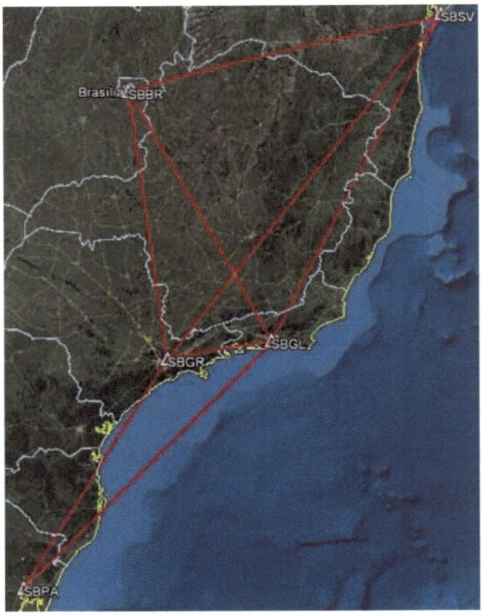

Fig. (7.8). Air Transport Network.

Table 7.4. Network Route Distances -Dij (nm).

Departure Airport (i)	Arrival Airport (j)				
	SBGR	SBGL	SBBR	SBPA	SBSV
SBGR	-	182	481	481	788
SBGL	182	-	507	640	595
SBBR	471	507	-	-	590
SBPA	481	614	-	-	-
SBSV	796	661	598	-	-

Table 7.5. Network Route Distances -Dij (nm).

Airport	(SBGR) São Paulo Intl/Guarulhos	(SBGL) Rio de Janeiro Intl/Galeão	(SBBR) Brasilia International	(SBPA) Porto Alegre	(SBSV) Salvador
Coordinates (Lat/Lon)	S23.432075/ W046.46951	S22.808903/ W043.243647	S15.863500/ W047.927583	S29.994428/ W047.927583	12.910994/ 38.331044
Elevation	2459ft	38ft	3497ft	15ft	64ft
Ref Temp	30°C	33°C	27°C	26°C	33°C
Magnetic Declination	20W	21W	20W	15W	23W

Table 7.6. Route Passenger Demand per Day and (Average Load factor).

Departure Airport (i)	Arrival Airport (j)				
	SBGR	**SBGL**	**SBBR**	**SBPA**	**SBSV**
SBGR	-	3547 (0.85)	1011 (0.80)	987 (0.80)	2007 (0.85)
SBGL	3500 (0.70)	-	999 (0.85)	4990 (0.80)	2997 (0.80)
SBBR	1000 (0.80)	1490 (0.80)	-	-	1540 (0.70)
SBPA	3020 (0.85)	1990 (0.80)	-	-	-
SBSV	3000 (0.90)	2010 (0.80)	2040 (0.75)	-	-

Table 7.7. Operation parameters of airlines.

#	Symbol	Parameters	Value
1	DU	Average Daily Aircraft Utilization	12
2	TA	Average Turn Around Time	30
3	TOFA	Takeoff and Initial Climb out Fuel allowance (kg)	200
4	TOTA	Takeoff and Initial Climb out Time allowance (min)	3
5	AFA	Approach and Landing Fuel allowance (kg)	100
6	ATA	Approach and Landing Time allowance (min)	2
7	GAFA	Go Around Fuel allowance (kg)	200
8	GATA	Go Around Time allowance (min)	3
9	TOT	Average Taxi Out Time (from gate to runway threshold)	10
10	TIT	Average Taxi In Time (from runway exit to gate)	5
11	PAXWT	Total Passenger Weight (85kg+25kg baggage)	110
12	ATP	Average Ticket Price (US$)	250
13	ID	Average Inflight Delay Cost (US$/min)*	30
14	Cf	Fuel Cost (US$/kg)	1.00
15	K1	Total Operational Costs/Direct Operational Costs ratio	1.3
16	K2	Total Revenue/ Ticket Revenue ratio	1.1
16	CaptSAL	Average Captain Annual Salary (US$)	100,000
17	FOSal	Average First Officer Annual Salary (US$)	85,000
18	FASal	Average Flight Attendant Annual Salary (US$)	65,000

Propulsion

Aircraft manufacturers select the type of powerplant based on several factors, but the cruising speed is one the relevant conditions which must be considered. As the design speed reaches 450 miles per hour turbojet and turbofan engines become a suitable propulsion solution. The turbofan utilizes a fan and larger air intakes to process much more air in comparison with standard turbojet engines. As a result, the turbofan operates at slower velocity and reduced temperature reaching higher thrust with less noise [36].

At the present study, the propulsion module was implemented in MATLAB® and it is based on the thermodynamic model proposed by Benson [37], developed for turbojet and turbofan engines. It is adapted from open source code developed by NASA Glenn Research Center [38]. The output parameters from the computation are fuel flow (fuel consumption in kg per hour) and net thrust for given altitude, Mach number, ISA deviation, Compressor Pressure Ratio, Fan Pressure Ratio, Fan Diameter, Turbine Inlet Temperature and throttle position (Fig. **7.9**). The classical one-dimensional thermodynamics modeling is the basis of the calculation procedure embedded in the code. The engine model is build up in two steps: the design step is where all engine characteristics are raised at a given design point (a cruise condition with 98% throttle setting) and an analysis module, where it is possible to calculate the engine thrust and fuel flow rate from the geometric characteristics obtained in the design step. Engine weight was calculated using the own methodology using data from Jane's Aero-Engines [39]. Calculated engine parameters are used in the noise module, with the noise signature being determinated at the three ICAO reference locations: fly-over, sideline, and approach. Other parameters are employed in the emission module.

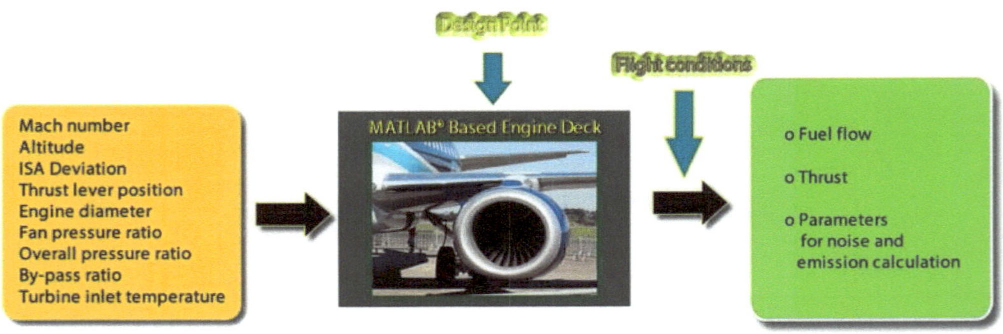

Fig. (7.9). EngineSim Model.

To verify the methodology that was implemented for the engine deck, the graph in Fig. (**7.10**) displays the thrust ratio number against Mach number. Fig. (**7.10**) also shows typical trends of thrust *vs*. speed for turbojets and turbofans with varying bypass ratio at sea level and all curves are in very good agreement with the literature [40].

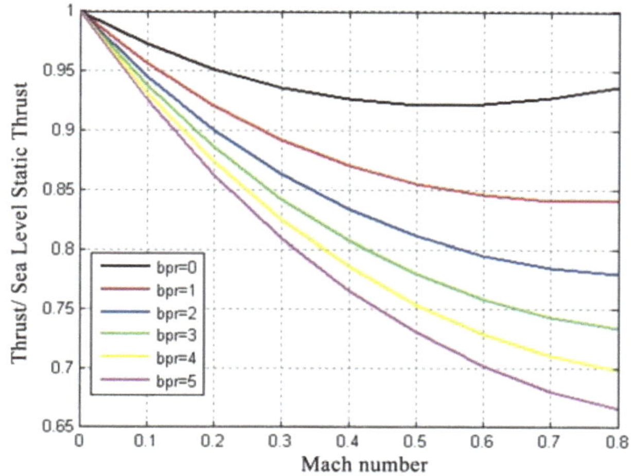

Fig. (7.10). Left: Thrust ratio *vs*. Mach number for several by-pass ratios values. Right: – Typical trend of thrust *vs*. speed for turbojets and turbofans with varying bypass ratio at sea level.

An updated version containing compressor efficiency obtained from a compressor map modeled with radial basis function from MATLAB® has been recently implemented in the airplane calculator but was not employed in the present design simulations.

Aerodynamics

Aerodynamic analysis in the aircraft conceptual design phase is usually carried out with numeric tools and wind-tunnel testing. The complexity of fluid flow is well demonstrated in many scientific papers and experiments. Most phenomena of fluid flow, such as shock waves and flow separation, are essentially nonlinear in nature and the variety of turbulence scales in the flow pattern is huge. Nowadays, computational fluid dynamics (CFD) is widely employed as a key tool for aircraft design (Fig. **7.11**). Reynolds Average Navier-Stokes (RANS) solutions are a common tool, as well as Euler and full potential formulations. Fig. (**7.12**) shows a hierarchy of several simplifications of the Navier-Stokes equations.

The length scale of the smallest persisting eddies in a turbulent flow can be estimated as of order of $1/Re^{3/4}$ in comparison with the macroscopic length scale. The solution of such scales for a complex aircraft configuration is still prohibitive. For this reason, simplified formulations are used in the aircraft industry. A computational grid with million cells are usually required for an external flow solution over a completed airplane configuration employing the RANS formulation.

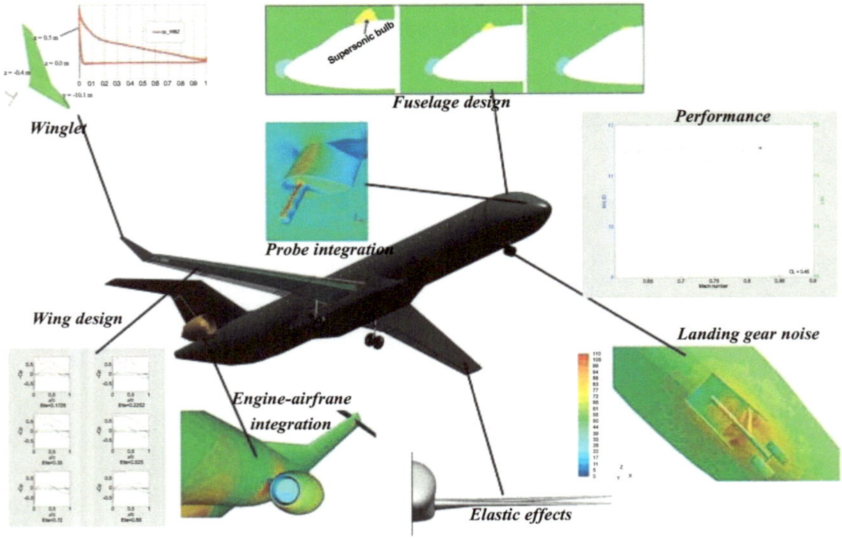

Fig. (7.11). Some CFD applications in aircraft design.

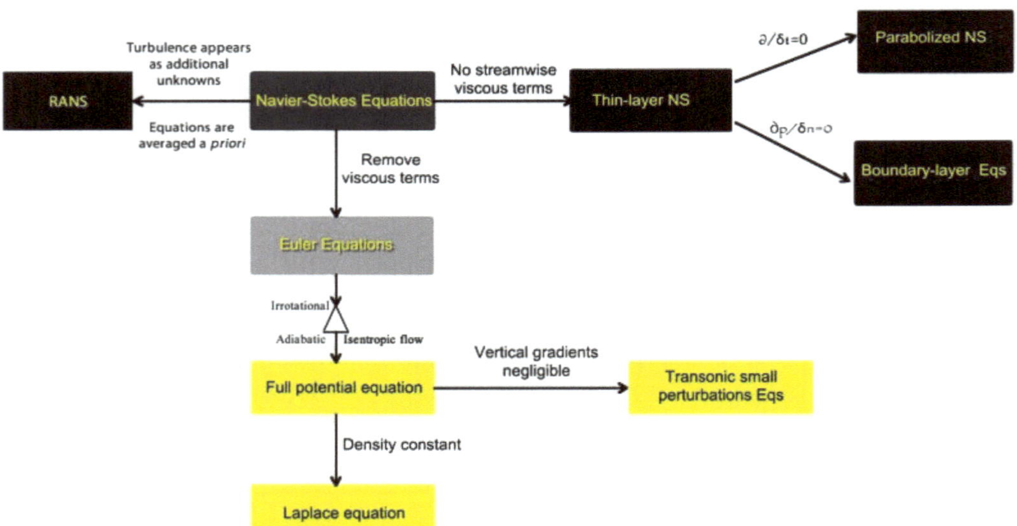

Fig. (7.12). Formulations for numerical flow analysis.

A viable alternative for MDO computations is the utilization of full potential codes with viscous corrections. Their cost benefit makes this formulation very attractive for higher fidelity aerodynamic computations in a MDO process, which requires extensive calls of the flow analysis codes for performance, load, and stability calculations. However, the extreme sensitive nature of transonic flow regarding airplane geometry, in which variations in the order of boundary-layer thickness or lower lead to significant changes in pressure distribution, makes mandatory that integral boundary-layer routines to be coupled with the transonic potential codes. Besides delivering satisfactory profile drag values, the viscous coupled calculation shall also be able to handle shock-boundary layer interaction.

A comparison between a RANS code and a full-potential one [33] was carried-out for a twinjet airliner with rear-mounted engines (Fig. **7.13**). The RANS simulation employed the SST k-ω turbulence model and the hexhedral mesh that was created for the simulation was composed of approximately 2.1 million cells [41]. Making use of an implicit scheme for time marching, the convergence was reached after all residuals dropped to values below $1x10^{-4}$, which consumed 5675 iterations. Each iteration demanded in average 84 secs on a desktop computer fitted with an Intel® Core™ i7-3820 processor. The full potential solution for the wing-fuselage combination took 25 secs to converge on the same machine. Fig. (**7.14**) shows a comparison between the results from the RANS and the full potential codes. There, Cp distributions for two wing stations of the airliner of Fig. (**7.13**) are shown. The agreement between the related Cp distributions is very good.

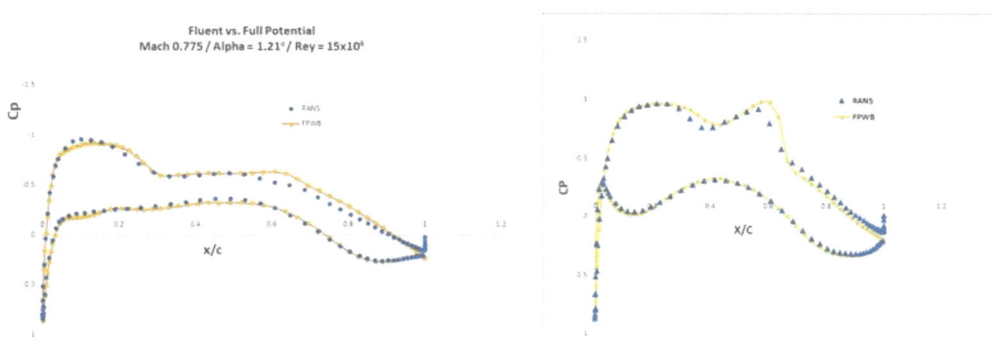

Fig. (7.13). Streamlines leaving the wing for the ITA50ADV airliner (Mach = 0.775, α=1.21°, Re=15x10^{6}).

The module that was developed in MATLAB® language is based on the model proposed by Secco and Mattos [30] to determine wing-body aerodynamic coefficients by an artificial neural network methodology. The output parameters from the computation are parasite drag (C_{D0}), wave drag (C_{Dw}), induced drag (C_{Di}) and lift coefficient (C_L). Besides airfoil parameters, flight condition and wing geometric parameters are required. Wing parameters are the typical ones such as aspect ratio, sweepback angle, taper ratio, incidence of definition stations, dihedral angles of inboard and outboard wing, fraction of wingspan where the break station is located (Fig. **7.15**). In this study, the airfoils used were results of previous aerodynamic optimization as explained in a preceding section, where a database of 14 airfoils was used to linearly obtain a profile geometry.

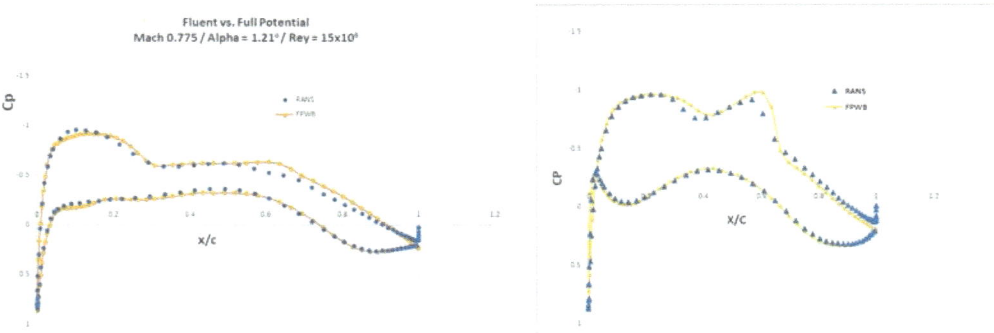

Fig. (7.14). Cp distributions obtained with a RANS code and a full potential one for the ITA50ADV airliner. At left, station a 22% of semispan; right, station located at 50% of semispan (Mach = 0.775, α=1.21°, Re=15x10^6).

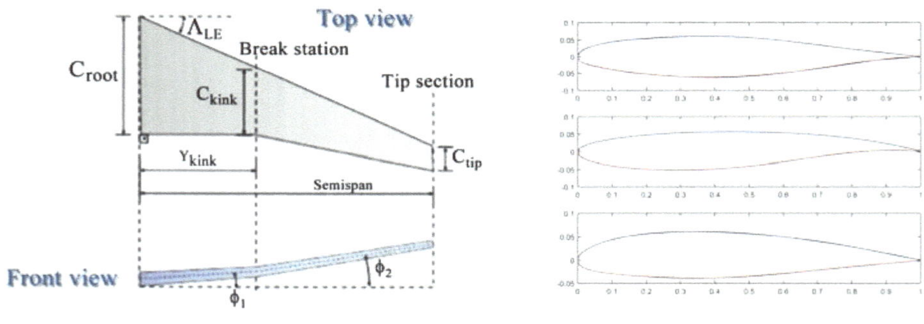

Fig. (7.15). *Left* - Wing Geometric Parameters. *Right* - root, kink and tip airfoils (not in same scale).

A multi-layer neuron network type was used for the aerodynamic surrogate model, consisting of three layers on feed forward configuration (50-50-1), hyperbolic transfer function and back propagation algorithm. The ANN was trained with 110,000 different wing geometry airfoil configurations with wing reference areas ranging from 50 to 200 m^2. A full potential aerodynamic code coupled with an integral boundary-layer module was employed for the aerodynamic coefficient calculations that provided data for the ANN training. A verification of the accuracy and capability of the ANN prediction of the drag divergence is shown here. For this purpose, two airplane configurations that were not used in the training phase were selected and their drag variation with the

Mach number can be seen in Fig. (**7.16**). Although the database contains not so many examples at Mach number above 0.80, Fig. (**7.16**) shows that the delay of the drag divergence with the increase of the wing sweep angle was correctly captured by the drag-predictor ANN.

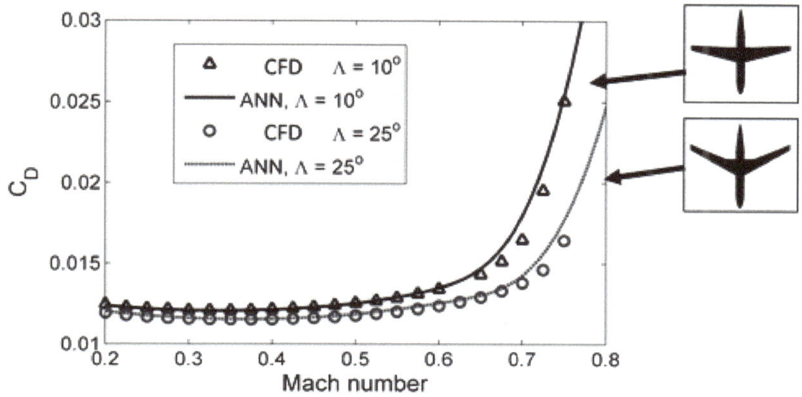

Fig. (7.16). Comparison between ANN overall drag predictions and CFD results for two airplanes with different wing sweepback angles. Altitude=10.5 km, $\alpha = 1°$.

In addition, an airliner with 93.5 m^2 wing reference area was chosen also to evaluate the accuracy of the designed ANNs in predicting drag and lift coefficient. Planform characteristics and flight condition information are given in Table **7.8**; three-view of the airplane are shown in Fig. (**7.17**).

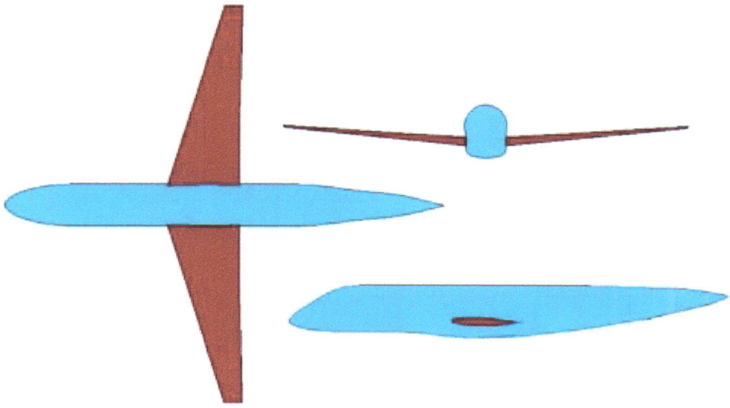

Fig. (7.17). Three-view of the airliner considered for test case.

Table 7.8. Data for test case with an airliner at cruise condition.

Parameter	Value
Incidence angle at root station	2°
Incidence angle at break station	0°
Incidence angle at tip station	-2°
Wing reference area	93.5 m^2
Wing aspect ratio	8.43
Wing taper ratio	0.235
Quarter-chord wing sweepback angle	17.5°
Mach number	0.77
Angle of attack	1°
Cruise altitude	10,500 m
Location of break station (fraction of semispan)	0.39

The coordinates of the three basic airfoils used in the wing definition of the airplane under consideration were read from files. The root, break, and tip station airfoils present a maximum relative thickness of 12.3, 12.3. and 10.9%, respectively. There is then a need for an optimization problem to fit Sobiesczky polynomials to these geometries. This was carried out with the *fsolve* optimization tool from MATLAB® [42 - 44]. Fig. (**7.18**) shows the original airfoil geometry and those approximated using Sobiesczky polynomials. Some small discrepancies exist between the original and calculated geometry of the tip airfoil.

Table **7.9** contains a comparison between the ANN and CFD results. The overall drag differs by one drag count only. The wave drag coefficient recorded the highest difference between the neural network and the full potential code, which was of three drag counts. The ANN drag estimation provided average error of 3 drag counts when compared with the full potential code results.

At the flight condition shown in Table **7.9**, the streamlines on the wing upper side as calculated by the full potential code indicates attached flow close to the fuselage and at the wingtip. However, there is a large separation region close to the trailing edge along a great portion of semispan, caused by shock waves. It is observed that in some wing parts the flow experiences a reattachment and suffers another separation. This is indeed a complex flow pattern, which was well captured by the ANN prediction. This example is an excellent boost for the ANNs designed in the present work. Despite the complexity of the airflow at the cruise condition over the test case airliner, ANNs could predict the drag coefficients.

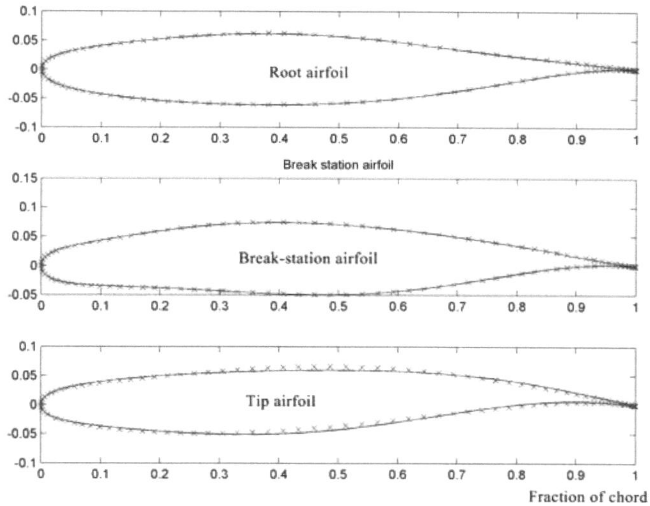

Fig. (7.18). Three-view of the test case to validate ANN prediction accuracy.

Table 7.9. Predicted and calculated coefficient values by ANN and full potential code, respectively. Drag coefficients given in counts.

Predicted Coefficient	ANN	Full Potential Code
C_{D0}	65	66
$C_{D\,ind}$	55	56
$C_{D\,wave}$	69	66
C_D	189	188
C_L	0.367	0.382

High-lift performance has an enormous impact on sizing, economics and safety of any airplane [45]. Navier-Stokes analysis are very timing consuming due to the complex nature of the flow in combination with complex geometries.

Several analytical methods that both account for stall effects and enable the prediction of the maximum lift coefficient were discussed and a trade-off between the methods was conducted in Ref [46]. From this trade-off, it was found that both the pressure difference rule and the so-called Critical Section are good option in terms of accuracy and versatility.

The Critical Section Method was incorporated XFOIL panel code [47] for determining an airfoil's maximum lift coefficient with a wing-fuselage full potential code with viscous corrections [34]. Within this method, stall is reached when the lift coefficient distribution along the semispan, obtained from the full potential code, locally equal the wing section's maximum lift coefficient. The pressure difference rule on the other hand, determines wing stall by implementing an empirical chordwise pressure difference criterion. Thus, wing stall is established when the wing section's chordwise pressure difference, at an angle of attack, equals to the critical pressure difference which is empirically derived and depends on both the Mach- and Reynolds number.

Singh [46] validated both the pressure difference rule and critical section method against wind-tunnel experiments, both for wing only samples and wing + fuselage models. The approximation of clean maximum lift coefficient showed to be in good agreement, about 3% error, a very good figure. A MATLAB® code was elaborated for automatically run XFOIL (Fig. **7.19**) until airfoil is reached for some sections on the wing at the local Reynolds number (Fig. **7.20**).

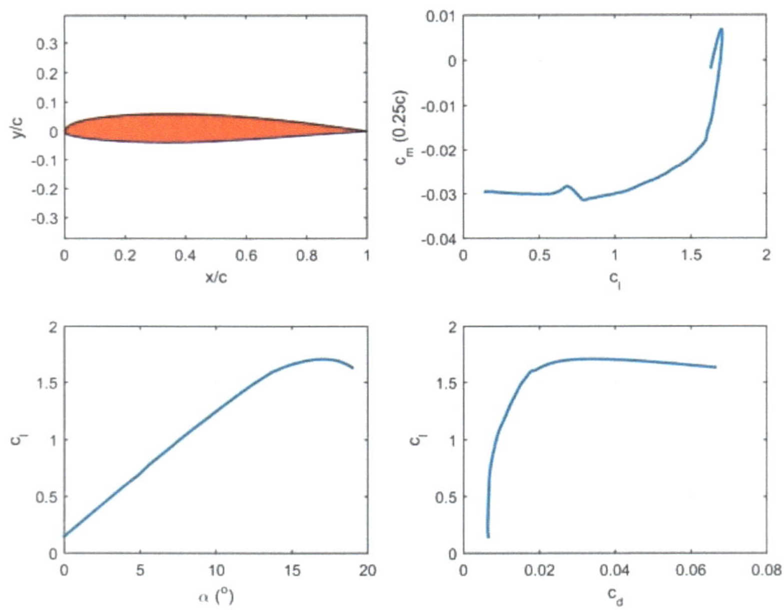

Fig. (7.19). A MATLAB® code automatically runs XFOIL a desired condition for a wing section and outputs the maximum lift coefficient and other aerodynamic characteristics.

Weight Estimation

In this calculation weight of pylons, fuselage, empennage, systems, landing gear and engines are calculated separately using Class II methodology. The wing weight is calculated by sizing the wingbox to withstand loads calculated with a full potential code in some few maneuvers in the flight envelope; the secondary structure being estimated by empirical methods. All these weights are considered for the determination of the Operational Empty Weight (OEW). With the weight of each component, it is also possible to obtain the center of gravity (CG) of the aircraft and its variation with fuel consumption and different payloads. The Maximum Takeoff Weight (MTOW) and Maximum Landing Weight (MLW) are estimated interactively using the mission analysis module and the calculated OEW assuming a design range of 2000 nm.

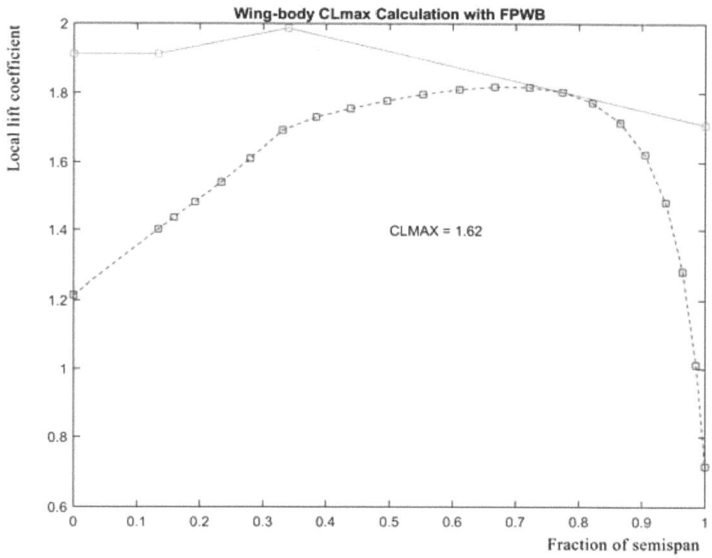

Fig. (7.20). The critical section method is employed for $C_{L_{max}}$ estimation.

Cabin Cross Section

A MATLAB® code was developed to design the cross section of the passenger cabin (Fig. **7.21**). A considerable sort of cargo containers can be incorporated into the configuration. The code has input such as seat width, aisle width, cabin height and other considered important to the fuselage sizing.

Design Diagram Verification

Before the Mission Performance module is activated, the airplane under consideration is checked concerning five operational performance requirements. This module was developed with MATLAB® and a geometrical CAD representation is created and wetted areas and other geometric parameters are calculated. A plot encompassing Thrust over Weight ratio (T/W) and wing loading is elaborated and the airplane characteristics are inserted into it.

The following conditions are verified (Fig. **7.22**):

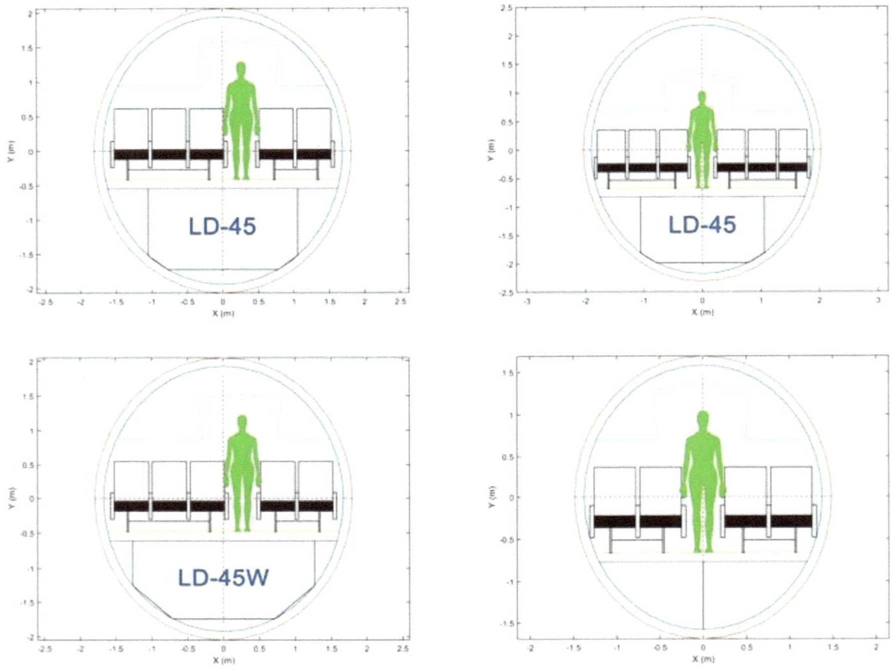

Fig. (7.21). Module for sizing of the fuselage cross section.

1. Takeoff field length of 1,450 m at Maximum Takeoff Weight (sea level, standard atmosphere).
2. Second segment climb gradient 2.4% with one engine inoperative (FAR 25.111 [35] requirements).
3. Missed approach conditions (FAR 25.121 [35] approach climb and FAR 25.119 [35] landing climb requirements).
4. Cruise at Maximum Operational Mach Number (MMO).
5. Residual rate of climb of 300 ft/min at maximum certified ceiling.
6. Landing at Maximum Landing Weight (sea level, standard atmosphere and landing field length of 1500 m).

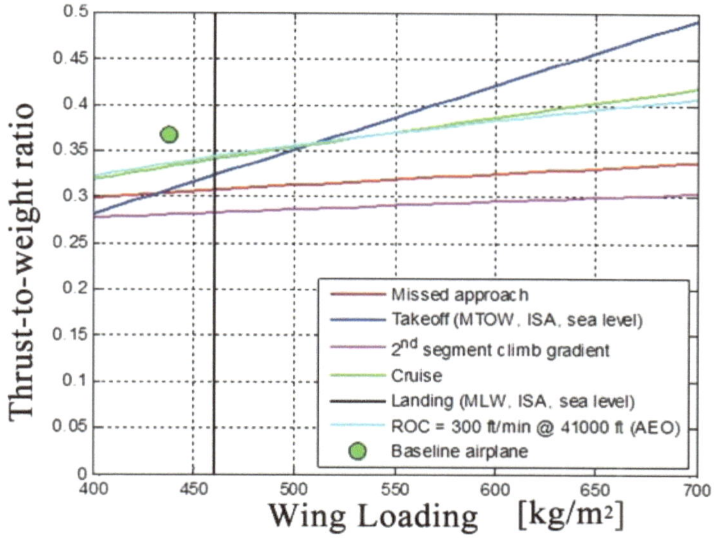

Fig. (7.22). Design Diagram Check.

If the actual T/W does not satisfy any of these conditions the related aircraft design is not considered in the optimization and the calculation does not proceed.

Tail Sizing

Most MDO frameworks still make use of the tail volume coefficients method for the sizing of horizontal and vertical tailplanes. Tail volume coefficient method is based on historical aircraft data and it does not consider configuration particularities like wing sweepback angle and tail topology. A methodology based on static stability and controllability criteria was then elaborated and integrated into a MATLAB® application conceived for airplane design. Immediate advantages with the present methodology are the design of realistic tail surfaces and properly sized airplanes.

The present calculation of the HT and VT areas by a higher fidelity method than that offered by the tail volume approach considers static stability and controllability criteria. The VT area is obtained by taking the larger area from that calculated employing both criteria, while the HT area is obtained with integration of the two criteria (Fig. **7.23**). The permissible areas of emphasis are now located between the straight lines from the controllability and the stability requirement minus the degree of stability. The necessary center of gravity range of 0.22 MAC (for this example) can now be fitted between these lines, resulting in the ratio between the HT and wing reference areas.

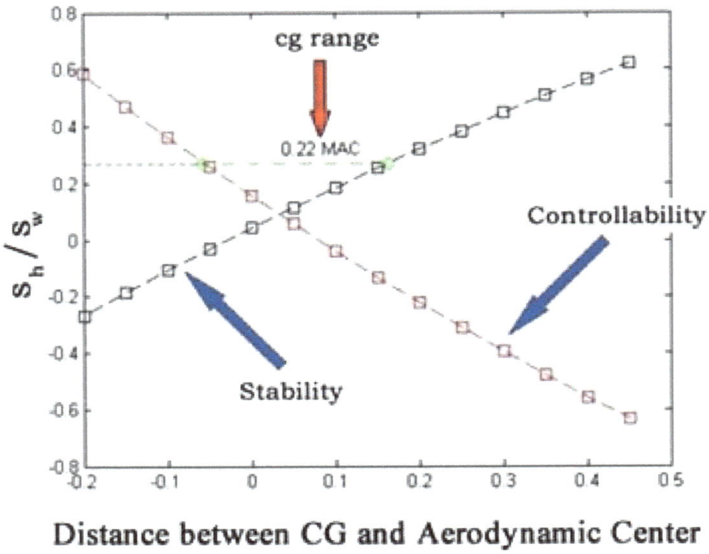

Fig. (7.23). HT sizing methodology.

Engine failure at takeoff poses a critical condition for the VT design. In this case, the remaining engine (or engines) must provide enough thrust to maintain the required rate of climb with the additional drag caused by rudder and aileron deflections. Trim drag due to rudder deflection and to a lesser extent aileron deflection may be critical in meeting FAR.121 climb requirements for the second segment, especially for twin-engine airplanes.

Considering that takeoff is a critical condition for the design of tailplanes some relevant aspects of this flight phase are described here. Fig. (**7.24**) illustrates the takeoff segments for airplanes. V_1 is the takeoff decision speed, V_R the rotation speed, V_{Lof} velocity of liftoff, and V_2 is the flight speed over a hypothetical 35-ft obstacle. During the initial phase of the takeoff path, the airplane must be accelerated on the ground to V_{EF}, at which point the critical engine must be made inoperative and remain inoperative for the rest of the takeoff. V_1 means the maximum speed in the takeoff at which the pilot must take the first action (*e.g.*, apply brakes, reduce thrust, deploy speed brakes) to stop the airplane within the accelerate-stop distance. V_1 also means the minimum speed in the takeoff, following a failure of the critical engine at V_{EF}, at which the pilot can continue the takeoff and achieve the required height above the takeoff surface within the takeoff distance. According to FAR 25.149 V_{mca} is the calibrated airspeed at which

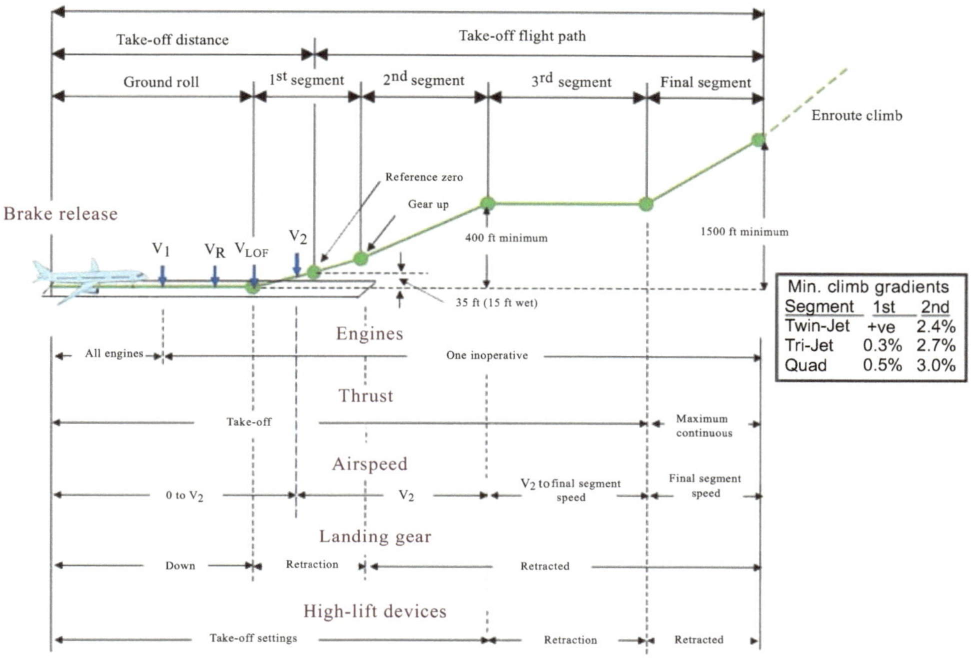

Fig. (7.24). Illustration of take-off segments and required FAR climb requirements.

- Critical engine suddenly becomes inoperative
- Control of the airplane is possible to maintain
- Maintain straight flight
- Bank angle shall be lower than 5°
- V_{mca} may not exceed $1.2xV_s$

The conditions for determination of for V_{mca} are:

- Maximum takeoff thrust on remaining engines
- Most unfavorable cg (usually aft cg, where the tail moment arm is the shortest)
- Aircraft trimmed for takeoff (takeoff flap setting)
- Maximum TOGW
- Most critical takeoff configuration existing along the flight path, except for landing gear retracted.

V_{mca} is used in determining the minimum V_R and V_2. The V_2 must also be chosen to satisfy the second segment climb requirement. V_{mca} must be obviously lower than the V_2 and considering its importance for aircraft performance and safety operation it was calculated after the tail surfaces were obtained.

Stability derivatives that are needed for the calculation of HT and VT areas were obtained with the AVL code from MIT (Fig. **7.25**). Initial estimated values are required to start iterative processes for the HT and VT calculation. This MATLAB® tool is used to find out the areas because they are dependent of several parameters and variables such as wing location along the fuselage.

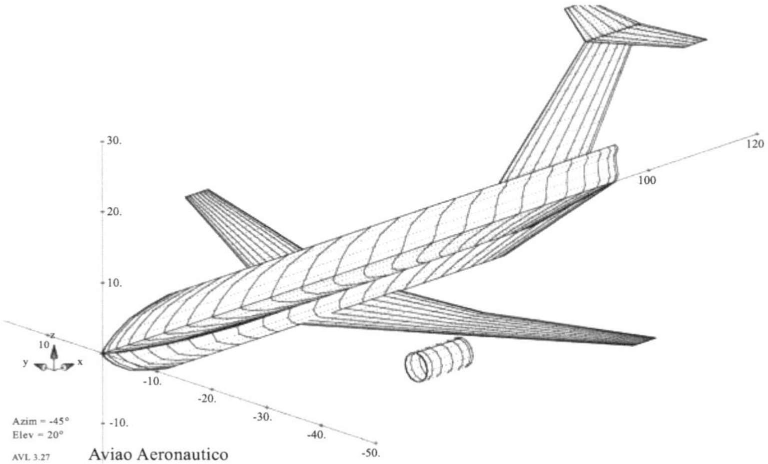

Fig. (7.25). Example of AVL model for the calculation of stability derivatives.

The incorporation of a more sophisticated methodology for the tailplane sizing poses a more complex task in the interactive process for MTOW calculation. The determination of the cg location is needed not only for the tailplane area calculation, but for the positioning of the wing, and the main and nose landing gears, which are also dependent on the overall cg location. CG location will guide the wing placement in the configuration. Fig. (**7.26**) shows an iterative process involving the sizing of the tailplanes. Ref [32] provides more details about the methodology adopted for the HT and VT sizing.

Mission Performance

This module was implemented in MATLAB® language embedding the aircraft performance calculations necessary to determine trip fuel (W_f) and time (T) for each sector, afterwards used to compute the Network DOC and Yield. Inputs from the aerodynamics (C_D, C_L) and propulsion (net thrust and fuel flow) modules are necessary for the application of mass point equations to determine delta fuel and time at integration steps, at a given performance state (weight and environmental conditions at altitude) and operational flight profile. Environmental conditions (pressure, density and temperature) at each integration point, as function of pressure altitude, are calculated as per the International Standard Atmosphere isentropic model [36]. Zero wind, standard atmospheric pressure and 10°C ISA deviation from standard temperature are assumed in this study.

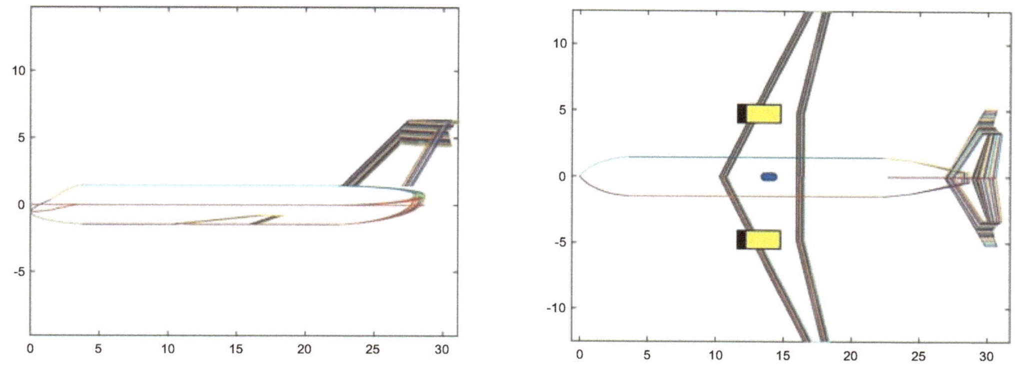

Fig. (7.26). The sizing of HT and VT are carried out interactively due to cg variation that leads to repositioning the wing.

Along the flight path the longitudinal and vertical equations of motion are numerically integrated considering steady states segments in climb, cruise and descent according to **Eqs. 1** and **2**:

$$T - D = W.\sin(\gamma) + \frac{W}{g}.\frac{dV}{dt} \tag{7.1}$$

$$L + \frac{W}{g}\frac{d\gamma}{dt} = W.\cos(\gamma) \tag{7.2}$$

The operational flight profile is shown in Fig. (**7.27**) and defined as follows:

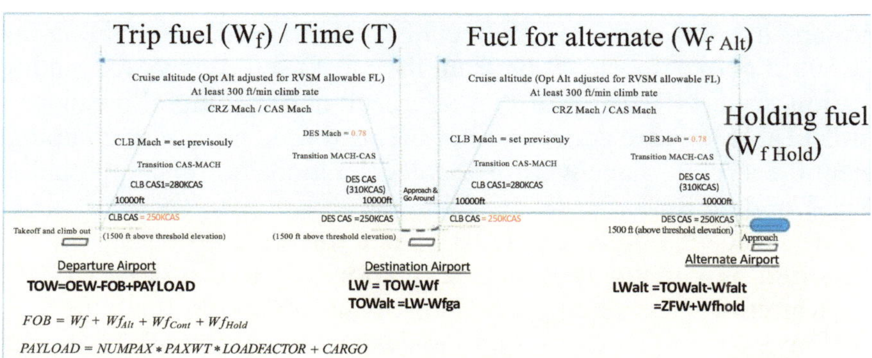

Fig. (7.27). Mission Profile.

1. The trajectory computation starts at a pressure altitude of 1500 ft above the elevation of the most used runway for takeoff. Because of that a takeoff and initial climb out allowances for fuel and time (Table **7.7**) are added to total fuel and time trajectory computations to represent the aircraft maneuvering and accelerations from takeoff run, lift off and initial climb out.
2. From the point at 1500ft, the aircraft climbs maintaining 250kt calibrated airspeed (CAS) until 10000ft (respecting Air Traffic Control speed restriction for Airspace Classes A, B, C and D under Instrument Flight Rules as per air traffic regulations [37]), where then accelerates to 280kt CAS and maintain this speed until the Mach-Crossover Altitude or Cruise Altitude is reached, whichever is lower. The Mach-Cross Over Altitude is the true altitude where the current Mach Number reaches the proposed Cruise Mach Number, defined as 0.78 for this study.
3. The cruise altitude is determined as the Optimum Altitude adjusted to the suitable flight level as per the Reduced Vertical Separation Minima (RVSM) air traffic rules [38], based on the average magnetic course between origin and destination airports (computed using Vincenty's direct solutions for geodesics on WGS84 ellipsoids [39] based on coordinates of origin and destination airports and respective magnetic declinations). Optimum Altitude is calculated as the minimum of: maximum certified ceiling, maximum specific range altitude (for the considered takeoff weight and environmental conditions), maximum altitude where 1.3g buffet margin (stall at 40° bank angle in clean configuration, given by Equations **3**, **4** and **5**) is obtained and maximum altitude where the residual rate of climb is 300ft/min.
4. The cruise phase is computed with constant Mach number, selected as 0.78.
5. The descent phase is performed with constant Mach Number until the CAS-Crossover altitude, defined as the true altitude where the calibrated airspeed reaches the selected constant calibrated airspeed, herein defined as 310 kt. After this altitude, constant CAS (310 kt) is maintained until 10,000 ft where the airplane in decelerated to 250 kt calibrated airspeed, maintaining this speed until 1,500 ft above the elevation from the most used runway for landing at the destination airport. Because of that approach and landing allowances for fuel and time (Table **7.7**) are added to total fuel and time trajectory computations to represent the aircraft maneuvering and decelerations on final approach to touch down and landing run.
6. The total fuel loaded on board (FOB) is determined considering the minimum fuel required as per the Brazilian regulations (RBAC 121.645 [40]) for jet transport aircraft, representing the sum of the following quantities:
   a. Fuel necessary to fly from origin to destination airport (W_f) considering the operational profile described on items (1) to (4);
   b. Fuel necessary to fly from destination to alternate (or diversion) airport

considering the operational profile described on items (1) to (4). In this study, the alternate airport is chosen as the closest airport from the destination airport in the network, considering that all airports in the company network have the capacity available and handling infrastructure to absorb the demand ($W_{fAlternate}$);

c. Fuel burn related to 10% the trip time determined in (1) to be used as contingency for route deviations and adverse weather conditions ($W_{fContingency}$);

d. Consideration of 30 minutes of holding at 1500ft height over the alternate airport elevation at suitable holding speed. In this study, the holding speed is selected with as the maximum L/D speed or 1.3 g margin to stall speed (ensuring a protection of 44° maximum bank angle to stall) in clean configuration, whichever is higher, considering weight estimated at the alternate airport.

$$\delta = \frac{2}{CLmax} \cdot \left(\frac{W}{S}\right) \cdot \frac{1}{a_0{}^2 . M^2} \cdot \frac{1}{\cos(\varphi)} \quad \textbf{(7.3)}$$

Below Tropopause upper limit ($\delta \geq 0.2234$):

$$Hmax_{Buffet} = 44330{,}7673(1 - \delta^{0{,}190263}) \quad \textbf{(7.4)}$$

Above Tropopause upper limit ($\delta < 0.2234$):

$$Hmax_{Buffet} = 11000 + 153{,}8462 . DISA - 6341{,}58 . \ln(4{,}47706 . \delta) \quad \textbf{(7.5)}$$

Considering the statements above the following equations are used in the mission performance calculation algorithm with the objective to determine trip fuel (W_f):

$$TOW = OEW + FOB + PAYLOAD \quad \textbf{(7.6)}$$

$$TOF = Wf + Wf_{Alternate} + Wf_{COntingency} + Wf_{Holding} \quad \textbf{(7.7)}$$

$$FOB = TOF + Wf_{taxi} \quad \textbf{(7.8)}$$

$$PAYLOAD = NUMPAX * PAXWT * LOADFACTOR + CARGO \quad \textbf{(7.9)}$$

$$LW = TOW - Wf - Wfapp \tag{7.10}$$

According to Fregnani *et al.* [41], the following payload-range diagram related limitations shall be respected when considering mission performance calculations:

$$TOW < MTOW \tag{7.11}$$

$$TOW < MZFW + FOB \tag{7.12}$$

$$TOW < MLW + Wf \tag{7.13}$$

$$FOB < MAX\ FUEL\ CAPACITY \tag{7.14}$$

The trip fuel and time determination routine is constructed considering the aircraft departing with a certain takeoff weight (TOW) from the origin airport, computing the forward sequence of the trajectory (climb, cruise and descent order). An interactive Flight Profile Algorithm is implemented to adjust the TOW to determine the top of descent point to match the sum of climb, cruise and descent distances with the total route distance of the whole profile, as shown in Fig. (**7.28**). For the complete mission calculation, it is necessary to adjust the TOW and payload for the Payload-Range envelope checks and perform the alternate fuel calculation (W_{falt}) considering the TOW as estimated landing weight minus a go-around fuel allowance (Table **7.7**) at the destination airport. The complete mission calculation algorithm is shown in Fig. (**7.29**).

The Direct Operational Cost (DOC) calculation for each sector is based on Roskan's methodology [42] and utilizes empirical formulas expressed in terms of Maximum Takeoff Weight (MTOW), trip time(T), trip fuel (W_f) and number of crew. Five cost components of costs are calculated: Flight Costs (crew, oil, fuel and insurance), Maintenance Costs (airframe labor, engine labor, airframe material and engines material), depreciation costs (airframe, engines and avionics), fee costs (Navigation, Airport and Register) and financial costs (airframe and engines leasing). The mission DOC related to a single sector *i* is then expressed by:

$$DOCi = DOCi_{flt} + DOCi_{maint} + DOCi_{depr} + DOCi_{fee} + DOCi_{fin} \tag{7.15}$$

Algorithm for Flight Profile Calculation

```
Function Flight Profile [Wf,T]=function (GW, T, ISADEV)
  Load aircraft&engine parameters
  Calculate OptAlt and Maximum Altitude (GW, ISA, aircraft& engine parameters, airport parameters)
  Determine Cruise Altitude =Min (RVSM FL, MaxAlt, OptAlt)
  Calculate Climb Wf, T and Dist_climb (GW, ISA,aircraft parameters, airport parameters)
  Dist_cruise=TOTALDIST-Dist_climb; GW_toc=TOW-Wf_climb; delta=1E9; tolerance=0.05
  Do While delta>tolerance
     Calculate Cruise Wf and T (Dist_cruise,GW_toc, ISADEV,aircraft parameters, airport parameters)
     GW_tod=GW_toc-Wf-cruise
     Calculate Descent Wf, T and Dist_descent (GW_tod, ISADEV,aircraft parameters, airport parameters)
    dtot=Dist_climb+Dist_Cruise+Dist_descent; delta=dtot-TOTALDIST;
    if delta>tolerance the Dist_cruise=Dist_cruise-delta
    Wf=Wf_climb+Wf_cruise+Wf_descent
    T=T_climb+T_cruise+T_descent
  End While
End
```

Fig. (7.28). Flight Profile Algorithm (Calculation of Trip Fuel and Time).

Algorithm for Mission Calculation

```
Procedure Mission Calculation
   PAYLOAD=NUMPAX*LOADFACTOR*PAXWT;
  Var init: ZFW=OEW+PAYLOAD; GW=ZFW+MAXFUELCAP (initial estimate);Tolerance=50; delta=1E9
  Do While delta>tolerance
     Calculate Wf and T: Flight Profile [Wf,T] = function (TOTALDIST, GW, ISADEV)
     LW=TOW-Wf; Wfcont=Wf*CONTPCT%
    Calculate Wf_alt and T_alt: Flight Profile[Wf_alt,T_alt]=function (ALTDIST, LW-Wfga,ISADEV)
    Calculate Wf hold (LW-Wfalt-Wfga,aircraft&engine parameters, airport parameters)
     RES=Wfalt+Wfhold+Wfcont; ZFW=LW-RES; TOF=Wf+RES; FOB=TOF+taxifuel
     PAYLOAD_calc=GW-FOB-OEW
     adjust payload: IF PAYLOAD_calc<PAYLOAD then PAYLOAD=PAYLOAD_calc;
      MLW check: If LW>MLW the delta1=LW-MLW else delta1=0
      ZFW check: If ZFW>MZFW the delta2=ZFW-MZFW else delta2=0
      MAXFULCAP check: If FOB>MAXFUELCAP then delta3=FOB-MAXFUELCAP else delta3=0
     MTOW check: If GW>MTOW the delta4=GW-MTOW
     delta=Max(delta1,delta2,delta3,delta4)
    GW=GW-delta
  End While
End
```

Fig. (7.29). Complete Mission Calculation Algorithm.

The mission analysis is applied used on each sector of the given transport network. The Total Network Direct Operational Cost (US$/nm) and Network yield (US$/Passenger. nm) are calculated considering the Network Parameters (Table **7.4**) and Airline Operations Parameters (Table **7.7**) on Eqs. **16** to **22** as follows:

$$TB_{ij} \ = T_{ij} + TA + TOT + TIT + DD_i + ADj \tag{7.16}$$

$$WBij = Wf_{ij} + TOFA + AFA \tag{7.17}$$

$$f_{ij} \ = int(\frac{DEM_{ij}}{MAXPAX.LF_{ij}}) \tag{7.18}$$

$$Nacft = \ int(\frac{\sum_{i=1}^{N}\sum_{j=1}^{N} TB_{i,j}}{DU}) \quad \text{for } i \neq j \tag{7.19}$$

$$NPAX = \sum_{i=1}^{N}\sum_{j=1}^{n} MAXPAX.LF_{ij}.f_{ij} \quad \text{for } i \neq j \tag{7.20}$$

$$NDOC = \sum_{i=1}^{N}\sum_{j=1}^{N}(DOC_{i,j}.f_{i,j} + ID * (DD_i + AD_j)) \quad \text{for } i \neq j \tag{7.21}$$

$$NYIELD = \ k1\frac{ATP}{\sum_{i=1}^{N}\sum_{j=1}^{N} D_{i,j}} - k2\frac{NDOC}{\sum_{i=1}^{N}\sum_{j=1}^{N} MAXPAX.LF_{i,j}.f_{i,j}} \quad \text{for } i \neq j \tag{7.22}$$

Optimization Features

In this study, the genetic algorithm MOGA-II (Multi-objective Genetic Algorithm) was employed for the proposed Multi-objective and multi-disciplinary problem. It is proposed to use the Uniform Latin Hypercube sampling [46] to generate the Design of Experiment (DOE) used as starting point for the GA optimization. The Design of Experiment (DOE) is methodology proposed by Fisher [47] with the objective to maximize the knowledge of experimental data, eliminating redundant observations allowing the analysists to extract as much as information as possible through a limited use of runs. In the ULH method, the design space is constructed in such a way that each of the dimensions (design variables) is divided into equal levels and that there is only one sample at each level. A random procedure is used to determine the point locations. The test points locations are then uniformly distributed inside the DOI providing reasonable space-filling properties at reasonable computational costs. In this study, 40 designs are initially created in the Latin Hypercube DOE to support the first generation of airplanes to be evaluated by the genetic algorithm that was chosen for the optimization runs.

All concepts exposed before were implement in a modeFrontier® workflow that is shown in Fig. (**7.3**). The multi-objective and multi-disciplinary optimization problem targeted the minimization of DOC and the maximization of network yield.

Besides the constraints of the flight conditions described in Section Design Diagram, other were also imposed:

- Fly-over noise < 84 dB.
- Divergence Mach number > MMO
- Mission fuel must be accommodated in the wings.

The Pearson correlation coefficient is a measure of the linear correlation between two variables X and Y. It has a value between +1 and −1, where 1 is total positive linear correlation, 0 is no linear correlation, and −1 is total negative linear correlation. It is widely used in the sciences and was employed in the preset work to measure the relation and design variables and some important parameters like takeoff noise and DOC. Pearson's correlation coefficient is the covariance of the two variables divided by the product of their standard deviations. The form of the definition involves a "product moment", that is, the mean (the first moment about the origin) of the product of the mean-adjusted random variables; hence the modifier product-moment in the name.

$$PCC_{A,B} = \frac{cov(A,B)}{\sigma_A \sigma_B} \quad \textbf{(7.23)}$$

The formula for $PCC_{A,B}$ can be expressed in terms of mean (μ) and expectation (*E*), considering that the *cov(A, B)* is

$$cov(A,B) = E[(A - \mu_A)(B - \mu_B)] \quad \textbf{(7.24)}$$

Then Eq. **23** becomes

$$PCC_{A,B} = \frac{E[(A-\mu_A)(B-\mu_B)]}{\sigma_A \sigma_B} \quad \textbf{(7.25)}$$

RESULTS AND DISCUSSION

Approximately 250 generations were carried out with the genetic algorithm MOGA-II implemented in modeFrontier®. Fig. (**7.30**) shows the resulting Pareto front. The unfeasible designs that arose during the computations are not shown in the figure. Table **7.10** contains important characteristics of the individuals present in the Pareto front that resulted from the optimization task.

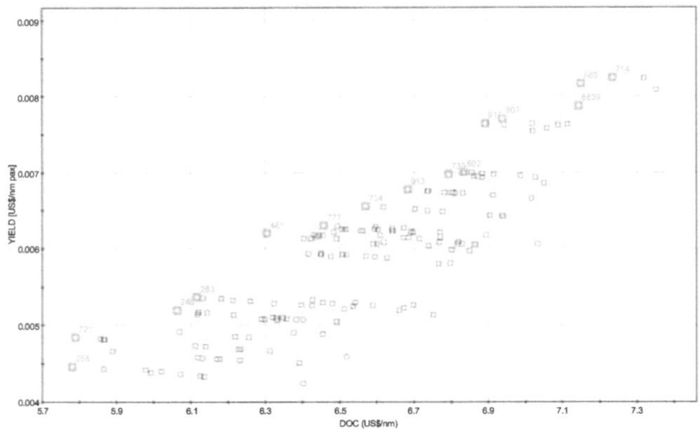

Fig. (7.30). Pareto Front of the two objectives adopted in the design simulations.

The relative position of the baseline airplane, whose characteristics are shown in Table **7.3**, to the Pareto front is shown in Fig. (**7.31**). Despite the excellent characteristics of the baseline airplane and its outstanding performance in great part thanks to its airfoils, it could be possible to improve it even further. The airplane with the same network yield in the Pareto front presents a considerable lower DOC.

Table 7.10. Some characteristics of individuals belonging to the Pareto front that resulted of the optimization task..

Design ID	Typical Seating	Seating Abreast	wS $[m^2]$	wAR	ebypass	ediam [m]	MTOW [kg]	DOC [US$/nm]	Yield [US$/(nm.pax)]	Takeoff Noise [EPNdB]
252	78	5	82	8.26	5.35	1.28	34,488	6.03	0.00511	83.3
262	79	4	78	8.08	6.04	1.42	34,929	6.09	0.00528	79.6
296	70	5	78	7.78	5.86	1.35	32,089	5.75	0.00437	80.0
461	87	6	86	8.36	5.71	1.34	36,835	6.27	0.00611	81.1
582	109	6	96	8.93	5.64	1.43	43,930	7.12	0.00808	82.4
623	107	5	96	9.54	6.49	1.46	44,685	7.11	0.00779	79.1

(Table 7.10) contd.....

Design ID	Typical Seating	Seating Abreast	wS [m ^{2}]	wAR	ebypass	ediam [m]	MTOW [kg]	DOC [US$/nm]	Yield [US$/(nm.pax)]	Takeoff Noise [EPNdB]
692	100	5	95	8.19	6.50	1.50	41,187	6.80	0.00692	78.5
714	112	5	96	7.66	5.32	1.43	42,253	7.20	0.00816	83.2
721	74	5	78	9.07	6.19	1.28	32,920	5.76	0.00476	79.0
734	95	6	91	7.6	5.76	1.38	38,573	6.54	0.00647	81.9
739	98	5	95	7.6	5.53	1.42	40,877	6.76	0.00686	81.7
777	92	6	91	7.81	6.27	1.40	37,991	6.43	0.00622	83.2
807	106	6	96	7.98	5.87	1.43	42,141	6.91	0.00762	81.2
913	96	6	94	7.60	5.62	1.40	39,238	6.65	0.00669	82.4
917	103	6	94	8.09	5.73	1.42	41,551	6.86	0.00756	81.2
998	109	6	96	8.93	5.64	1.43	43,930	7.12	0.00808	82.4

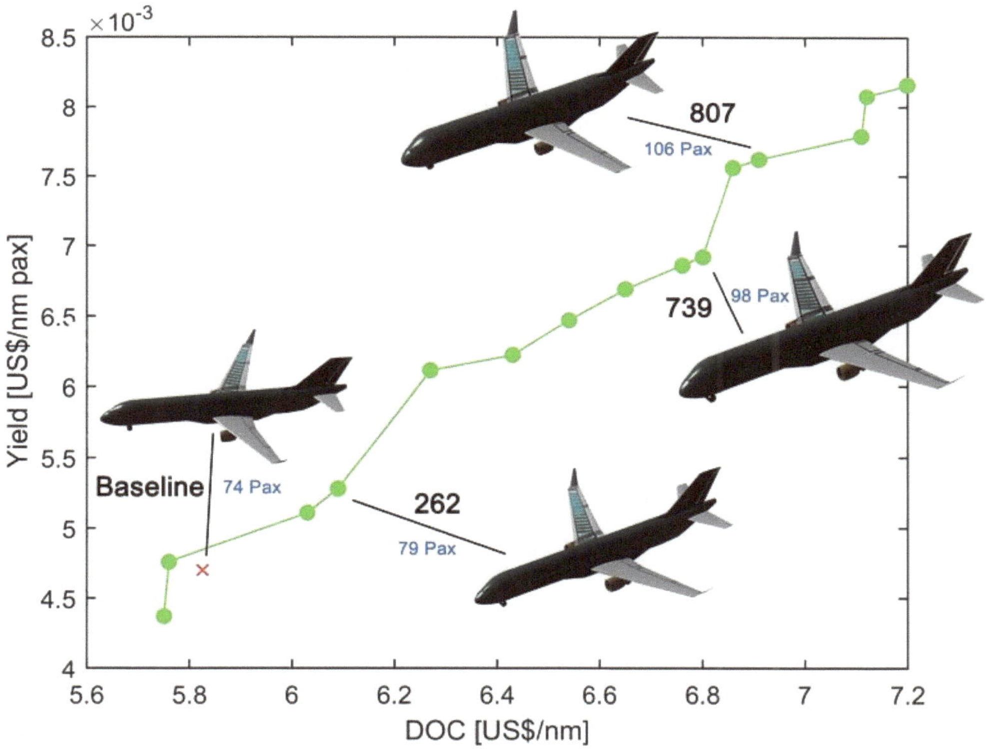

Fig. (7.31). Relative position of baseline airplane to the Pareto front.

Fig. (**7.32**) provides an overview of the Pareto front variation regarding the wing area and wing sweepback angle.

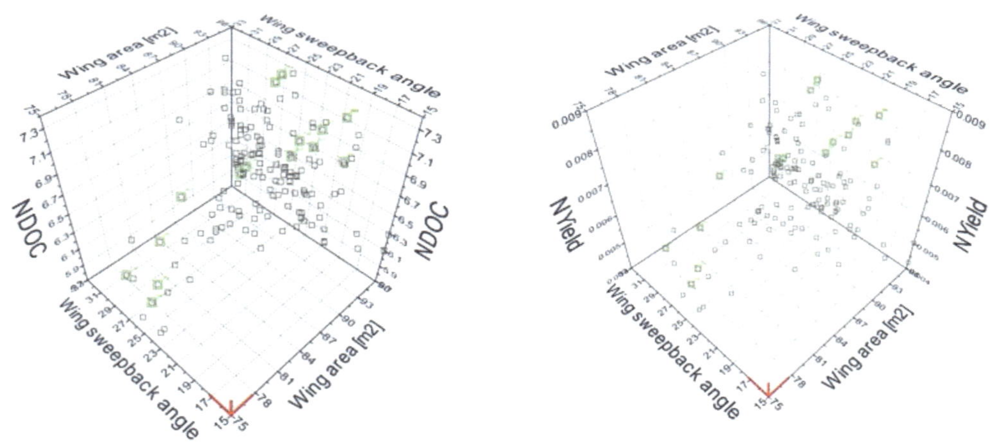

Fig. (7.32). DOC and Yield as function of Wing Area and Wing Sweep Angle.

Figs. (**7.33** and **7.34**) show the probability density distributions of the objective functions obtained in both algorithms (green bars are related to the Pareto front designs).

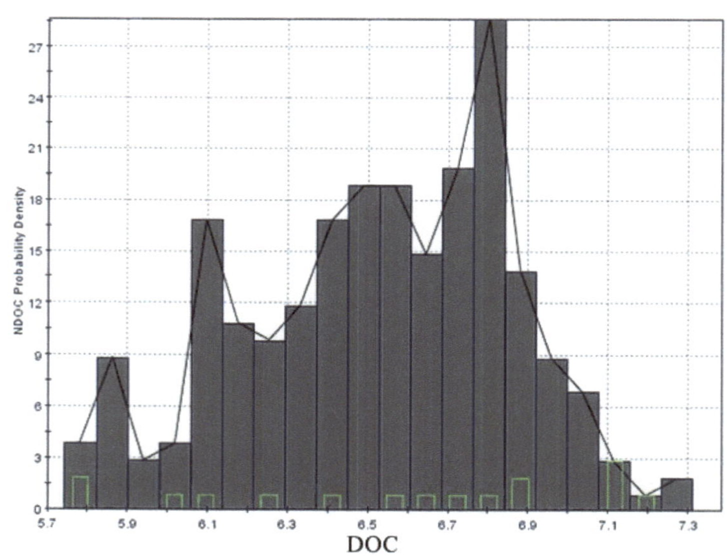

Fig. (7.33). Network Direct Operational Cost Probability Density Distribution.

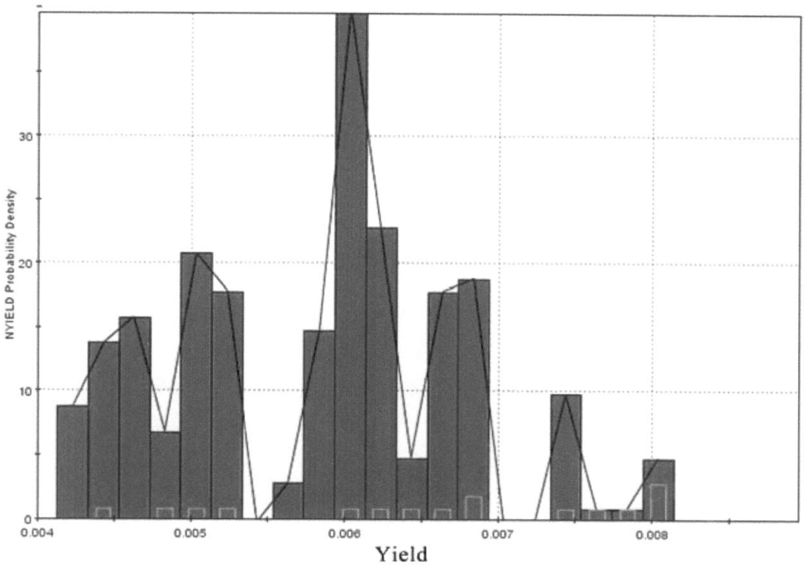

Fig. (7.34). Network Yield Probability Density Distribution.

The Pearson correlation matrix is shown is Fig. (**7.35**). As expected, the takeoff noise is heavily dependent on engine diameter and engine by-pass ratio.

The Pareto front analysis shows that there are two remarkable design extremes: the configuration presenting the maximum yields (approximately 0.00816 US$/nm.pax); and the point related to the minimum DOC (approximately 5.75 US$/nm). It can be noticed that the design related to the minimum Network Direct Operational Cost (NDOC) led to the maximization of specific range, considering that the flight speeds along all flight profile are fixed parameters and the airfoils are the same all airplanes. Therefore, under this perspective, both algorithms consistently converged to some drastic aerodynamics and engine performance improvements from the baseline aircraft: approximately slight increase in wing area or the design presenting the lower DOC; 26% for the design with highest network yield. An aspect worth mentioning is that the wing aspect ratio was kept within reasonable boundaries; the highest value was 9.54. For the class of airplane, with passenger capacity topping 130 seats and 2000-nm range, no high-tech concepts such as extremely flexible wings or truss-braced configurations seem to be necessary. Wing sweepback angle higher than the baseline design is present in most of the Pareto front inhabitants. Engine by-pass ratio above 5.5 revealed to be necessary.

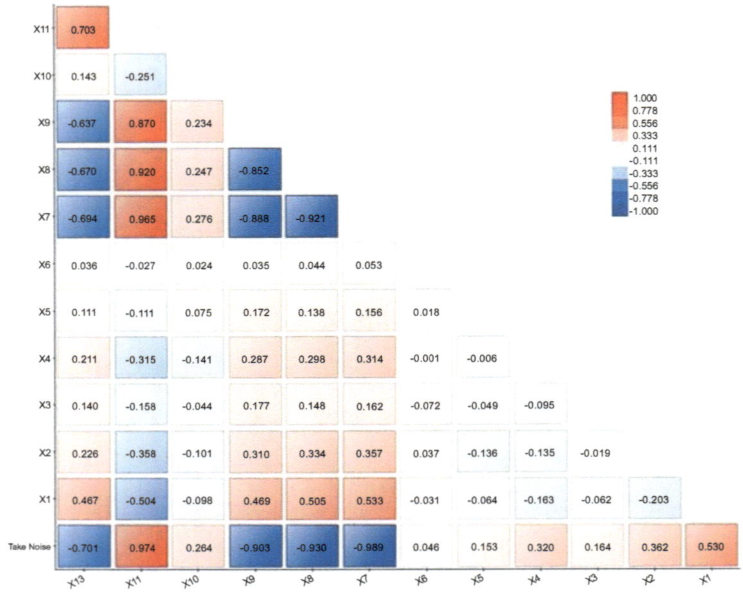

Fig. (7.35). Pearson correlation matrix.

In the Pareto Front's extreme point related to the maximum network yield (NYIELD), the optimization task provided solutions towards the increase of aircraft capacity, close to 110 but still below the 130-seat boundary. This maximizes the trip revenue considering the given fixed average ticket price. Once the number of isles is fixed to a unit, this produced a stretched aircraft when compared with the baseline aircraft. Considering that, the trip yield is also dependent on DOC, some aerodynamic and engine improvements are present in both algorithms, trying to maximize the specific range: increase in wing area by 9%/14%, wing sweep angle by 42%/45%, engines by-pass ratio by 17%/11% and fan diameter by approximately 5%. Because of the bigger aircraft size, the number of required aircraft to transport the given passengers demand in the network decreased from 11 to 7, representing a possible opportunity for the airline on reduction of maintenance and spare parts costs. Both methods, however, produced a significant increase in total Network Yield (approximately 80%) regarding the baseline aircraft, as expected by the optimization.

CONCLUDING REMARKS

This study proposed the development of an aircraft multidisciplinary design optimization inserted in each air transport network, using MOGA-II as optimizer and considering 3 design disciplines (aerodynamics, propulsion and mission performance), with design certification diagram check. Two objective functions were considered: maximization of network yield and minimization of network direct operational cost. The final designs converged on both objective functions to aerodynamic and propulsion solutions related to the optimization of specific range, considering the fixed speed schedule and given airfoils on tree different wing stations (root, kink and wing). Under this solution, the neural network utilized in the aerodynamics module led to wing designs with increased sweep angles, suggesting convergence towards the minimization of wave drag (the airfoils were in fact originally optimized on wings designed for lower Mach numbers). Also under this objective, more efficient engines were obtained with larger bypass ratios and fan diameters, suggesting the improvement in the thrust specific fuel consumption in the final design. The design associated to the minimum network DOC converged to a smaller aircraft close to the lower seating capacity limit, with the maximum yield to a bigger aircraft close to the upper limit of seating capacity, considering the given demands on this specific network.

In the Pareto front, two design extremes were identified (Maximum Network Yield and Minimum Network DOC), producing the following average results when compared with the baseline aircraft: 80% increase in the network yield and 2.5% reduction in network DOC. Although the classical approach on aircraft design frequently considers the minimization of DOC [4, 5, 15, 24], this study suggests that the Network Yield may be considered a suitable candidate in the design objectives, due to its larger impact on the baseline optimization. In fact, yield is an economic parameter that has been used in the air transport industry as the measurement of profitability and has special significance on finance decisions rather that DOC. However, its optimization suggests producing bigger aircraft designs (towards maximum seat capacities) which may bring other non-operational finance impacts for the airlines, such as increase in the inventory costs and airport infra-structure and compatibility issues.

FUTURE DEVELOPMENTS

With the objective to improve the proposed MDO framework we propose future researches to be conducted on the introduction of the optimum route structures and hub allocations in the cycle, considering the given demand flows between airports (network optimization). Under this process, the mission speed profile could also be optimized, *via* surrogate model, using the cost index concept. The introduction of structural analysis and tail design discipline, besides flight qualities check, are also suggested to be developed to refine even more the suitable designs produced in the Pareto Front.

ACRONYMS AND SYMBOLS

a0	= Sound speed at International Standard Atmospheric conditions
AFA	= Approach and landing fuel allowance
ASM	= Available Seat Mile
ALTD	= Alternate Airport distance
ANN	= Artificial Neural Network
ATA	= Approach and landing time allowance
ATP	= Average Ticket Price
Aw	= Aisle width
BuffMGN	= Buffet margin measured in g force
CaptSAL	= Average captain annual salary
Cf	= Fuel cost
CH	= Cabin height (m)
CLmax	= Maximum wing-body lift coefficient
Cp	= Pressure coefficient
D	= Drag force
DEMij	= Daily demand from airport i to airport j
DICi fin	= Financial costs (airframe and engines leasing)
Dij	= Route Distance from airport i to airport j
DISA	= International Standard Atmosphere temperature deviation (C)
DOCi	= Direct Operational Cost related to sector i (US$/nm)
DOCi depr	= Depreciation Costs (airframe, engines and avionics) - US$/nm
DOCi fee	= Fee Costs (Navigation, Airport and Register) - US$/nm
DOCi flt	= Flight Costs (crew, oil, fuel and insurance) - US$/nm
DOCi maint	= Maintenance Costs (airframe labor, engine labor, airframe material, engines material) - US$/nm
DU	= Average Daily Aircraft Utilization
ebypass	= Engine by-pass ratio
ediam	= Engine fan diameter
Eopr	= Engine overall pressure ratio
Ep	= Engines Position (1=below wing, 0=tail)
epsilon	= camber line angle at trailing edge
FASal	= Average Flight Attendant Annual Salary
FOSal	= Average First Officer Annual Salary
FusDiam	= Fuselage diameter

FusHeight = Fuselage height

FusWidth = Fuselage width

HTAR = Horizontal tail aspect ratio

HTArea = Horizontal Tail Area

HTSweep = Horizontal tail sweep angle

HTTR = Horizontal tail taper ratio

ID = Average Inflight Delay Cost

Inc_kink = Wing Kink incidence angle

Inc_root = Wing Root incidence angle

K = Direct Operational Cost/ Total Operational Costs ratio

K1 = Total Operational Cost/Direct Operational Cost ratio

K2 = Total Revenue/ Ticket Revenue ratio

Kink_semispan = Position of wing break station

KS = Kink Semispan position (%)

LDA = Available landing runway

Lf = Fuselage length

Lfij = average load factor form airport i to airport j

Maxalt = Max certified altitude

MAXFUEL = Maximum fuel capacity

MAXPAX = Passenger Capacity

MAXRATE = Maximum Engine Thrust at sea level @ ISA conditions (lbf)

MinCRZt = Minimum Cruise Time

MLW = Maximum Landing Weight

MMO/VMO = Maximum Operational Mach number/Maximum Operational Speed

MZFW = Maximum Zero Fuel Weight

N = Number of airports in the transport network

Nacft = Total aircraft number

NCorr = Number of aisles

ncrew = Number of crew

NDOC = Total Air Transport Network's Direct Operational Cost (US$/ nm)

ne = Number of engines

Nseat = Seating abreast

NYIELD = Total Network Yield (US$/passenger. Nm)

PAXWT = Total Passenger Weight (85kg+25kg baggage)

PCC = Pearson Correlation Coefficient

phi	= Thickness line angle at trailing edge
r0/c	= Leading edge radius ratio
RROC	= Residual rate of climb
SPDLIM	= Speed Limit Below 10000 ft
SW	= Seat width
t/c	= Airfoil thickness ratio
TA	= Average turnaround time
TIT	= Average Taxi In Time (from runway exit to gate)
TOFA	= Takeoff and Initial Climb out Fuel allowance
TORA	= Takeoff Runway Available
TOT	= Average Taxi Out Time (from gate to runway threshold)
TOTA	= Takeoff and Initial Climb out Time allowance (min)
V	= True airspeed
W	= Aircraft mass
wAR	= Wing Aspect Ratio
wS	= Wing reference area
wSweep	= Wing sweepback angle
wTR	= Wing taper ratio
wTwist	= Wing twist angle
δ	= Atmospheric Pressure Ratio (actual static pressure / standard sea level pressure)
ϒ	= Flight-path angle
ϕ	= Bank angle

REFERENCES

[1] R. Doganis, *Flying Off Course IV: Airline economics and marketing.* 1st ed. Routledge, 2010, p. 352.

[2] U.S Department of Transportation, "Bureau of Transportation Statistics - Bottom-Line Statistics: 2000-2005", *Mai,* 2017.

[3] G. Burghowt, *Airline Network in Europe and its Implication for Airport Planning.* Ashgate: Burlington, 2007.

[4] E. Torenbeek, *Advanced Aircraft Design.* John Wiley & Sons, 2013. [http://dx.doi.org/10.1002/9781118568101]

[5] C. Taylor, and O.L. Weck, "Integrated Transportation Network Design Optimization", *47th AIAA/ASME/ASCE/AHS/ASC Structures, Structural Dynamics, and Materials Conference,* 2006 [http://dx.doi.org/10.2514/6.2006-1912]

[6] C. Taylor, *"Integrated Transportation System Design Optimization"*, PhD Thesis, Massachusetts Institute of Technology, Cambridge, MA, 2007.

[7] C.A. Coello, G.A. Lamont, and D.A. van Veldhuizen, *Evolutionary Algorithms for Solving Multi-Objective Problems.* Springer, 2007.

[8] S.N. Sivanandam, and S.N. Deepa, *Introduction to Genetic Algorithms.* Springer, 2007.

[9] M.D. McKey, R.J. Beckman, and W.J. Conover, "A Comparison of Three Methods for Selecting Values of Input Variables in the Analysis of Output from a Computer Code", *Technometrics,* vol. 42, no. 1, pp. 55-61, 2000. [http://dx.doi.org/10.1080/00401706.2000.10485979]

[10] G.C. Bower, and I.M. Kroo, "Multi-Objective Aircraft Optimization for Minimum Cost and Emissions over Specific Route Networks", *26th International Congress of Aeronautical Congress, Anchorage*

[11] L.V. Cabral, P. Paglione, and B.S. Mattos, "Multi-Objective Design Optimization Framework for Conceptual Design of Families of Aircraft", *44th AIAA Aerospace Sciences Meeting and Exhibit, Reno,* 2006

[12] P.C. Magalhães, and B.S. Mattos, "Conceptual optimal design of environmentally friendly airliners: a review of available methodologies and their integration into a consistent framework for everyday use", *16th AIAA/ISSMO Multidisciplinary Analysis and Optimization Conference, Dallas,* 2015

[13] L. Siqueira, B.S. Mattos, and V. Loureiro, "The Suited Airliner for an Existing Airline Network", *50th AIAA/ASME/ASCE/AHS/ASC Structures, Structural Dynamics, and Materials Conference, California,* 2009

[14] "Genetic Algorithms in Engineering Systems", In: *The Instituion of Electric Engineers*, 1997.

[15] D. Kalyanmoy, A. Pratap, S. Agarwal, and T. Meyarivan, "A Fast and Elitist Multiobjective Genetic Algorithm: NSGA-II", *IEEE Trans. Evol. Comput.,* vol. 6, no. 2, 2002.

[16] R.J. Balling, and J. Sobieszczanski-Sobieski, *Optimization of coupled systems - A critical overview of approaches.* vol. Vol. 34. AIAA Journal, 1996.

[17] N.V. Queipo, R. Haftka, S. Shyy, T. Goel, R. Vaidyanathan, and P.K. Tucker, "„Surrogated Based Analysis and Optimization", *Prog. Aerosp. Sci.,* pp. 1-28, 2005. [http://dx.doi.org/10.1016/j.paerosci.2005.02.001]

[18] A.T. Isikveren, *Quasi-Analytical Modelling and Optimisation Techniques for Transport Aircraft Design," Royal Stockholm of Technology.* KTH: Stockholm, 2002.

[19] J. Cavalcanti, B.S. Mattos, and P. Paglione, "Optimal Conceptual Design of Transport Aircraft", *11th AIAA/ISSMO Multidisciplinary Analysis and Optimization Conference,* 2006 Portsmouth

[20] R. Henderson, *"Multidisciplinary Design Optimization of Airframe and Engine for Emissions Reduction"*, Master Thesis, Uniersity of Toronto, Toronto, 2009.

[21] W.A. Crossley, and M. Mane, "System of Systems Inspired Aircraft Sizing Applied to Commercial Aircraft / Airline Problems", *AIAA 5th Aviation, Technology, Integration, and Operations Conference (ATIO),* 2005 Arlington [http://dx.doi.org/10.2514/6.2005-7426]

[22] N. Davendralingam, and W. Crossley, "Concurrent Aircraft Design and Variable Resource Allocation in Large Scale Fleet Networks", *9th AIAA Aviation Technology, Integration, and Operations Conference (ATIO),* 2009

[23] G. Roth, and W. Crossley, "Commercial transport aircraft conceptual design using a genetic algorithm based approach", *7th AIAA/USAF/NASA/ISSMO Symposium on Multidisciplinary Analysis and Optimization, Multidisciplinary Analysis Optimization Conferences,* 1998 St. Louis

[24] A.W. Crossley, T.M. Eric, and D.W. Fanjoy, "A multiobjective investigation of 50-seat commuter aircraft using a genetic algorithm", *1st AIAA, Aircraft, Technology Integration, and Operations Forum, Aviation Technology, Integration, and Operations (ATIO) Conferences,* 2001 West Lafayette [http://dx.doi.org/10.2514/6.2001-5247]

[25] R. Satradu, and W.A. Crossley, "An EGO-like Optimization Framework for Simultaneous Aircraft Design and Airline Allocation", *57th AIAA/ASCE/AHS/ASC Structures, Structural Dynamics, and*

Materials Conference, AIAA SciTech Forum, 2016 San Diego.

[26] S. Roy, K. Moore, J.T. Hwang, J.S. Gray, and W.A. Martins, "A Mixed Integer Efficient Global Optimization Algorithm for the Simultaneous Aircraft Allocation-Mission-Design Problem", *58th AIAA/ASCE/AHS/ASC Structures, Structural Dynamics, and Materials Conference, AIAA SciTech Forum* Ann Arbor.

[27] N. Davendralingam, and W. Crossley, "Concurrent Aircraft Design and Airline Network Design Incorporating Passenger Demand Models", *9th AIAA Aviation Technology, Integration, and Operations Conference (ATIO),* 2009.

[28] N. Davendralingam, and W. Crossley, "Robust Approach for Concurrent Aircraft Design and Airline Network Design", *J. Aircr.,* vol. 51, pp. 1773-1883, 2014. [http://dx.doi.org/10.2514/1.C032442]

[29] J.T. Hwang, and J.R. Martins, "Allocation-mission-design optimization of next-generation aircraft using a parallel computational framework", *57th AIAA/ASCE/AHS/ASC Structures, Structural Dynamics, and Materials Conference, AIAA SciTech Forum,* 2016 San Diego. [http://dx.doi.org/10.2514/6.2016-1662]

[30] N.R. Secco, and B.S. Mattos, "Artificial neural networks to predict aerodynamic coefficients of transport airplanes", *Aircr. Eng. Aerosp. Technol.,* vol. 89, no. 2, pp. 211-230, 2017. [http://dx.doi.org/10.1108/AEAT-05-2014-0069]

[31] B.S. Mattos, and N.R. Secco, "An Airplane Calculator Featuring a High-Fidelity Methodology for Tailplane Sizing", *Journal of Aerospace Technology and Aerospace Management,* vol. 4, pp. 371-386, 2013.
[http://dx.doi.org/10.5028/jatm.v5i4.254]

[32] ESTECO, "Optimization with modeFrontier", *ESTECO,* 2017. http://www.esteco.com/modefrontier/optimization-modefrontier.

[33] B.S. Mattos, *"Numerischer Entwurf von transsonischen Flügeln und Tragflügelprofilen unter Anwendung des AF2-Algorithmus zur Lösung de vollständigen Potentialgleichung",* Universität Stuttgart, PhD Thesis, Stuttgart, 1995.

[34] Brazilian Airspace Control Department, "Aeronautical Information Publication – Enroute Charts H1-H2", *Institute of Aeronautical Cartography, Rio de Janeiro,* .

[35] G.F. Newell, "Airport Capacity and Delays", *Transport. Sci.,* pp. 201-241, 1979. [http://dx.doi.org/10.1287/trsc.13.3.201]

[36] D. Lombardo, *Advanced Aircraft Systems.* 1st ed. McGraw-Hill Inc, 1993, p. 359.

[37] T. Benson, "An interactive educational tool for turbojet engines", *31st AIAA Joint Propulsion Conference and Exhibit,* 1995 San Diego. [http://dx.doi.org/10.2514/6.1995-3055]

[38] V. Loureiro, and B.S. Mattos, "Powerplant as Design Variable Into Multi-Disciplinary Design Optimization of Transport Airplane", *27th AIAA Applied Aerodynamics Conference,* 2009 San Antonio. [http://dx.doi.org/10.2514/6.2009-4108]

[39] Jane's, "Jane's Aero-Engines", *IHS,* 2017. http://janes.ihs.com/janes/home.

[40] J.D. Mattingly, *Elements of Gas Turbine.* Mc Graw Hill Education Private Ltd: New Delhi, 2013.

[41] ANSYS Inc, *ANSYS 14 Fluent User Guide.* ANSYS Inc.: Canonsburg, PA, 2011.

[42] M. Levenberg, *A Method for the Solution of Certain Problems in Least-Squares.* Quartely Applied Mathmatics, 1944, pp. 164-168.

[43] D. Marquardt, *An Algorithm for Least-squares Estimation of Nonlinear Parameters.* SIAM Journal Applied Mathmatics, 1963, pp. 431-441.

[44] M.J. Powell, "A Fortran Subroutine for Solving Systems of Nonlinear Algebraic Equations", In:

Numerical Methods for Non-linea Algebraic Equations, P. Rabinowitz, Ed., , 1970.

[45] G.W. Brune, and J.W. McMasters, "Applied Computational Aerodynamics", In: *Progress in Aeronautical Series,* P.sA. Henne, Ed., American Institute of Aeronautics and Astronautics, Inc: Washington, D.C., 1990.

[46] B. Singh, *A Medium-Fidelity Method for Rapid Maximum Lift Estimation.* Delft University: Delft, 2017.

[47] M. Drela, "XFOIL: An Analysis and Design System for Low Reynolds Number Airfoils", *Massachusetts Institute of Technology, Cambridge,* 2014. http://www.airlines.org/Pages/Annual-and-Per-Minute-Cost-of-Delays-to-U.S.-Airlines.aspx.

CHAPTER 8

Flight Operations and Environment

Abstract: Despite efforts to optimize the design of airframes and engines with the objective to produce more fuel-efficient aircraft, flight operations may also have a key role in fuel consumption and emission reductions. The cost of the adoption of operational procedures related to fuel conservation is relatively less than the investment in modern technologies and designs, involving most of the times training efforts adopted by the operational staff. A series of techniques is adopted by airlines with this objective, such as flight planning, dispatch and in-flight techniques, leading to improvements of about 6% in fuel efficiency. The automatic speed control and management provided by the development of Flight Management and Autothrottle systems permitted the adoption of the Cost Index concept, thus enabling the operators to further optimize the flight path and therefore minimize fuel and time costs. In addition, the adoption of aircraft conditioning monitoring programs may point to drag and engine-degradation patterns, which may be corrected through simple maintenance actions, with potential to recover up to more than 4% of fuel consumption. Considering the integration of the aircraft with the airspace system and network, an additional 12% improvement may be achieving through the adoption of common Air Traffic Management practices, supported by Communication, Navigation and Surveillance emerging technologies. Therefore, efficient flight operations have the potential to provide almost half of the necessary emission reductions required to be achieved by 2050, which should correspond to at least half of the levels in 2005.

Keywords: Air traffic management, Aircraft condition monitoring, Cost index, Cost optimization, Flight operation engineering, Performance engineering.

THE ROLE OF FLIGHT OPERATIONS

As stated in Chapter 1, the aviation industry is committed to reducing GHG emissions by 50% by the year 2050, based on the total amount recorded for 2005. World traffic is estimated to grow at an average 5% for the next decades, despite potential economic crises. This means it is an immense challenge to reduce fuel aviation fuel burn.

Several initiatives have been considered to develop efficient aircraft configurations, with the focus on the development of innovative airframe technologies and engine improvements.

Bento S. de Mattos, José A. T. G. Fregnani & Paulo Eduardo C. S. Magalhães

As fuel emissions are directly proportional to fuel burn (*i.e.*, every kg of JET A1 fuel burnt represents approximately 3.16 kg of CO_2 in the atmosphere), initiatives to reduce fuel burn also lead to emission reductions.

The global airline industry's fuel bill topped US$ 180 billion in 2015, accounting for 27% of operating expenses at US$ 55/barrel Brent of oil [1]. Since the 1970s, oil crises and barrel price variations have been influencing airline economics. Therefore, fuel conservation programs have been developed to optimize fuel related costs. This has been a key factor for the survival of many airlines in the last decades, mainly because the operational margin of the airline industry from the start has been very narrow. Data regarding the year 2014 show that the world average operational margin has been verified as 3% only. Besides the environmental aspect, the economical push for fuel burn emission reductions is a significant factor to take into consideration.

In the present work, it has also been shown that technological improvements and advanced design techniques may lead to approximately 25%-30% reductions in fuel burn, mainly dependable on the research pace related to engines and aerodynamics technologies. Therefore, it is likely that such initiatives will not be sufficient to achieve the industry targets in the mentioned time frame. This poses the question as to what other options remain.

The first study performed by the Intergovernmental Panel on Climate Change specific for aviation [2] suggests that the adoption of operational procedures has potential to reduce emissions from 2% to 6%. In fact, inadequately operated aircraft may nullify all technological investments. It is worth mentioning that operational procedures have generally lower costs of investment for airlines than new technologies. However, such an initiative depends heavily on the implementation of company policies and staff training, which are sometimes prone to experience various complications due to cultural aspects and resistance to change.

There are many people from different departments related to aircraft operations from ground or flight staff: pilots, engineers, dispatchers, handing operators, mechanics, schedulers, aircraft and maintenance, and mainly, operation management. Thus, the adoption of fuel conservation programs may take some time to show its effectiveness, depending on the ability of higher management levels to implement the necessary changes.

In addition to airline operational procedures, Air Traffic Management initiatives also have the potential to improve fuel efficiencies up to 12% [2], twice as much as operational procedures. This area may be considered as the ultimate enhancement of flight operation initiatives as technological developments in this area have a direct impact on the operations of aircraft. The integration of onboard and ground systems (related to CNS/ATM technologies) has been greatly driving the efficiency of the airspace, considering all stakeholders (airlines, airports and air navigation service providers). The main objective here is to reduce the delays associated with airspace capacity and infrastructure constraints. The more delays aircraft experience while maneuvering, the more fuel is burned. Thus, the minimization of flight time (from shocks out to shocks in) means less fuel burnt and therefore diminished emissions.

In the flight operation domain, the adoption of flight operation procedures is expected to lead to fuel burn reductions by the magnitude of a one-digit percentage. Although this seems to be in small numbers related to a single flight, the impact on the whole network served by a fleet throughout a year is significant. For example, 1% of fuel burn reduction for a Boeing 737NG fleet (which is realistically achievable by – for example - using a short alternate selection) for a typical Low-Cost Carrier (LCC), considering 13 hours of daily utilization, represents savings between 47.5 tons of fuel per year per aircraft. A fleet of 120 aircraft, typically large LCC, would result in annual savings of 5.7 Million USD for this airline, considering the world average fuel price of 1.00 USD/kg.

Therefore, it can be asserted that improvements in the order of 1% or less of individual operational fuel savings techniques are generally small but the network multipliers are significant, thus leading to significant savings for airlines specially when fuel prices soar. Because of this, fuel conservation programs and associated initiatives are always emphasized in the operation´s domain, especially in a competitive industry such as air transport, where profit margins generally do not reach two-digit percentages [3].

FUEL CONSERVATION PROGRAMS

Fuel conservation programs have been implemented and run by airlines, assisted by aircraft manufacturers, since the early 70´s, initially conceived to overcome the effects of the international oil crisis. With aircraft performance significantly impacted by technological developments over the last three decades (mainly engines, Flight Management Systems and aerodynamics improvements), several operational procedures have been developed and are being continuously improved with the focus on this area. However, it is important to mention that these procedures are mostly developed to improve the efficiency of a single aircraft maneuvering into the airspace and the effect into the network is therefore a consequence. Such procedures are not designed to consider the integration and impact of the aircraft operations into the whole airspace and interaction between other operational stakeholders as well. This integration would lead to an improved capacity of the whole system in a collaborative environment, leading to synergetic savings for all stakeholders.

Fuel management programs have been developed with focus on two areas: Operational Techniques and Condition Monitoring, both (related to engines and structures influence on drag and fuel flow) of the airplane. The main objective, of course, is to minimize the fuel used on every flight of a single aircraft. Although this approach is focused on aircraft, airlines adopt this as initial methodology, considering that there is no dependence on external resources to manage their own costs.

OPERATIONAL TECHNIQUES

These techniques are most of the times implemented with the help of airline policies and generally do not involve significant amounts of investments in technology for airlines. Training and standardization applied to all flight operation stakeholders are the key for the success of implementation. Mainly pre-flight planning and in-flight techniques are adopted to minimize fuel burn as described below:

Reduction of Landing Weight

The landing weight reduction represents the most direct (and obvious) technique adopted by airlines for fuel savings. The basic statement shows that less weight in the aircraft means less fuel burned. In general, it can be assumed that 1% of reduction in the landing weight corresponds to 0.5% to 1% of reduction in the trip fuel, depending on aircraft/engine combinations and the type of mission. Table **8.1** shows the percentage reduction in trip fuel for every 1000 kg of reduction in landing weight based on some Boeing aircraft types for typical missions.

Table 8.1. Fuel burn reduction for each 1000kg landing weight reduction.

B717 200	B737 300/400/500	B737 700/800/900	B757 200/300	B767 200/300/400	B777 200/300	B747 400
2.0%	1.5%	1.3%	1.1%	0.7%	0.4%	0.4%

Considering that the landing weight corresponds to the mass of aircraft at the destination airport after burning the trip fuel, the following may be expressed according to Eq. **8.1**:

$$LW = OEW + PLD + RES + ADL \quad \textbf{(8.1)}$$

Where:

LW: Landing Weight (kg)
OEW: Operational Empty Weight (kg)
PLD: Payload (kg)
RES: Reserve Fuel Required (kg)
ADL: Additional Fuel loaded- not used (kg)

Except for the payload, which is related to the airline revenue and which is interesting to maximize, all other parameters from this equation can be reduced by adopting adequate company policies. The following strategies may be adopted.

OEW Management

The Operational Empty Weight (also called Dry Operating Weight or Basic Operating Weight) is the weight of the aircraft ready to fly without fuel and payload. It includes the weight of the whole structure of the aircraft plus the emergency equipment, navigation kit, system fluids, trapped fuel, entire crew (including baggage), catering, passenger service items, passenger entertainment items, empty cargo and baggage containers and excess potable water. Many of these items have been optimized by airlines as the examples below show:

a. Navigation bags substituted by electronic flight bags (laptops or tables loaded with operational manuals and applications), submitted to local regulations. Each bag, full of paper manuals, may weight up to 30kg.
b. Catering quantity customized per flight length, passenger class or even eliminated in short sectors.
c. Elimination of galley equipment such as ovens and coffee makers, restricting passenger in-flight services.
d. Elimination of unnecessary emergency equipment according to the type of operations (*i.e.* no rafts or lifejackets when operating over land areas).
e. Elimination of newspapers, folders and magazines onboard.
f. Load potable water quantity as function of flight sector. In this case, statistical data is required to manage the exact quantity to be loaded at each station.
g. Use of lightweight aluminum containers in the cargo compartments.

Experience has shown that LCCs have been able to manage most of these items, reducing the OEWs up to 5% related to the same aircraft type and similar configuration operated by legacy airlines.

Reserve Fuel Management

The Reserve Fuel herein defined is the one related to each flight, as the remaining fuel in the aircraft while landing at the destination airport, after burning the trip fuel. The appropriate amount of reserves must ensure a safe flight and meet local regulatory requirements, generally expressed as follows (Eq. **8.2**):

$$\text{RES} = \text{ALT+CONT+HOLD} \tag{8.2}$$

The components of this equation and opportunities for such reductions are described below:

a. Alternate Fuel (ALT). This is the trip fuel required to fly from the destination to alternate airports, including the fuel for the go around maneuver at destination (kg). The quantity is highly dependable on the company policy regarding the selection of the alternate airport. Obviously, the shorter distance from destination to alternate airport is normally the first criterion for alternate airport selection. However, some other strategic factors may also be considered such as: emergency/navigation infrastructure, presence of maintenance/handling facilities (company base or not), presence of passenger terminal facilities, weather history and company base.
b. Contingency Fuel (CONT). Does the amount of fuel loaded for eventual deviations from the planned flight route correspond to the one stated for regulatory requirements? The CONT normally corresponds to a certain percentage of the trip fuel from the origin to destination or the related fuel considering a certain percentage of total time from origin to destination (kg), depending on the applicable operational regulations. For example, under FAA operational rules [4] the contingency fuel for international operations is the amount correspondent to 10% of the trip flight time (from liftoff to touchdown) using the top of descent fuel flow. In European operational regulations [5], the contingency fuel corresponds to 5% of the total trip fuel burned.
c. Holding Fuel (HOLD). This refers to the fuel loaded correspondent to holding patterns executed at a certain altitude at the alternate airport during a certain time according to most regulatory requirements [6]. International regulations [6], for example, require 30-minute holdings at 1500 ft above field elevation.

Some operational regulations permit the reduction of this percentage if the airline demonstrates that it is capable to control statistically the contingency use of each route. For example, under European rules [5], the contingency fuel may be reduced below the 5% threshold limit and may use the correspondent 95% or 99% confidence interval instead. Also under this regulation, if the airline has implemented an aircraft condition monitoring program (where drag and engine degradations are determined per tail number and flight plans adjusted accordingly) the limit value may be reduced to 3%.

Another widespread practice to reduce the contingency is to adopt the redispatch technique, allowed by some operational regulations, particularly beneficial on long haul flights where trip fuel and time are significant. Defined by a percentage of flight time or planned fuel burn, the contingency may be reduced by splitting a flight plan into two different calculations: one from the departure airport to an airport that is closer than the intended destination, and another from a decision point on the route of flight to the planned destination (Fig. **8.1**). Each calculation requires contingency fuel over the flight´s entire distance, but each is less than the total that would be required for the entire flight to the planned destination. The actual flight must carry the greater of the contingency fuels for the two scenarios. The optimal flight plan places the decision point in a location where the contingency fuels for the two scenarios are exactly equal. Outside the decision point the required fuel increases for one scenario or the other. The minimum contingency fuels are obtained when the diversion points are placed at around 80% of the total route distance. Using this technique, the contingency fuel may be reduced from 2% to 5% of the trip fuel depending on the choice of the route alternate.

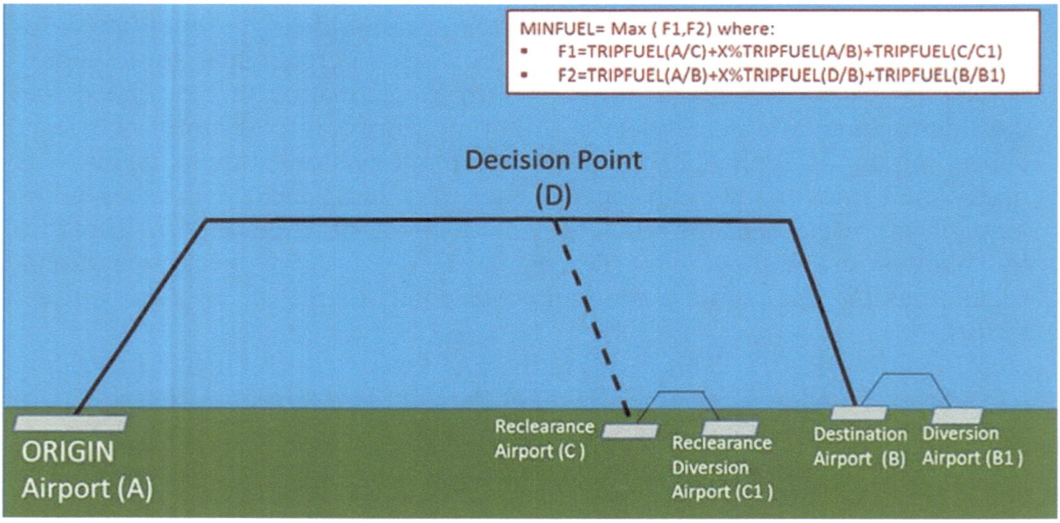

Fig. (8.1). Redispatch Airports Selection.

Theoretically the lowest fuel to be loaded should be the one considering maneuvering at minimum fuel flow speed, usually very close do maximum *L/D* speed. However, in modern jet transport aircraft this speed may be close to stall speed (between 5 to 10 kt indicated airspeed) and therefore a widespread practice adopted by airplane manufacturers is to define the holding speed as the maximum

L/D speed added to a safety margin. This margin is normally designed to protect the aircraft from inadvertent stall while turning under moderate turbulence in the holding maneuver. The holding speed is therefore determined as the stall speed considering a load factor correspondent to 40° bank angle (25° normal bank angle from autopilots + 15° overshoot, corresponding to a 1.3 g margin over stall) or the maximum L/D speed whichever is higher. This speed is published in the operation manuals and available in the FMS for pilot's selection. Any holding planned above these speeds may increase the holding fuel. In modern jet transport aircraft for every 10kt above the recommended holding speed, 1% of extra fuel consumption is expected.

Flight Planning and Dispatch

The operational flight plan is required to ensure that an airplane meets all the operational regulations for a specific flight, providing flight crew with all information to conduct the flight safely, and in coordination with air traffic control. Computerized systems for calculating flight plans have been widely used since the early 80s, but not all systems are similar. There are advantages to selecting a more capable system and using all its analytical and optimal capabilities. While flight plan calculations are necessary for safety and regulatory compliance, they also provide airlines with an opportunity for cost optimization by enabling them to determine the optimal route, altitudes, speeds and amount of fuel to load on an airplane. The optimization process may be challenging because it involves a wide range of different elements. An optimized flight plan must not only consider the correct airplane performance and weather forecast but also route restrictions from Air Traffic Control and all relevant regulatory restrictions.

The mathematical nature of these constraints and the overall size of the calculation combined make it a challenging problem, even by modern optimization standards. Some of the equations that describe the behavior are nonlinear and discontinuous, and the airplane state is dynamic. As a result, innumerous calculations and demanding working hours are required for a single flight.

The Optimal Flight Plan

An optimal flight planning scenario for saving fuel (and emissions) involves calculating multiple routes or operating approaches for each flight, ranking these scenarios with regards to total cost and then choosing the scenario that best accomplishes the airline´s cost objectives while providing summaries of the other scenarios for operational flexibility.

While the scenario chosen by the system might be used most of the time, dispatchers at an airline control center may choose another scenario to meet the airline operational goals, such as routing of airplanes, crews, and passengers.

The best route to fly depends on the actual conditions of each flight. These include the forecast upper air winds and temperatures, the amount of payload, and the time-based costs that day. The time-based costs are especially dynamic, driven by the value of the payload and the schedule and operational constraints for the crew and the airplane. Winds can have a significant impact on the optimal route: They can be very far from the great circle "direct" route (Figs. **8.2** and **8.3a&b**). Flight planning systems use international wind forecasts (*i.e.* Wide Area Forecast Center produced by the U.K. Meteorological Office), updated between one to six hours, to include the winds in every flight plan calculation.

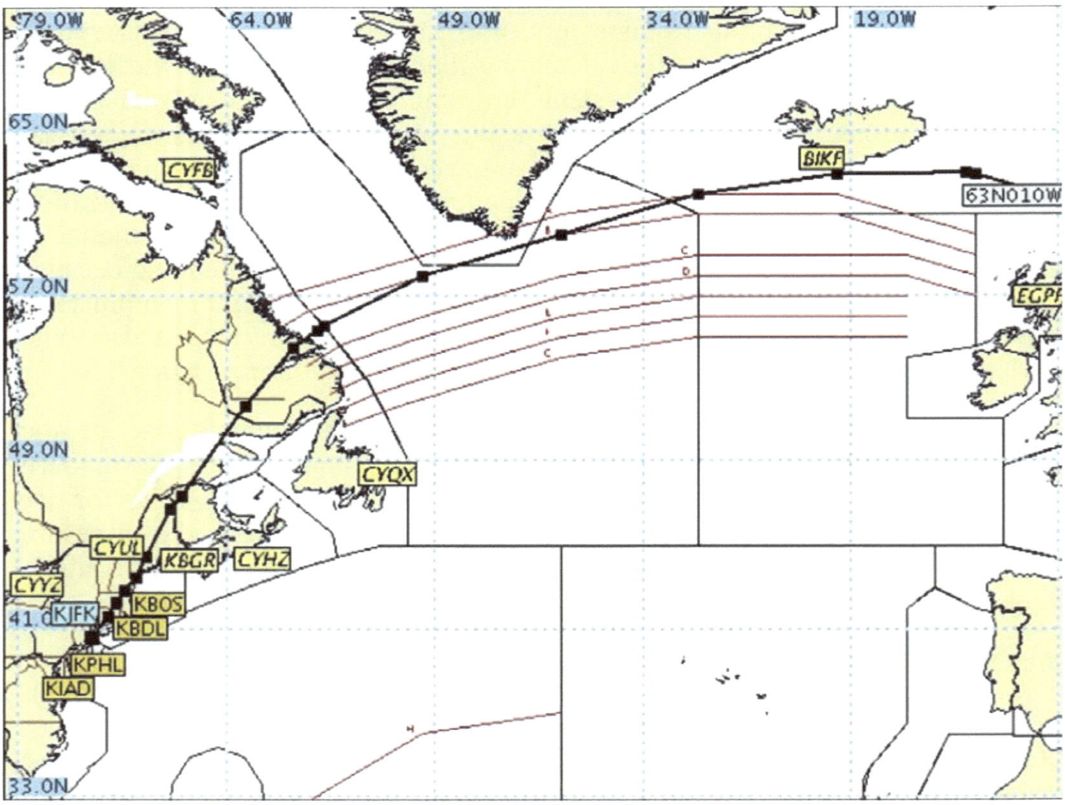

Fig. (8.2). Optimized Routes for North Atlantic (Computerized Flight Plan).

While nearly all computer flight planning systems can optimize routes, many airlines still mainly use fixed "company routes." One reason that the adoption of dynamic route optimization has been limited is that Air Traffic Control (ATC) organizations, overflight permissions, and company policies place restrictions on routing in certain areas. An effective flight planning system contains models of all these restrictions, which are then applied as constraints in the numerical optimization process. This allows the flight plan to be optimized with the dynamic data on winds, temperatures, and costs while still complying with all restrictions.

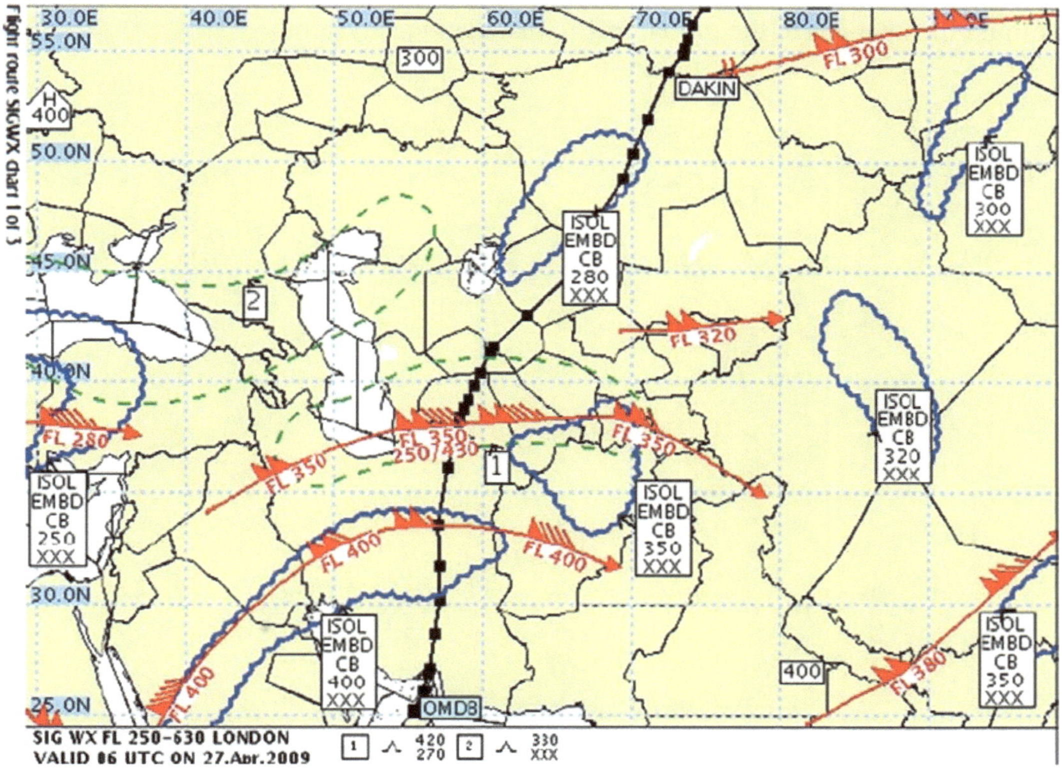

Fig. (8.3a). Flight Plan lateral profile optimized with wind forecast.

The advanced flight planning systems can also recalculate the flight plan while the airplane is already in flight, the so-called rerouting. Winds, temperature, convective weather, and ATC congestions have a sizeable impact on the optimal 4D path for an airplane. Over a long-flight course, this information may change significantly, and the predeparture flight plan may no longer be optimal. The airline operation center has more information about weather and traffic far ahead of the airplane, as well as about the dynamic costs associated with other flights -

related to crew, airplane, and passenger connections, so the flight planning system can find better solutions than those from the flight crew working with the flight management system in an isolated manner. The new route and latest forecast winds can interact directly to the FMS, minimizing crew workload and fuel consumption. Briefly, altitude, and speed optimization will also be made possible by 4D trajectory-based approaches, such as predicted in the Next Generation Air Transportation System, which is FAA's plan to modernize the national airspace system through 2025, and the Single European Sky Air Traffic Management Research Programme (SESAR) [7]. Ongoing research goes beyond compliance with novel approaches, identifying opportunities for improved optimization that build on the changes to the global traffic management system.

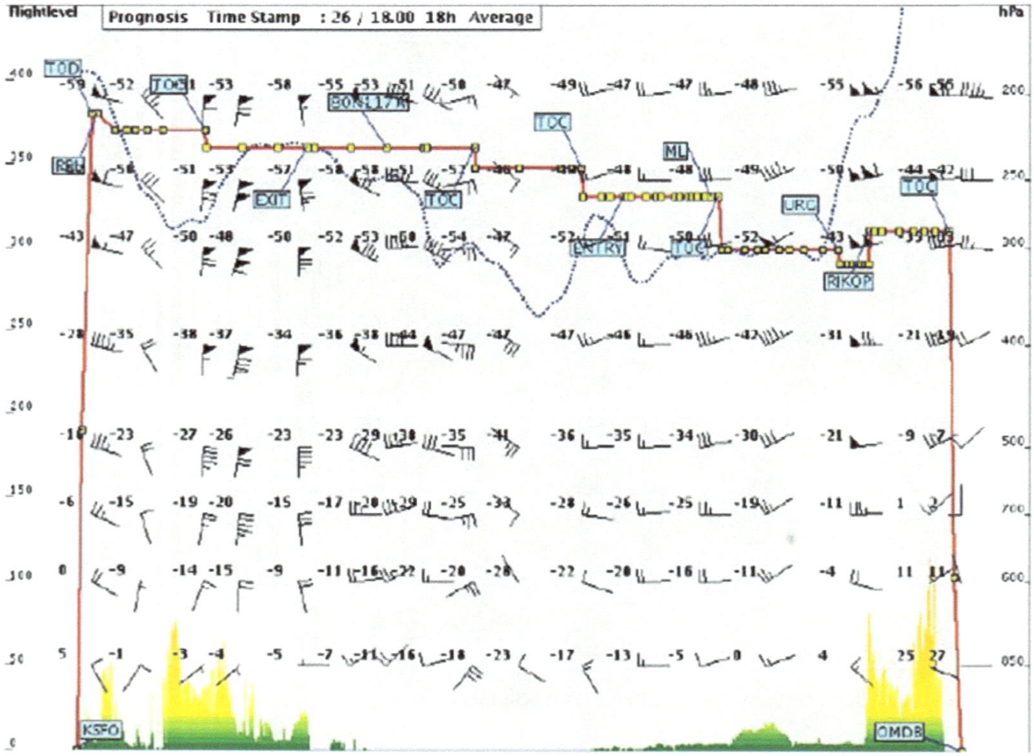

Fig. (8.3b). Flight Plan vertical profile optimized with wind forecast.

The future of flight planning optimization is attempting to provide a deep integration with other flight operation efforts, such as disruption recovery, integrated operations control, and collaborative decision-making widely adopted by air traffic management. Current systems are already able to evaluate different costs for arriving at separate times. These costs, however, will not be independent from a single flight anymore, but related to the decisions made for all flights of an airline's network. For instance, cost for passengers, crew, and the airplane itself to arrive at a specific time depending on when the next flights will depart or arrive. Combining the different operational decisions and optimizing them will lead to better solutions considering the multiple constraints in the operations.

Center of Gravity Management

During the dispatch phase, the location of the center of gravity (CG) needs to be precisely calculated, especially at the beginning of the flight. Looking at the longitudinal stability perspective, it can be established that: the more forward the CG is, the more stable the aircraft is and therefore the less submitted to turbulence and gust effects it is.

At the aft center of gravity, the lift required for static equilibrium at the tail is reduced due to the reduction of the distance between the lift generated at the wings and the weight. Therefore, a smaller angle of attack is necessary to generate a lower lift at the wings for the speed. If the angle of attack lowers, less drag is generated and therefore less thrust is required at cruise conditions. Less thrust implies smaller fuel flows and therefore the conclusion is that aft CG means less fuel consumption (Fig. **8.4**). For large-jet transport aircraft if CG is moved 1% afterwards, approximately 0.1-0.2% of fuel consumption per hour is reduced.

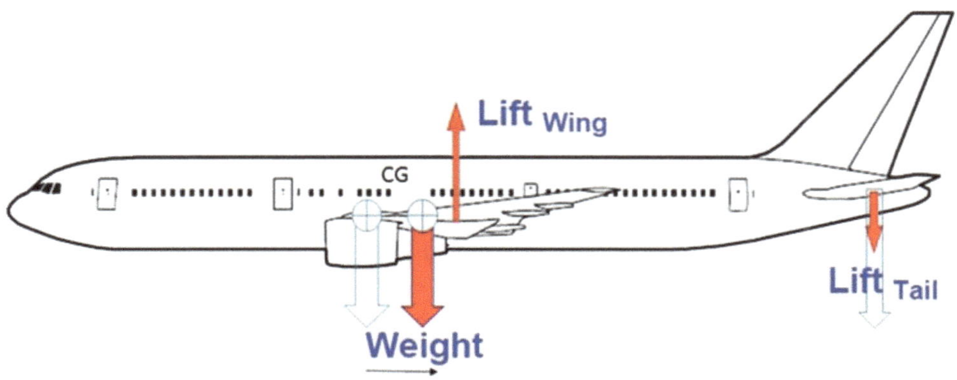

Fig. (8.4). Moving the CG aft unloads the horizontal stabilizer resulting into lower drag for the configuration.

In terms of longitudinal stability, the lower the static margin is (distance between the aerodynamic center and CG) the more unstable, more maneuverable and more sensitive to turbulence and gusts the aircraft is. Therefore, for the design of modern airplanes, small static longitudinal stability is usually the goal, frequently referred to as relaxed static stability to capture the benefit of improved fuel efficiency. Modern jetliners are designed to be aerodynamically efficient, and stability is augmented artificially so that stick force gradients will meet certification requirements.

Augmented stability provides better cruise performance with no increase of workload and no adverse effects due to flight with aft CG. This technology also allows for a smaller tail size, which further reduces drag and weight. For example, Boeing 777 uses redundant digital flight control computers to provide positive (static longitudinal) stability and enhances that stability with airspeed feedback. The MD-11 uses computers to provide neutral speed stability. In other words, the CG of the MD-11 appears to be at the neutral point transferring fuel from tail to wing tanks and vice versa during all the flight.

A simple operational procedure is frequently adopted by airlines to guarantee the lowest possible fuel consumption, despite the presence of stability augmentation systems: dispatchers always have the main goal to equalize the cargo and passengers load as aft as possible, respecting the CG-weight envelope. This will ensure that at least during the first phases of the flight the fuel consumption is optimized.

In-flight Strategies

After dispatch, operating and maneuvering the aircraft using all recommended operational techniques provided by the manufacturer as well as all technological resources available is the secret for efficient operations and therefore operational cost reductions. The main goal is always to perform as close as possible to the planned flight path (predicted by the dispatch process) and, through tactical initiatives in-flight, optimize the fuel burn and flight time even more.

Since the mid-eighties, with the improvement of computational capabilities, the Flight Management System has been helping flight crews to optimize the vertical and lateral navigation of the computerized flight plans. Lateral navigation tactical decisions, such as route shortcuts, may reduce ground distance significantly and have the largest potential to reduce fuel and time. Practical experiences show that the fuel savings may reach up to 10% using only "direct to waypoint" navigation strategy in cruise phase, in synergy with ATC initiatives [8, 9].

The adoption of flexible airspace structures and Performance Based Navigation (PBN) being more and more implemented enroute since the year 2000 have helped to improve gains with computerized systems. Global Navigation Satellite System based operations permit more direct routings, independent from any ground navigation infrastructure. However, the management of the vertical navigation has been explored as the new computational technologies evolved.

Up to the seventies fixed speed schedules had to be continuously manually adjusted by the flight crew (as function of weight and environmental conditions), thus increasing their workload, making them operate frequently under suboptimum conditions. Normally the main objective of the airlines was to minimize fuel burn (and therefore emissions) and, as a second priority, time management was the focus. However, with the increase of the traffic worldwide after the liberalization of many markets at the beginning of the eighties, the congestion of the airspace started to become critical for airlines, since ground delays, expanded taxi times and holdings were common as strategy for terminal area flow management adopted by the Air Traffic Control (ATC). Time also became a critical factor and therefore was another variable to be optimized besides fuel on flight operations. It is remarkable that minimizing in-flight delays also directly minimizes fuel burn and therefore emission reductions.

The development of the FMS and Auto Throttle Systems represented natural technological solutions adopted by the aircraft manufacturers to minimize fuel consumption and time simultaneously, with the objective of lowering direct operational costs of flights. Since the early eighties, flights were then conducted with variable speed schedules (adjusted automatically) with this same objective. Consequently, the crew workload was minimized which was one of the drivers that led to the removal of the flight engineer of the cockpit (representing also a reduction of the operating costs of airlines).

THE COST INDEX CONCEPT

The minimization of the direct operational cost of an airline flight, and therefore the adoption of a variable speed schedule along all the profile, was only possible with the introduction of the COST INDEX concept and its implementation in the FMS speed management and vertical navigation algorithms. To understand this concept, it is first necessary to identify the Direct Operational Costs of operations of a flight. This may be generically expressed through the following E.q **8.3**:

$$DOC = Cfix + Ct.T + Cf.Wf \quad \textbf{(8.3)}$$

Where:

Cfix: fixed costs ($)
Ct: Time Related Costs ($/hour)
T: Total Flight time (hours)
Cf: Fuel related costs ($/kg)
Wf: Total Fuel Burned (kg)

The COST INDEX (CI) is then defined as the ratio (E.q **8.4**):

$$CI = Ct/Cf \tag{8.4}$$

Notice that Eq. **8.3** is function of flight speed over flight time (T) and trip fuel (W_f) is directly dependable on this parameter for a given range. Also, Ct and Cf are constants which depend exclusively on the airline cost management structure. Considering that $T=R/V$ (where R is a given range and V is the true airspeed and Vw is the direct wind component) the Equation 1 may be rearranged as (E.q **8.5**):

$$\frac{\mathbf{DOC}}{\mathbf{R}} = \frac{\mathbf{Cf.(CI+FF)}}{\mathbf{V+Vw}} \tag{8.5}$$

The ratio DOC/R represents the Direct Operational Cost per distance unit of a given flight, and the dependence of this quantity on flight speed and fuel consumption per unit of time (fuel flow, which is also a function of flight speed). It can be noticed that the Direct Operational Cost is minimized when the ratio (CI+FF)/V is minimum. This only happens when the flight is conducted at the so-called economic speed (V_{econ}), as shown in Fig. (**8.5**). This speed is determined by derivation of **Eq. 8.5** equaling it to zero. In this case - for reasons of simplification - a parabolic drag polar and a constant specific fuel consumption is assumed (TSFC), where V_{econ} is obtained solving the following E.q **8.6**:

$$\frac{CI}{W*TSFC} = C_{D0} * \left(\frac{(Vecon+Vw)^2}{V*^2}\right) - 3 * K * \left(\frac{V*^2}{(Vecon+Vw)^2}\right) \tag{8.6}$$

Where:

$V *= \sqrt{\frac{2*W}{\rho.S}}$ (m/s);
CI: Cost index (kg/s);
W: aircraft weight (N);
TSFC: Thrust specific fuel consumption (Kg/h/N);
S: Reference wing area (m^2);
ρ: air density (kg/m^2);
V_w: direct wind component (m/s);
Vecon: Economic cruise speed (m/s);
C_{D0}: Zero Lift Coefficient;
K: Induced drag coefficient;

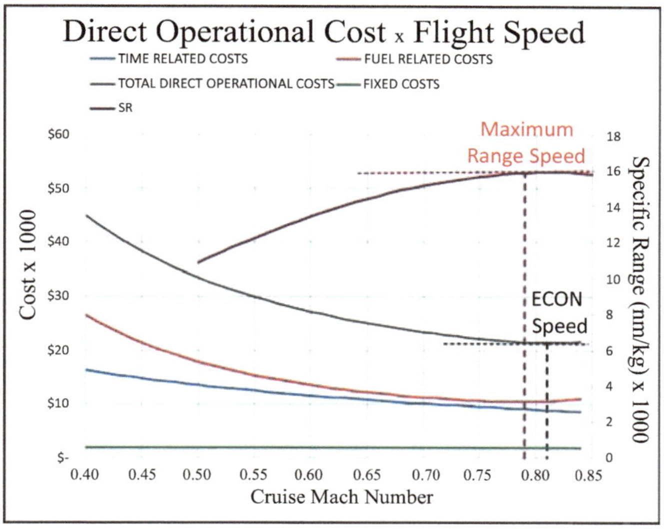

Fig. (8.5). Economic Speed Selection (example on cruise phase).

Notice that when CI →0 (*i.e.* fuel related costs are much more significant than time) V_{econ} tends to the maximum range speed obtained analytically (considering zero direct wind component) as $\mathbf{Vecon_{CI=0}} = \mathbf{V} *. \sqrt[4]{(\frac{3K}{C_{D0}})}$, for jet transport aircraft. On the other hand, if the time related costs are relatively larger than the fuel costs, (for example in lower fuel cost scenarios or when hourly labor rates are expressively high), flight time is a critical factor and shall be reduced as much as possible. This is achieved by accelerating flight speeds, limited to the maximum certified structural values (VMO or MMO) minus a certain margin (normally 5 kt or Mach number of 0.005). In this case, fuel consumption - and therefore emissions - is increased.

It is important to mention that while using the COST INDEX technique, winds are part of the cost optimization equation and therefore the flight speed must be adjusted depending on the direct wind component to minimize the cost function (expressed by **Eq. 8.5**), while maintaining the relative proportion of time and fuel costs. For example, the FMS will increase the economic speed in case of headwinds, and decrease in case of tailwinds. Thus, the selected economic speed will vary as a function of winds, even if the COST INDEX zero is held (maximum-range speed).

In addition, the regular setting of the modern FMS does not allow the flight speed to drop below the maximum specific range speed in cruise. Although possible in terms of performance (holding speed is lower than COST INDEX zero speed) flying on the left side of the specific range curve may lead to the backlash region of the drag polar where the aircraft may experience an undesired deceleration trend in case of turbulent air penetration.

LEGACY FUEL CONSERVATION TECHNIQUES IN VERTICAL PROFILE

As mentioned before until the eighties airlines adopted manual speed adjustment in all flight phases, which were not optimized and managed automatically *via* FMS or planned *via* a computerized flight planning system. At that time (right after the seventies oil crisis) a set of techniques has been developed by manufacturers with the sole objective to save fuel. The COST INDEX idea, minimizing fuel and time costs, has already been elaborated but it remains a complex matter to be implemented without an automated speed management system.

Typical techniques developed to save fuel in the vertical profile are described in the following sections.

Cruise Techniques

As shown in Fig. (**8.5**), in theory, the best speed to save fuel (and therefore reduce emissions) would be the one correspondent to the maximum range, which maximizes the ratio $M\,{}^{L}/_{D}$ in cruise. However, this speed is generally slower when compared with typical cruise values managed by ATC, also causing longer flight times. To reduce the time delays, operators generally choose to fly at the so-called Long-range Cruise (LRC) during the cruise phase, which represents the speed correspondent to the 99% of the maximum specific range. This selection provides an increase up to approximately 30-40 kt (or 0.1-0.2 Mach number increase at typical cruise altitudes) over maximum range cruise speed (MRC) representing a -1% penalty on the best fuel consumption schedule, taking advantage of the flatness of the specific range curve near the maximum specific range region. Until the implementation of the FMS, this was the airlines speed strategy used to minimize fuel consumption in cruise. Manufacturers then provided in the flight operations manuals dedicated tables to be used by crews to constantly perform manual adjustments on thrust levers to achieve the correct LRC speeds. It is important to notice that the LRC regimes do not have any dependence on direct wind effects, looking only at the specific range curve, and therefore the direct operational cost is most of the times sub-optimized while selecting this flight regime. In addition, depending on the cruise length (*i.e.* weight variation impact on C_L not significant in such a way that cruise Mach variation is less than 0.01, typically expected on flight lengths below 4 hours), LRC could be replaced by a fixed speed. This represented a significant simplification on dispatch calculation and crew workload.

The initial cruise altitude was set to be correspondent to the best specific range for a given weight, cruise speed (LRC) and atmospheric conditions. After that, the best strategy to save fuel during the cruise phase is to fly LRC while continuously tracking the Optimum Altitude. However, this procedure represents a challenging strategy since the Optimum Altitude constantly increases as fuel burns and the aircraft weight decreases, thus also changing the *L/D* condition. Typically, optimum altitude rates of climb are between 10 to 20 ft/min for jet transport aircraft, which are very hard to follow even with the current autopilot technology. The solution adopted since the beginning of the jet aviation is to proceed with discrete climb steps of 4000 ft (or 2000 ft in Reduced Vertical Separation Minima –RVSM airspace) around the Optimum Altitude, restricted to ATC flight level rules (Fig. **8.6**).

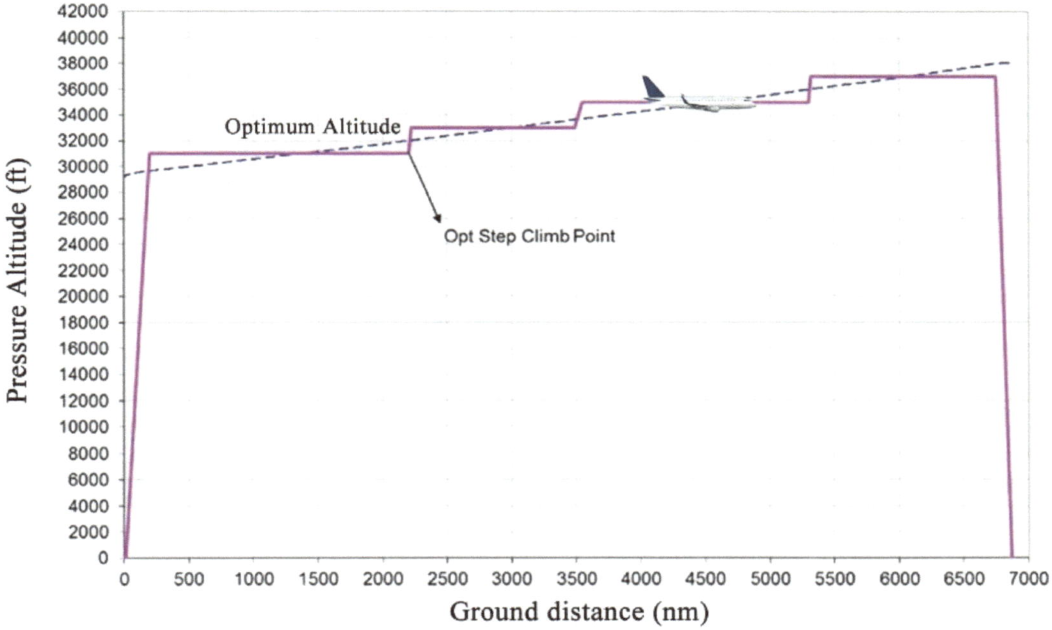

Fig. (8.6). typical step climb profile (2000ft steps on RVSM airspace).

The technique consists of performing the flight at a constant cruise altitude which is 2000 ft (or 1000 ft in RVSM airspace) below the optimum altitude. At such a point, a climb to the next allowable altitude is executed (2000 ft or 4000 ft above the current altitude). This is the so called "step climb technique", often used during long international flights. It is remarkable that step climbs are feasible only after each 150-200 minutes of levelled cruise flights, typically used above 1000-nm flight legs.

Climb and Descent Techniques

In the past, climb and descent speeds were also normally selected with the main objective to minimize fuel consumption, which in the tactical scenario sometimes needed adjustment to comply with ATC requirements. With this objective, in theory, climb speeds should be initially selected as near as possible to the maximum rate of climb speed Vy (at constant IAS) since this minimizes climb time to the cruise altitude. Regardless of ATC constraints, this speed (in terms of indicated airspeed) was generally maintained until the altitude when the cruise Mach number is intercepted (normally above 20000 ft when air compressibility starts to influence performance). Afterwards, Mach number is kept constant until the capture of the cruise altitude. Typical *Vy* speeds for jet transport aircraft were selected from 230 to 280 KIAS, depending on weight.

During the descent phase, the speed schedule strategy was set in an analogous manner as carried out for the climb. The initial descent speed was set normally to the cruise Mach flown up to a selected indicated airspeed which was maintained down to the approach or ATC constraints. To save fuel, at least in theory, the minimum fuel speed should be set as close as possible to the maximum *L/D* speed (best glide speed), which is also very slow considering ATC requirements (typically between 180 kt to 230 kt indicated airspeed for jet transport aircraft). These airlines usually adopted faster speed schedules during the lower phases of the descent to minimize the delays. Considering that the aircraft is most of the times at idle thrust at this phase, the difference in fuel consumption between the max L/D speed and any other selected speed below 250 KIAS is normally not significant. Therefore, in the descent phase speed was normally planned considering the minimization of delays rather than fuel consumption. Typical descent speeds for jet transport aircraft were selected between 280 and 310 KIAS, depending on weight.

It is worth mentioning that either in climb or descent profiles, the 250 KIAS restriction below 10,000 ft needs to be respected in most of the controlled airspaces in the world - airspaces class A, B and C according to ICAO classification [10], turning the fuel optimization during these phases even less efficient.

In summary, without the FMS and Autothrottle assistance for speed management, fixed-speed schedules were normally set at climb and descent phases, and manually by crews during the cruise phase, in this case LRC settings. This was convenient for crews and dispatchers (who were beginning to receive assistance by computerized systems, using mostly manual processes to plan the flights). Fig. (**8.7**) shows a typical legacy fuel conservation vertical profile operation. However, this strategy generally does not correspond to the minimum cost of operations, which involves also time as the parameter of optimization.

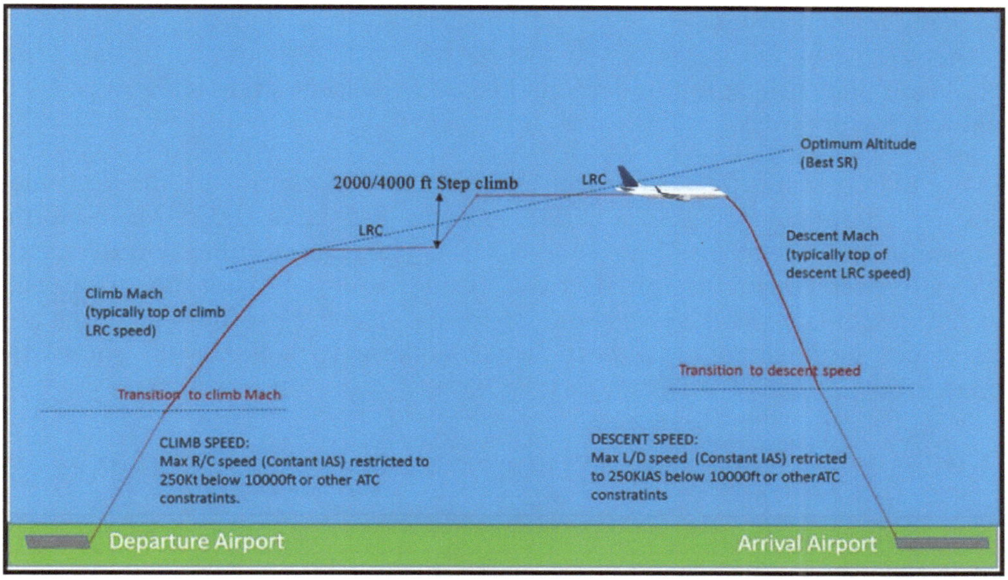

Fig. (8.7). typical "legacy" profile on early fuel conservation operation.

The Enhanced Cost Optimization Technique in Vertical Profile

After the development and enhancement of the FMS and Auto throttle systems, it was finally possible to implement the cost index concept in a reliable and efficient manner, permitting the flight speed to be fully managed in the whole vertical profile with the objective to minimize the total direct operational costs. The first aircraft to have a robust and complete cost index algorithm were the Boeing 757 and 767, followed by the Airbus A300/310 series, certified in the early eighties.

Time and fuel were now simultaneously optimized in a successful way. Economic speeds (in terms of IAS and Mach), based on the cost index concept, are now calculated and managed by the FMS in synchronization with Auto throttles and refreshed at short intervals of time. Therefore, variable speeds are commanded during all the flight, driven by cost index algorithms. As already mentioned, since time is now involved, wind effects could significantly affect the flight speeds.

An interesting fact to remark on, is that at cost index zero (where time related costs are negligible) the FMS commands the minimum fuel consumption profile, but now also adjusted to wind effects. In this case, the following pattern is attained:

- Climb speeds are driven to the maximum rate of climb;
- Cruise speeds at maximum range cruise (MRC);
- Descent speeds to best glide angle in case of zero direct wind component, like the legacy flight profiles.
- The net result in the trajectory is the shortest intercept of the initial cruise altitude and the earliest top of descent, since the descent angle is correspondent to the shallower profile.

At a very high cost index (where time related costs are significant), the maximum speeds are commanded within a certain margin (3-5 kt or 0.005 Mach) to the maximum operating speeds (VMO and MMO). The net result in the trajectory is the longest intercept of the initial cruise altitude and the latest top of descent, since the descent angle is correspondent to the steepest profile. All other cost index values produce trajectories in between these two. Fig. (**8.8**) shows the difference in profiles of different cost indexes.

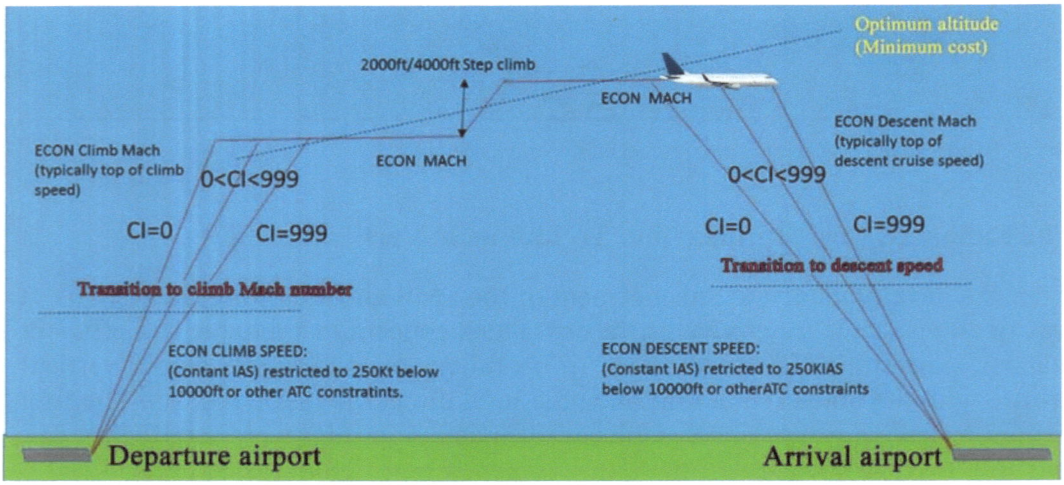

Fig. (8.8). economic speeds vertical profiles for operational cost optimization.

At the same time, the computerized flight planning systems also evolved considering the dispatch calculations with updated wind forecasts along the route and economic speeds based on cost index. Step climb points may be calculated by the flight planning systems now considering the minimum cost altitudes, instead of maximum specific range. Thus, the aircraft could be dispatched more accurately and many times more efficient than based on FMS predictions. It is important to emphasize once again that the economic speeds profile will always produce the lowest operational cost for the airline (optimizing time and fuel simultaneously), while the "legacy" fuel conservation profile will produce the lowest fuel burn only.

The Cost Challenge

After the cost index algorithms implementation, the biggest challenge for the airlines changed from accurate speed management with focus on fuel conservation to the accurate determination of the cost coefficients (Ct and Cf) since they were now the key factors to ensure the optimal vertical profile leading to the lowest direct operational costs.

The fuel related costs (Cf) are relatively easy to determine, since their value depends on external supplier contractual deals. However, the time related costs are the challenging component of the Direct Operating Costs. It is generally not easy for airlines to identify what operational costs are variable with time due to the complexity of operations and cross dependence of the departments. For example, maintenance costs (one of the most difficult to raise) may be divided by some airlines into labor and airframe costs. The latter is related to the component repair, which may incur in cycles, flight time or even through a failure condition event. Also, engines, auxiliary power units, and airplanes can be leased by the hour or owned by a private person, and maintenance costs can be accounted for an airplane by the hour, by the calendar, or by cycles. As a result, each of these items may have a direct hourly cost or a fixed cost over a calendar period with limited or no correlation to flight time. Crews may be paid by the hour, fixed salaries or a combination of both, *etc.*

This poses the question of how to identify and control the time relation of this kind of costs. Some airlines divide the total maintenance costs by block hours, others prefer to determine exactly this value by tracking each component. A wide discussion on airline strategies as how to determine the time related costs can be found in Doganis [3].

Therefore, due to the complexity involved in Ct determination many airlines use the average value of the COST INDEX determination for each route, which depends only on the fuel cost variation at every station. Another option might be the use of average Cf and Ct of a single COST INDEX for all routes, typically used for networks where the routes are short with small fuel price variations. However, with the improvements and integration of the finance computer systems with other departments (such as maintenance), airlines are more enthusiastic in determining the exact value of Ct and Cf for each route and then ultimately minimizing the direct operational costs.

AIRCRAFT CONDITION MONITORING

Overview

The condition of the airframe and engines have a direct impact on aircraft fuel consumption. Therefore, the monitoring of the aircraft performance is an essential activity that airlines developed to ensure that the drag and engines degradations are kept as low as possible with the objective to reduce fuel burn and emissions. With the objective to help airlines with this task the aircraft manufacturers developed the so-called Aircraft Performance Monitoring Programs (APM).

The first step to start monitoring the aircraft condition is the definition of the aircraft book-performance status. This represents the fleet average of brand new airframe and engine levels, established through mathematical models in advance of the production process and it is the reference for the determination of the aircraft deterioration over time. The nominal scatter of brand new aircraft leads to individual performance above or below the book value. The performance levels are then measured in their variations from book performance over time which may be used on statistical analysis of resulting trends, used by operators in various departments to perform corrective actions to maintain a satisfactory aircraft airworthiness. It is worth mentioning that the actual aircraft performance deterioration originates from two main causes: engine performance degradation (increase of fuel consumption at a given thrust) and airframe deterioration (seals, doors, slats and flaps rigging, spoilers rigging, surface roughness, *etc*..) linked to the zero lift drag. Therefore, the performance degradation is primarily measured in terms of drag and fuel flow deviation from the book performance.

Once the book performance and degradation levels are defined, a starting point is required to evaluate trends in performance deterioration. The baseline level is an aircraft performance level retained as a reference to get the trend of aircraft performance deterioration. Most of the times the baseline is established at the aircraft entry into service during the first flight or delivery flight which may be above or below the book level because of above-mentioned scatter. The APM Program is then set as a process to determine the airframe and engine degradation for single aircraft (or a fleet of aircraft) to analyze the trends of the performance degradation over time with the objective to identify patterns and apply the necessary corrective actions in maintenance (*i.e.* need for engine washes, flight controls rigging or surface polishing).

From the flight operation perspective, the results of the aircraft performance monitoring are used to adjust the flight plans and FMS to calculate the most accurate fuel burn, permitting a better planning and fuel predictions for each flight. Flight plans are therefore more reliable and permit the right planning of the fuel loaded on board when such adjustments are applied. However, the adjustment is made by the so-called "performance factor" which is calculated as a composition of the average drag and fuel flow degradations into a single number which is directly applied to the fuel burn predictions on either FMS or Flight Planning systems. The performance factor may be determined from the drag and fuel flow degradation measured at each monitored flight by the following set of equations:

$$\mathbf{DFF} = \frac{1}{\mathbf{N}}\sum_{\mathbf{i=1}}^{\mathbf{N}}(\mathbf{FFi} - \mathbf{FFibook})/\mathbf{FFibook} \tag{8.7}$$

$$\mathbf{DDRAG} = \frac{1}{\mathbf{N}}\sum_{\mathbf{i=1}}^{\mathbf{N}}(\mathbf{DRAGi} - \mathbf{DRAGibook})/\mathbf{DRAGibook} \tag{8.8}$$

$$\text{DSR} = -(\text{DDRAG}+\text{DFF}) \tag{8.9}$$

$$\text{PF} = 1/(1+\text{DSR}) \tag{8.10}$$

Where:

N: number of data points monitored in stable cruise condition;
FFi: Actual fuel flow measured at data point *i*;
FFibook: Theoretical fuel flow calculated for data point I at the related operational conditions (weight, speed, altitude, environment, *etc*…);
DRAGi: Actual drag measured at data point *i*;
DRAGibook: Theorectical drag calculated for data point i at the related operational conditions (weight, speed, altitude, environment, *etc*…);
DFF: Average Fuel flow degradation (deviation from book performance);
DDRAG: Average Drag Degradation (deviation from book performance);
DSR: Average Specific Range Degradation;
PF: Performance Factor to be applied in the Flight Plan and FMS adjustment for fuel burn.

Several flight data parameters are supposed to be collected at stable cruise conditions to compute the actual drag (or thrust required) and fuel flow (Mach, pressure altitude, ambient temperature, power settings, linear/angular accelerations, heading, wind speed and direction are examples of basic parameters). Automatic data sets are collected *via* Aircraft Condition Monitoring Systems (ACMS) programmed on very straight stabilization criteria, defined for a certain time interval. For example, on the Boeing 777 the ACMS is normally programmed to define a stable cruise condition in a three-minute period where Mach Number cannot vary more than 0.004, pressure altitude by 80ft and heading change by 2 degrees (among others). Once the stabilization condition is satisfied, the set of flight parameters is saved on a solid-state memory which is downloaded later by ground maintenance for the APM analysis. Normally, few points achieve the complete stable criteria of each flight. On long range flights (more than 10 hours), three or four stable points are usually collected.

The minimum number of points to be collected for each aircraft to provide reliable results is related to the normal distribution. Therefore, samples beyond 20 elements are usually considered by airlines for APM analysis. Samples are generally very scattered. The larger the number of points collected, the better the quality of analysis is. Most airlines collect sufficient points for an airplane in as little as a month, ensuring that samples are large enough to compensate the scattering characteristics. Once collected, data are processed *via* a specific software designed to determine the drag and engine degradations and perform the historical data analysis. The interpretation of the performance degradation trends is the key to determine further actions to be applied on the aircraft (maintenance or operations). Fig. (**8.9**) shows the complete APM cycle for operational performance.

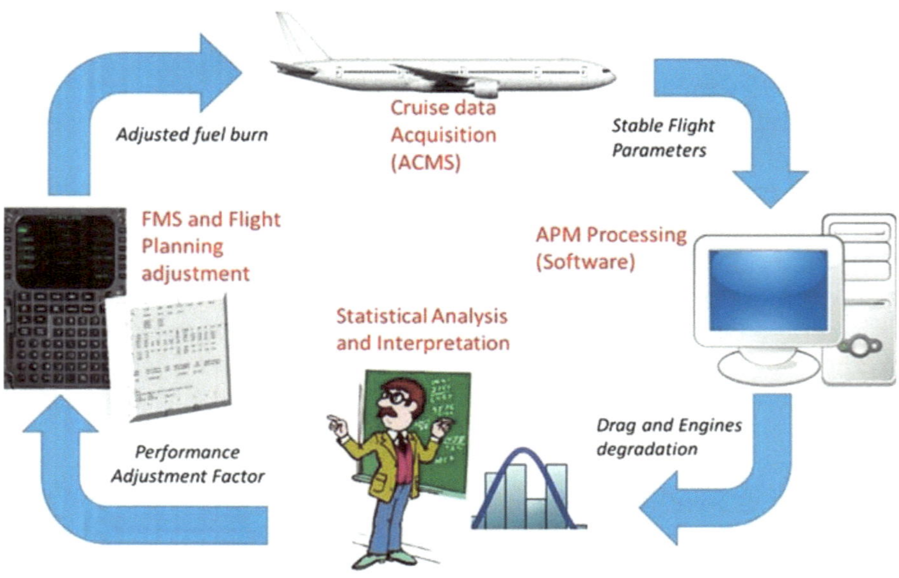

Fig. (8.9). APM Cycle for flight operations.

The adoption of an APM Program allows operators to perform various statistics about fuel consumption and as such is a good aid to define the operators' fuel policy. In addition, some regulations permit the reduction of the regulatory fuel contingency if the airline adopts such a program instead. For example, according to FAA ETOPS rules, the performance factor to be applied in the flight plan may be reduced to the computed performance factor instead of the required 5%.

So, what else can airlines do to reduce the impact of specific range degradation?

Drag Degradation

As discussed above, drag control is one of the key elements to maintain the aircraft performance as close as possible to "the book". It is observed that between 40%-50% of the total specific range degradation is related to drag increase.

As stated in almost all aerodynamics books, the total drag of the aircraft is composed of compressible drag, induced drag, and parasite drag (or C_{D0}). The latter is influenced by the boundary-layer skin friction coefficient and is highly dependent on the wet area and surface finishing.

The additional drag of the airplane due to the sum of all the deviations from smooth sealed external surfaces, the so-called excrescence drag, is responsible for a significant part of the total zero lift drag and usually lies in the 3-5% range of the total drag of the aircraft [11, 12]. This is the part of the drag that the airline may have control of and, if well managed, influences positively the performance of the aircraft, directly related to the roughness and irregularities of the aircraft skin (non-flush fasteners, gaps, waviness and surface finishing), internal airflow, air leakage, mismatched gaps and some discrete items (such as antennas, masts and lights).

Fig. (**8.10**) shows a picture of the EMB-111 Bandeirulha, a twin-turboprop maritime patrol airplane. By analyzing the airplane, some sources of excrescence drag can be easily recognized:

- Antennas;
- External radio cable;
- Navigation and anti-collision lights;
- Scoopers and naca inlets.
- Windshield wipers;
- Engine exhaust ducts;
- Wing fences;
- Deicing boots at wing and vertical tail leading edges;
- Rain rail above the rear door;

- Static electricity dischargers;
- Flap actuators;
- Current diverter strip of radome
- Search lights casing;
- Pitot probes.

Although there are many sources of excrescence drag of the airplane shown in Fig. (**8.10**), some drag reduction measures like the filling surfaces between the tip tank and the wing, and the wing and the fuselage can be observed. A great part of engine nacelle was placed below the wing, to avoid excess interference drag between these two aircraft components. In addition, tip tanks help to reduce induced drag.

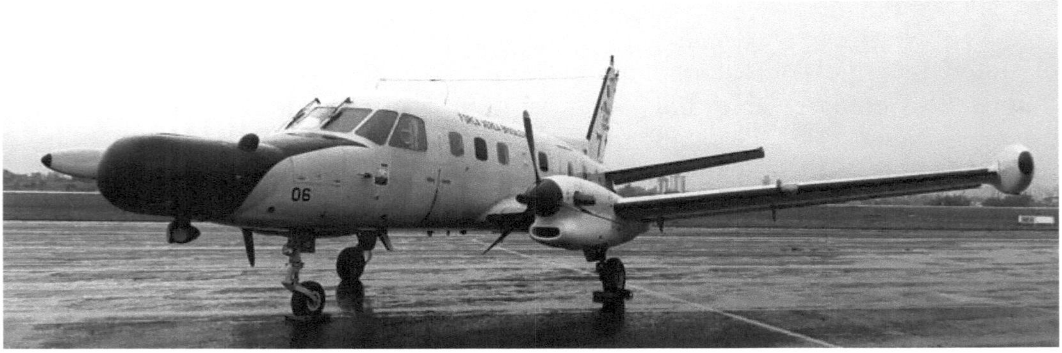

Fig. (8.10). EMB-111 Bandeirulha patrol airplane (Photo: ©2017 Bento Mattos).

Maintenance plans are therefore developed with tasks specifically related to drag assessment and recovery, which are mostly related to the excrescence drag minimization. Some examples of maintenance tasks with this objective are listed below:

- Flight control rigging (ailerons, spoilers, rudders and elevator offsets);
- Check items which are adjustable and could become misaligned after years of service such as adjustable panels and doors fitting (cargo, entry and landing-gear);
- Surface mismatch adjustments;
- Recovering of sealing to avoid air leaks;
- Rough surface paintings;
- Surface washing/cleaning/polishing and dirt removal (0.1% drag reduction);

Proper maintenance applied along the lifespan of the aircraft may present an excrescence drag increase. A well-maintained airplane should not exceed 0.5% drag increase over the new airplane level.

Engine Degradation

The other part of the specific range degradation is related to engine deterioration. However, differently from drag, recovery of degraded performance need to be balanced due to the cost of engine maintenance tasks, which are far more expensive than drag control tasks.

The most common maintenance actions are related to low and high-pressure turbines and compressors which make a major contribution to fuel flow recovery (thrust specific fuel consumption) and require longer maintenance stops on ground, with engine removals for shop deeper examination. Issues usually associated with these components are: blade rubs, thermal distortion of blades, blade leading edge wear, fan rubstrip wear, lining loss on high-pressure compressor, oil or dirt contaminations of compressors. Other contributions are related to seals, valves and cooling components of the engines such as: leak on thrust reverser seals, bleed and air conditioning valve leaks, fan air valves and turbine case cooling leaks.

On-wing engine wash is a relatively simple, quick and cheap task (few man hours are spent on overnight checks) that may be done during specific cycle intervals and may recover up to 1.5% of fuel flow degradation (Fig. **8.11**). Another simple procedure that can be performed are leak repair of bleed valves, providing up to 2.5% recovery of degraded fuel flow.

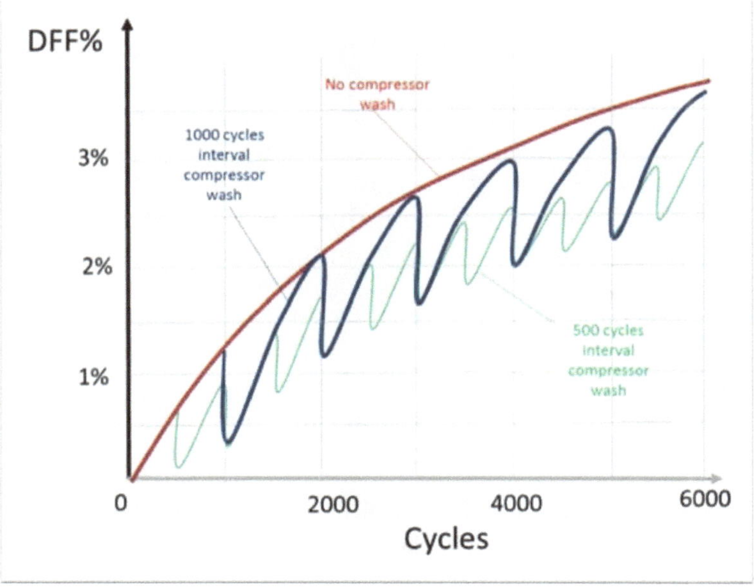

Fig. (8.11). Engine Wash impact on fuel flow degradation

A well-managed APM Program has the potential to provide operators with up to 4% of recovery of fuel efficiency, depending on the operational conditions and the adopted maintenance plan.

THE AIR TRAFFIC MANAGEMENT ROLE

Overview

Air traffic management (ATM) is the dynamic, integrated management of air traffic and airspace including air traffic services, airspace management and air traffic flow management (safely, economically and efficiently) through the provision of facilities and seamless services in collaboration with all stakeholders.

Significant fuel and emission savings can be achieved by employing an efficient ATM system and may lead up to 12% of fuel savings. To ensure the environmental and operational efficiency of air traffic management, the three basic elements of ATM should be addressed and optimized: airspace management, air traffic services and air traffic flow management.

New and established technologies and concepts of operations in Communications, Navigation, and Surveillance (CNS), such as data link, Performance-based Navigation (PBN), Automatic Dependent Surveillance (ADS), flexible use of airspace and Advanced Collaborative Decision Making (CDM) are opportunities to improve the efficiency of ATM. It is extremely important to match airspace planning initiatives with operational limitations and requirements. Airspace planners need to consider factors such as flight operational requirements, aircraft equipage, airspace capacity (including adjacent airspace sectors), location of adjacent airports and routes, interdependencies between arriving and departing traffic, areas of restricted airspace, runway capacities, terminal capacities, taxiway limitations, restrictive terrain and any local or regional environmental regulations or procedures. Each of these areas can influence the effectiveness of air traffic management and the resultant environmental impacts of aircraft operations.

It should be noted that operational efficiency solutions in one phase of the flight should be balanced with possible greater inefficiencies in another flight-phase. ATM procedures and measures must be considered by all operational stakeholders, including the civil and military aviation authorities, air navigation service providers, air traffic controllers, pilots and aircraft operators.

Although a perfect ATM system is a desirable goal many aircraft compete for the best profiles in limited volumes of airspace. Specific details of a fuel-optimized profile are highly dependent upon the aircraft type and the distance flown. Improved fuel efficiency can be achieved through improved aircraft energy management, which relies on the aircraft constantly changing speed and altitude. It is recognized that aircraft may not fly these trajectories for a number reasons, including the provision of safe separation, the existence of restricted airspace, delay management, pilot's accuracy and weather avoidance. However, reference to these profiles for comparison with current performance allows the identification of potential areas for improvement in fuel efficiency.

Opportunities to reduce fuel consumption and increase the safety and efficiency of air traffic operations can be identified through collaboration among all operational stakeholders. Since air traffic operations at any airport are unique due to local conditions, circumstances and limitations, enhancements can be achieved by the establishment of local forums that allow all stakeholders to assess and understand the airspace and its constraints and explore what can be done to improve the safety and efficiency of air traffic management. Under this scope the Air Traffic Control has a key role in operation efficiency and therefore several measures may be adopted under this focus as described in the following sections.

On-Ground Operation Management

The airport is critical to ATM efficiency and has the potential to contribute significantly to reducing delays and therefore fuel consumption (and emissions). Thus, it is critical to analyze the use of airport assets (runways, stands, taxiways and tugs, *etc.*) to ensure a balance between operational and environmental needs.

Technology offers the opportunity to advance the continuous improvement of ATM as for example the introduction of Collaborative Decision Making (CDM) processes, which brings together all airport data and shares it with all stakeholders. The use of CDM can improve the efficiency of ground operations at an airport and deliver fuel and emission savings and can also contribute to significant savings in the departure, enroute and arrival phases of a flight.

By acting collaboratively, airspace users, airports, airlines and other stakeholders can counter-balance known delays by holding aircraft on the ground rather than in the air, where delay or inefficiency leads to higher fuel burn penalties. Some practices may be adopted by the Air Traffic Control to minimize ground delays such as:

- At the departure gate/stand: ATC should keep flight crews informed of pushback and departure delays. This allows them to use the most efficient ground power source;
- If traffic permits, consider gate holds instead of taxi-holds;
- Early notification of departure sequence (*e.g.* "you are number x for take-off") allows the flight crew to safely and efficiently start an engine(s) shut down

during taxi, reducing fuel consumption and possibly reducing taxiway congestion caused by a late engine start or checklist completion;

- To the extent possible, arrange tactical ground aircraft movements and give timely taxi clearances which allow for uninterrupted taxiing and avoid stop-starts of aircraft;
- Prioritize moving aircraft to ground vehicles;
- Consider a marginally longer taxi to allow aircraft to depart on a runway more aligned with its direction of flight;
- If possible and authorized, allow rolling take-offs (enhancing runway capacity);

Departure Management

The climb-out is a critical phase of flight as aircraft can be at their maximum weight. It is particularly important for heavy wake turbulence category aircraft. Consequently, any restrictions on the aircraft's climb-out to an optimum enroute cruising level increase fuel burn and emissions.

A full load of fuel means that a heavier aircraft will burn more fuel to climb. This phase of flight is therefore important in terms of optimization - any efforts to reduce inefficiencies will result in higher fuel and emission savings. As the demand for aviation has grown, airspace around airports has become congested, resulting in increased air traffic complexity. To manage this complexity, airspace control has focused on ensuring that flows are strategically deconflicted by using additional track miles and periods of level flight for climbing and descending aircraft. This compromise has led to aircraft often climbing in a series of steps separated by periods of level flight, to keep them separated from arrival traffic flows and aircraft from other airports. If departures are required to level off at low altitudes or climb at a speed below of what is operationally efficient, the pilots must employ flap settings that will increase drag. Such flap settings require additional thrust to maintain operational control of the aircraft, which increases fuel burn and CO_2 emissions. One of the best potential Air Traffic Control solutions in the climb phase is to ensure that an aircraft can conduct an optimum continuous climb (Continuous Climb Operations) from the runway to cruise altitude without any intermediate steps.

Airspace design to strategically de-conflict arrival and departure flows can facilitate better achievement of continuous climb procedures and therefore delivers a better performance with lower fuel burn. Departure is a critical phase of flight as aircraft can be at their maximum weight. It is particularly important for heavy wake turbulence category aircraft. Consequently, any restrictions on the aircraft climb-out to an optimum enroute cruising level will increase fuel burn and emissions.

One potential ATM solution in the climb phase is to seek to ensure that an aircraft can conduct an optimum continuous climb from runway to cruise altitude. Airspace design to strategically de-conflict arrival and departure flows can facilitate better achievement of continuous climb procedures and therefore delivers better fuel burn performance.

Departure Noise *Versus* Emissions

In the departure phase, there may be significant trade-offs between providing noise relief and emission reductions. Noise abatement procedures were first developed in the 1960's in response to the widespread introduction of the first generation of turbojet air carrier aircraft. Since then, through the evolution of new engine technologies and ICAO noise standards, there has been considerable reduction in source noise. Consequently, the noise footprints of new jet aircraft are significantly smaller than those of the early generation jet aircraft they replaced.

Noise abatement procedures may come at the expense of additional fuel burn. The ICAO Standards for noise abatement [13] states that aircraft operating procedures for noise abatement shall not be introduced unless the regulatory authority, based on appropriate studies and consultation, determines that a noise problem exists. Additionally, aircraft operating procedures for noise abatement should be developed in consultation with the operators which use the aerodrome concerned. Therefore, it is recommended that Civil Aviation Authorities should routinely review noise abatement departure procedures and discontinue noise abatement procedures where they are not justified.

The need to avoid noise sensitive areas at low altitudes can lead to extra track mileage and fuel burn in the Terminal Areas. There is potential for Performance Based Navigation (PBN) departure routes to optimize the noise performance of departing aircraft while simultaneously reducing flight track miles at lower altitudes. They have the potential to allow aircraft to optimize fuel uplift. Carrying extra contingency fuel can significantly affect the weight of the aircraft and therefore its fuel burn performance. Airline industry flight planning tools are increasingly tuned to reduce carriage of extra fuel. Shorter PBN routes can enable less trip fuel.

Enroute Management

As previously mentioned the aircraft cruise performance varies, depending on factors such as weight, range, wind and weather conditions as well as airspace characteristics. Modern onboard Flight Management Systems (FMS) are now able to determine the most efficient cruise altitude and speed to optimize fuel burn or operational costs.

Air Traffic Control (ATC) may assist in this process by providing capacity in the enroute phase of flight that offers aircraft the cruise levels and speeds requested. Also, efficiency gains are enabled when ATC offers aircraft routing or altitude changes to take advantage of favorable wind conditions. As aircraft approach the end of their enroute phase of flight (top of descent), ATC can potentially offer improved streaming to enable continuous descents and required times of arrivals (RTA) managed by the FMS to improve the efficiency of flows and reduce holdings at Terminal Areas. Therefore, some common tactical actions performed by ATC to reduce fuel burn in cruise are:

- Allow cruise or step climbs at pilot's discretion when traffic permits;
- Offer higher altitudes when available, even when not requested by the pilot; Approve speed variances when requested;
- Cancel speed restrictions when no longer required;
- Offer direct or wind optimized routes where available;
- If a coordination mechanism is in place, offer direct routing through military airspace when not in use.

Descent Management

Opportunities for reductions in fuel burn and emissions in the descent phase through ATC facilitation may include: delaying the aircraft descent from cruise, where fuel burn rates are more optimal; using sophisticated arrival management tools to better sequencing and queueing of aircraft to minimize holdings. To achieve overall flight efficiency in the descent phase, a balance should be struck between expediting traffic, meeting airport capacity, and reducing flight times and distances, fuel burn, emissions and noise within the overall requirement for safe operations. When considering any solutions described for descent, it should be noted that these measures should not introduce or increase inefficiencies in another flight-phase. For example: between climbing and descending aircraft, integrating continuous departure procedures with other simultaneous descent operations and with operations using adjacent airspace or airports. Actions adopted by ATC controllers to minimize fuel use during descent include:

- For sequencing, if possible, offer speed control as far out as possible in lieu of radar vectoring;
- Allow 'path-stretching' (or linear holdings) in lieu of a standard holding, wherever possible;
- Allow continuous descent to the initial approach fix;
- Use RNAV/RNP STARs that have been designed for continuous descent;
- When traffic permits, allow pilot discretion descents, ideally from the top of

descent;

- Avoid late descent clearances, as height energy must be dissipated with drag;
- Minimize holding at low altitude and provide pilots with realistic holding times.

After landing, the following actions may be considered:

- Provide advanced taxi information to allow pilots to plan for fuel saving techniques with respect to the landing roll;
- Publish coded taxi route instructions for efficient runway exit and reduced ATC radiotelephony;
- If possible, assign the runway that is closest to the passenger terminal and minimize taxi time;
- Clear to vacate the runway *via* a high-speed taxiway.

Continuous Descent Operations

Descent operations, when performed from cruise flight levels at idle thrust settings to the final approach intercept (Fig. **8.12**) offer the opportunity for significant fuel savings, reduced emissions, quieter operations, as well as improved safety.

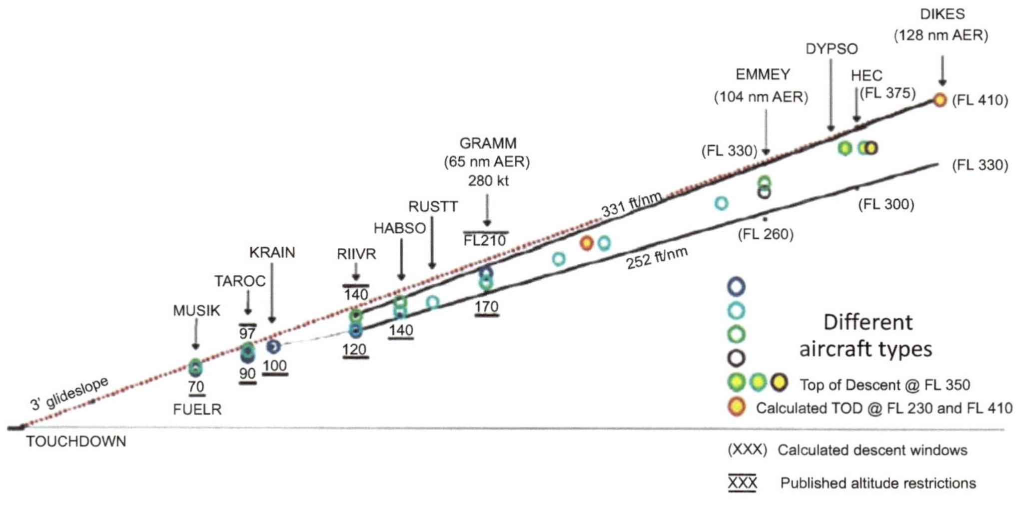

Fig. (8.12). Example of Continuous Descent and Approach simulation [14].

The optimum vertical profile takes the form of a continuously descending path, with a minimum of level flight segments only as needed to decelerate and configure the aircraft, or to establish the aircraft on the final approach segment. It should be tailored to the operating capability of the aircraft, with low engine thrust settings and, where possible, a low drag configuration.

Aided by appropriate airspace and procedure design, air traffic control (ATC) clearances will enable the execution of a continuous descent. Ideally, ATC should refrain from tactical interference in the lateral and vertical flight path during the execution of a continuous descent. When vectoring is unavoidable, providing timely and accurate distance-to-go information to the pilot will facilitate resumption or continuation of an optimum descent profile to the extent possible. A continuous descent typically saves 150-600 kg of CO_2 per arrival, depending on the aircraft model and engine combination. If a Standard Arrival (STAR) or instrument approach procedure does not specify a continuous descent, the same reduction of CO_2 emissions can be achieved, if the controller can authorize a descent clearance at the pilot's discretion, or provides a predictable flight path with distance-to-go information to the pilot, again allowing descent in a fuel-efficient profile.

A Harmonized ATM

Communication, Navigation, Surveillance and Air Traffic Management (CNS/ATM) Systems are known for the benefits they have delivered to civil aviation throughout the years. As CNS systems continue evolving they serve as key enablers in delivering to the aviation community a paradigm shift from an environment of Air Traffic Control (ATC) to that of Global Air Traffic Management (ATM).

The Global Air Traffic Management System is transitioning from a technology-based system to one driven by the provision of services. These services are based on the expectations and performance requirements of the aviation community. Such performance requirements are enabled by appropriate technologies, which in turn allow it to achieve the interoperability and seamlessness across all regions to meet safety and efficiency benchmarks during all phases of flight. As aviation is a global system, it is crucial that requirements and enablers support a global framework that is safe, efficient and environmentally responsible.

Considering the unique and diverse regional requirements, ICAO promotes regional implementation plans that fall within the global planning framework but are selectively prioritized and deliver benefits at the local and regional level, under the principle of 'Thinking Globally, Implementing Regionally." The ICAO Global Air Traffic Management Operational Concept (Doc. 9854) and the Global Air Navigation Plan (Doc. 9750) provide the guiding principles for States and ICAO Planning and Implementation Regional Groups (PIRG's) to improve the safety, efficiency and capacity of their ATM systems with the related environmental benefits.

ADVANCED IDEAS

Flying Airliners in Formation

Migrating birds fly in formation to benefit from each other´s wake vortex. This helps them to save approximately 3% in energy, which is significant as it can decide if some of them will live or die as their migration trajectories are extensive and strenuous.

Some researchers believe that this behavior of nature can be applied to long-haul airliners [15]. Formation flight are common practice in military operations. NASA performed flight tests with F-18 fighters and further studies concluded that fuel savings of up to 12% could be achieved if commercial airlines adopt a similar strategy [16].

Aiming for potential fuel savings, many studies were carried out to study the particularities of aircraft formation flight. To obtain drag minimization, Hanson and Ryan [17] presented a methodology for the in-flight optimization of lift distribution along wingspan. The usual optimal elliptical distribution for minimization of induced drag is not valid for the surfing aircraft in a formation flight. This is due to the asymmetric nature of the flow field, which is disturbed by the upstream airplane. According to the authors of the study, control surfaces along the trailing edge of the wing can be configured to obtain a non-elliptical profile that is more optimal in terms of minimum of an objective consisting of an induced and profile drag combination.

However, the flight formation approach faces a series of obstacles:

- A holding pattern of the airplanes is necessary to join them before they start heading to the long-haul flight destination. This requires additional fuel.
- An interlaced control system to avoid mid-air collisions. The system must detect possible turbulence in airplanes' path, mainly the clear-air turbulence.
- Passenger comfort will be impacted. There is need for additional system or reprogramming of existing ones to recover that comfort of solo flights.
- Coordination among air traffic controllers must be improved and updated.
- Change of present regulations which prohibit such flights is needed.
- Evaluation of how airplanes facing disturbed airflow must be designed to resist additional loads. Structural fatigue and distorted airflow entering engine intake are also big issues to be addressed.
- Usually the wake vortex downstream of an airplane descends 250 m with regard to its cruise altitude at a certain distance from the wing trailing edge. Thus, the surfing airplane must be positioned at lower altitudes to benefit from the vortex energy. Doing so, flying at a lower altitude than that of the preceding airplane,

means that it will burn more fuel, nullifying the gains provided by the formation flight.

Catapulting Airplanes

In the 1930s, Germany established post and passenger flights over the North and South Atlantic with seaplanes. Some of these regular flights were operated with aircraft like the Blohm und Voss Ha 139 (Fig. **8.13**) and Dornier Wal. With stops in the middle of the ocean, they were catapulted after refueling and serviced to continue the journey until destination.

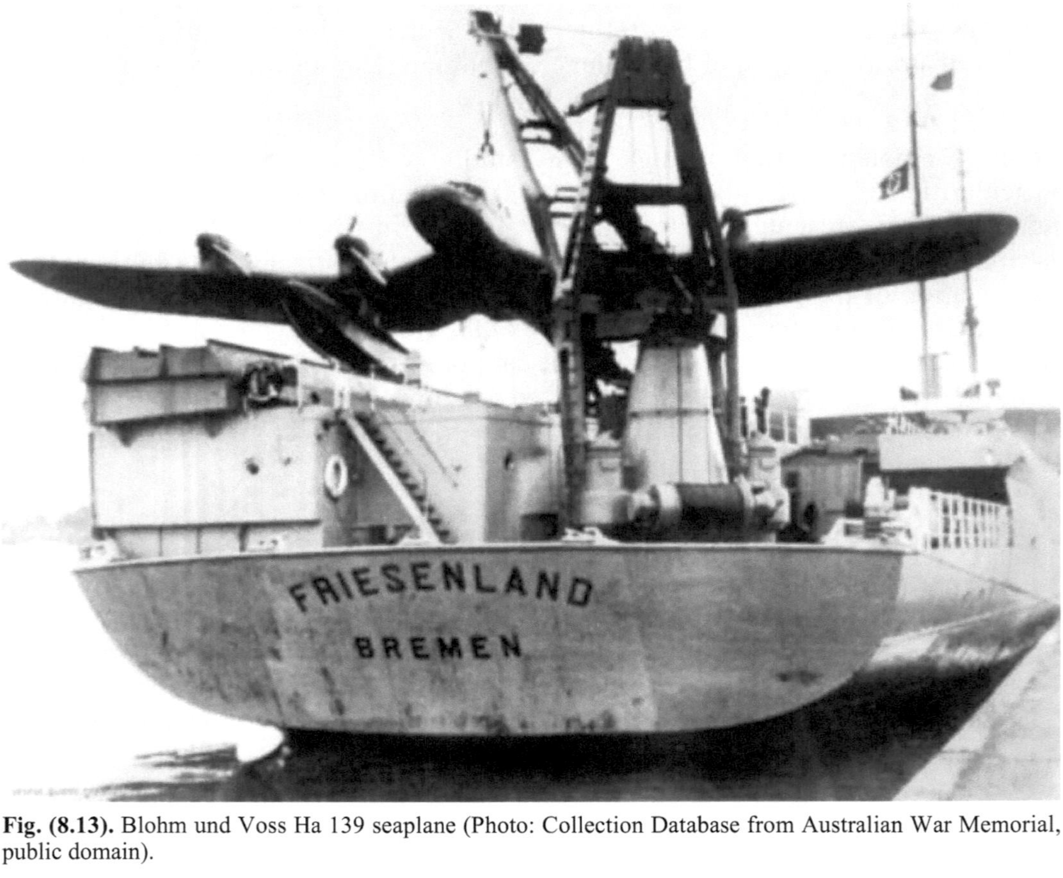

Fig. (8.13). Blohm und Voss Ha 139 seaplane (Photo: Collection Database from Australian War Memorial, public domain).

German warships were equipped with interceptor seaplane fighters, which took the skies by catapult systems. During World War II, Blohm und Voss BV 138 performed reconnaissance missions over the North Atlantic [18]. This German airplane was fitted with three 880-hp Jumo Junkers diesel engines. In addition to operating from bases ashore, BV 138 could operate from seaplane carriers with catapult systems (Fig. **8.14**). All exemplars of this impressive airplane could be fitted with assisted take-off rockets, and several sprouted FuG 200 Hohentwiel radar for shadowing convoys. Thanks to its diesel engines and catapulted takeoff, BV 138 could fly over 4000 km and stay airborne for 16 hours with full load.

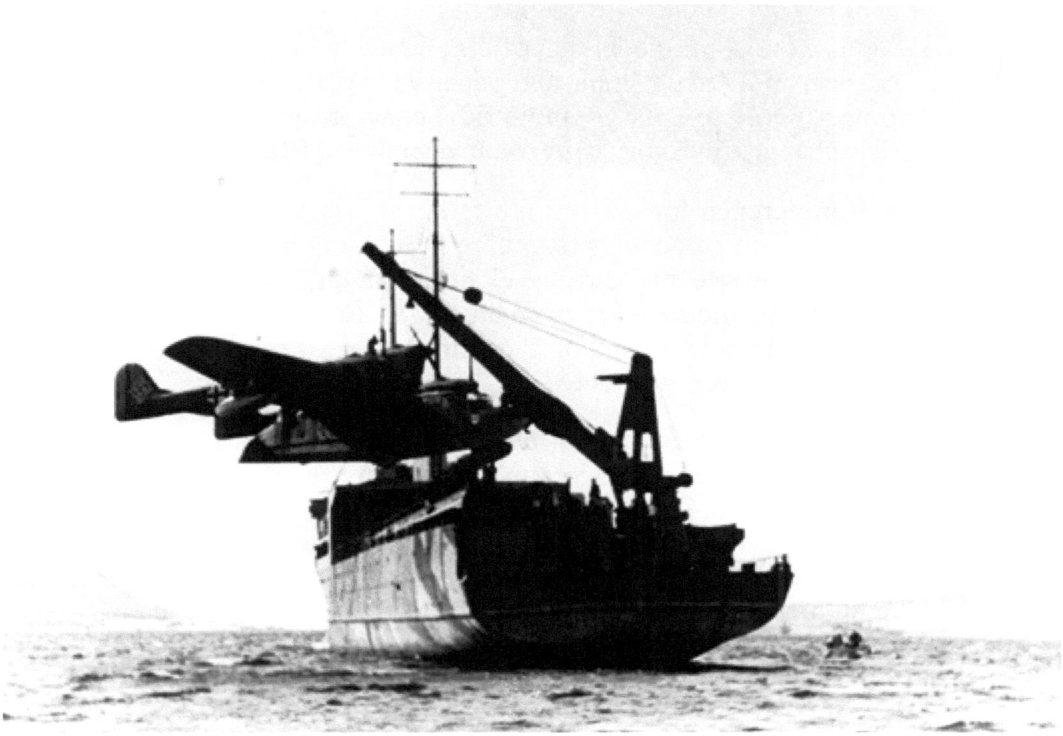

Fig. (8.14). German Blohm & Voss BV 138 seaplane being lifted aboard a German aircraft in World War II. This plane was put airborne by a catapult system (Photo: U.S. Navy, public domain).

In the case of the BV 138, another reason to catapult them was the better positioning in the aeronaval war theater of the North Atlantic. The useful life of military airplanes was not a major reason of concern before World War II. The civil flights with seaplanes before that war were intended to improve military operations for the war on the horizon.

High loads from a catapult launch shorten the useful life of the aircraft structure and introduce a set of safety concerns. Designing airliners to withstand such loads could nullify all benefits from using the system. Maintenance of such systems at airports could pose a very challenging and costly task. In addition, the safety regulations of the present days, would require a broad range of structural reinforcements and additional systems that would penalize the airplanes considerably. For similar reasons, seaplanes lost the quest for land-based airplanes. The ability to land and takeoff from calm waters degraded their performance and operational costs.

HIGH-SPEED TRAIN *VS.* AIR TRAVEL

High-speed train is a transport modal that offers some degree of competition to air transport in Europe and Asia (China and Japan) [19]. Research indicates that intermodal competition presents asymmetric behavior, with airlines quicker reacting to price changes introduced by train operators [19].

In regard to user preference for rail transportation services, collected data point for heterogeneity between passengers travelling in working hours and those doing so for leisure [20]. Price levels and travel times of high-speed train services dictate the share that this modal takes from air travel. According to some studies, there could be a considerable impact on the demand for air travel if new railway services being expected are implemented.

The advantages of high-speed trains decrease dramatically as the distance increases. Thus, due to the longer travel time, there is a loss of competitiveness in favor of air travel, especially in the business segment [21]. It is possible to conclude that the high-speed train may be considered as a truly competitive product over distances that may be covered in 3 hours, at most [21]. This is the case where the high-speed train may compete with the air transport, considering that for longer distances, the airplane is the preferred service [21].

Trips to or from work is a very particular travel segment, where decisive conditions differ considerably to that of other types of modals. Research in interurban contexts is scarcer and especially lacking in analyses where the plane or the high-speed train are presented as travel alternatives.

FINAL COMMENTS

Besides improvements of aircraft configuration designs, there are significant gains that can be obtained from aircraft operations. Due to the increasing airspace congestion, single-aircraft operations have demonstrated less significance than the airspace management. Individual operational techniques may be adopted, as described in the present chapter, but if airspace is not properly managed the in-flight delays due to airspace capacity constraints will jeopardize all savings obtained with such initiatives. Increasing data and information that can be exchanged among airborne aircraft, Air Navigation Service providers, and Airlines Operational Centers, more and more with the integration of the stakeholders will enable increased operational efficiency and therefore fuel savings. It is important to notice that individual aircraft procedures in synergy with condition monitoring techniques may reach up to a 10% improvement in fuel efficiencies. Since integrated ATM procedures have also the potential to save 12% in fuel burn, part of these gains would be provided by Flight Operations, based on the pace of the CNS/ATM related technology developments. The other part of the savings could come from technological improvements such as new airframe/engine concepts and adoption of biofuels as discussed in the previous chapters.

REFERENCES

[1] IATA, *Industry Economics Performance Dec 2015 – Briefing Notes,* 2015. http://www.iata.org/publications/economics/Pages/industry-performance.aspx

[2] IPCC, *Special Report on Aviation and Global Atmosphere.* IPCC: Montreal, 1999.

[3] R. Doganis, *Flying Out of Course. Airline Economics and Marketing.* Taylor&Francis Group: New York, 2010.

[4] Federal AViation Administration, *14 CFR 121 Operating requirements: Domestic, flag, and supplemental operations – 121.645 International Fuel Reserves.* Washington, 2015.

[5] European Comission, *Council Regulation (EEC) No 3922/91 as regards common technical requirements and administrative procedures applicable to commercial transportation by aeroplane.*Cologne, 2008.

[6] International Civil Aviation Organization, ICAO, *Annex 6 to the Convention on International Civil aviation – Operation of Aircraft.* ICAO: Montreal, 2014.

[7] Coordination Committee (CCOM) for the US–EU MoC Annex 1 High-Level Committee, *NextGen – SESAR State of Harmonisation* Publications Office of the European Union: Luxembourg, 2016.

[8] S. Altus, *Efficient Flight Plans.* Boeing AERO Magazine, 2009.

[9] M. Vogel, C. Thiel, and H. Fricke, "Assessing the Air Traffic Control Safety Impact of Airline Pilot induced Latencies", *Proceedings of ATACCS'2012,* 2012 London

[10] International Civil Aviation Organization, ICAO, *Annex 11 to the Convention on International Civil aviation – Air Traffic Services* ICAO: Montreal, 2014.

[11] M. Goldhammer, and B. Plendl, *Surface Coatings and Drag Reduction.* vol. 14-20. Boeing Aero Magzine, 2013.

[12] A.D. Young, and J.H. Peterson, *Excrescence Drag.* Technical Editing and Reproduction Ltd: London, 1981.

[13] International Civil Aviation Organization, ICAO, *Annex 16 to the Convention on International Civil aviation – Environmental Protection,* ICAO: Montreal, .

[14] International Civil Aviation Organization, ICAO, *Doc 9931 - Continuous Descent Operations Manual.* ICAO: Montreal, 2012.

[15] H. Shen, H. Perkins, K-C. Lin, and A. Zarmehr, "Energy-saving Formation Flight", *International Journal of Innovative Research in Technology & Science,* vol. 4, 2016.

[16] B. Dunbar, *F/A-18 Autonomous Formation Flight (AFF),* 2017. https://www.nasa.gov/centers/dryden/multimedia/imagegallery/AFF/EC01-0328-17.html

[17] C. Hanson, and J. Ryan, *Peak-Seeking Optimization of Spanwise Lift Distribution for Wings in Formstion Flight.* AIAA Guidance, Navigation, and Control Conference: Minneapolis, 2012.

[18] F. Kober, *BV 138 Der Fliegende Holzschuh* Podzun-Pallas Verlag: Friedberg, 1973.

[19] G. Abrate, G. Viglia, J.S. Garcia, and S. Forgas-Coll, "Price Competition within and between Airlines and High-speed Trains: the Case of Milan-Rome Route", *Tour. Econ.,* pp. 311-323, 2016. [http://dx.doi.org/10.5367/te.2016.0549]

[20] J. Bates, *Journal of Transportation Economics and Policy,* vol. 1, 1988.

[21] M. González-Savignat, "Competition in Air Transport", *J. Transp. Econ. Policy,* vol. 38, no. 1, pp. 77-107, 2004.

SUBJECT INDEX

A

B

Bento S. de Mattos, José A. T. G. Fregnani & Paulo Eduardo C. S. Magalhães

C

D

E

F

G

H

I

J

K

L

M

N

O

P

R

S

T

U

V

W

Y

Z

www.ingramcontent.com/pod-product-compliance
Lightning Source LLC
LaVergne TN
LVHW070944210926
848482LV00002B/92
* 9 7 8 1 6 8 1 0 8 3 2 8 5 *